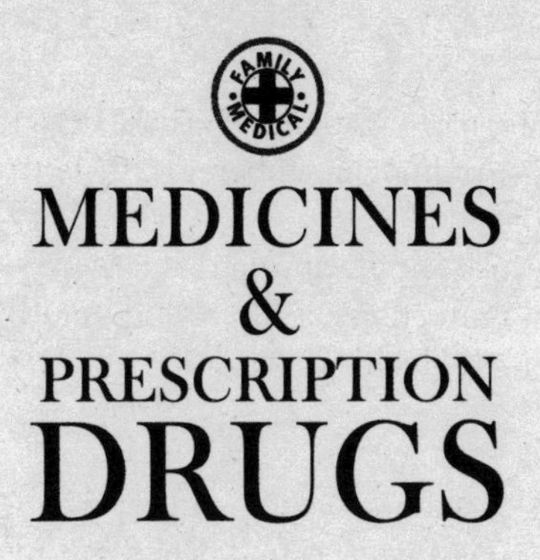


# MEDICINES & PRESCRIPTION DRUGS

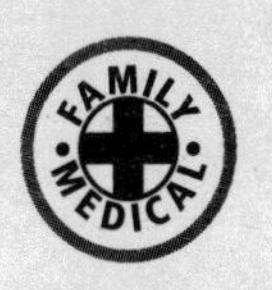


# MEDICINES & PRESCRIPTION DRUGS

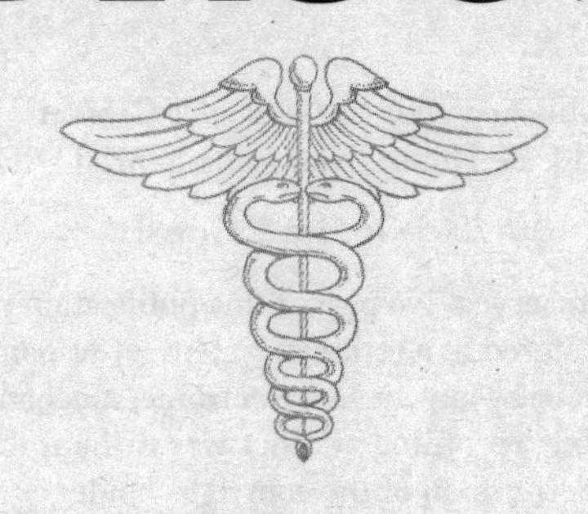

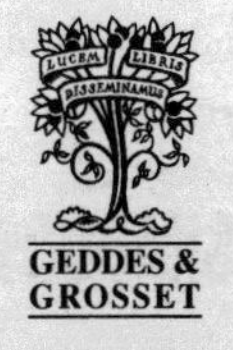


GEDDES & GROSSET

Published 2005 by Geddes & Grosset,
David Dale House, New Lanark, ML11 9DJ



ISBN 1 84205 520 8

Printed and bound in Poland

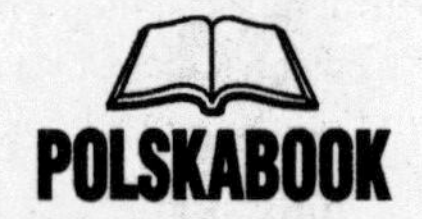

## Symbols Used in this Book

μg = microgram, one millionth of a gram
mg = milligram, one thousandth of a gram
g = gram, one thousand milligrams
ml = millilitre, one thousandth of a litre
kg = kilogram
iu = international unit
U = unit
mU = milliunit
mEq = milliequivalent
PhEur = European Pharmacopoeia
mmol = millimoles per litre, world standard unit for measuring glucose in blood.
mg/dl = (milligrams/decilitre) traditional unit for measuring glucose in blood

# A

## ACCUPRO

*Description*: a proprietary preparation of the antihypertensive drug, quinapril; used in conjunction with a diuretic or cardiac glycoside. Available as brown tablets (oval, round or triangular according to strength).

*Used for*: hypertension and congestive heart failure, especially after other treatments have been tried.

*Dosage*: in adults only, starts at 2.5mg per day usually increasing to 10 to 20mg per day. The maximum daily dose is 40mg.

*Special care*: all elderly patients, impairment of kidney function, haemodialysis, severe congestive heart failure, some types of vascular disease and in patients having anaesthesia.

*Avoid use*: children, pregnant and nursing mothers, some kidney and heart valve diseases.

*Possible interaction*: potassium-containing supplements, diuretic drugs, NSAIDs, tetracyclines.

*Side effects*: numerous including hypotension, abdominal, chest and muscle pains, headache, nausea, dizziness, rhinitis, upper respiratory tract infection and allergic reactions.

*Manufacturer*: Pfizer.

## ACCURETIC

*Description*: an ACE inhibitor and diuretic containing 10mg quinapril and 12.5mg hydrochlorothiazide in pink, oval scored film-coated tablets.

*Used for*: hypertension.

*Dosage*: 1 tablet daily (maximum 2). Not recommended for children.

*Special care*: patients with diabetes, kidney or liver disorders, severe congestive heart failure, collagen vascular disease (changes in connective and small blood vessels). Haemodialysis, surgery and anaesthesia. Kidney function, urinary protein and white cell count should be monitored before and during treatment.

*Avoid use*: pregnancy or lactation, anuria.

*Possible interaction*: potassium supplements, diuretics, tetracyclines, NSAIDs, ACTH (adrenocorticotropic hormone), tubocurarine and corticosteroids.

*Side effects*: coughing, headache, fatigue, dizziness, myalgia, gastrointestinal upset, chest pain, hypotension, chest infections, angioedema (a painless swelling usually on the face), pancreatitis, hyperlipidaemia, kidney disorders.

*Manufacturer*: Pfizer.

**ACEBUTOLOL *SEE*: SECTRAL.**

**ACECLOFENAC *SEE*: PRESERVEX.**

**ACEMETACIN *SEE*: EMFLEX.**

**ACETAZOLAMIDE *SEE*: DIAMOX.**

## ACETYLCYSTEINE *SEE*: ILUBE; PARVOLEX.

## ACEZIDE

*Description*: a combined diuretic/ACE inhibitor antihypertensive preparation. Contains captopril (50mg) and hydrochlorothiazide (25mg) in a white, scored tablet, code AZE 50/25.

*Used for*: mild to moderate hypertension.

*Dosage*: 1 tablet daily (maximum 2) (in patients who have first become accustomed to the two components given in the same amounts separately).

*Special care*: patients with renal disorders or undergoing haemodialysis.

*Avoid use*: in children, pregnant and breast feeding mothers, outflow obstruction of the heart, aortic stenosis and renovascular disease.

*Possible interaction*: NSAIDs, potassium-containing supplements, antihypertensives, vasodilatory and immunosuppressant drugs.

*Side effects*: protein in urine (proteinuria), rash, loss of sense of taste, fatigue, changes in constitution of the blood and, very unusually, a cough.

*Manufacturer*: BMS.

ACICLOVIR *See*: ZOVIRAX.

## ACT-HIB DTP

*Description*: a combined vaccine preparation; triple, inactivated surface antigen combined with aluminium hydroxide and toxoid vaccine. Contains at least 60iu of tetanus toxoid; 30iu diphtheria toxoid; 4iu of killed Bordetella pertussis toxoid, all per 5ml. Also, 10μg per 0.5ml of polysaccharide of Haemophilus influenzae type b conjugated to tetanus protein.

*Used for*: active immunisation against tetanus, diphtheria, whooping cough and infections caused by *H. influenzae* type b.

*Dosage*: for children aged between 2 months and 4 years only: 3 separate 0.5ml injections spaced at intervals at least 1 month apart; delivered intramuscularly or as deep sub-cutaneous injections.

*Special care*: history of epilepsy in recipient's family.

*Avoid use*: other age groups; fever or other acute illness, previous convulsions, neurological problems (including developmental defects), history of brain inflammation or cerebral problem as newborn, adverse reaction to previous injection.

*Side effects*: soreness at injection site, fever, crying and irritability, sleepiness, allergic reactions, general malaise, headache, possible neurological effects.

*Manufacturer*: Aventis Pasteur MSD.

## ACTILYSE

*Description*: a fibrinolytic (disperses blood clots) drug available as a powder for reconstitution and injection. It can only be used under close medical supervision.

*Used for*: thrombosis, embolisms and particularly myocardial infarction.

*Dosage*: a total of 100mg, given intravenously over a 2-hour period in adults only.

*Special care*: in patients with liver or kidney disease, diabetes or hypertension.

*Avoid use*: in children, pregnant and nursing mothers, those with any form of bleeding (e.g. menstruation), recent surgery including dental treatment, or haemorrhage, any condition likely to bleed, e.g. active peptic ulcer or case of pancreatitis. Should not be administered to those having allergic reactions to streptokinase and anistreplase (no longer available) or who have recently been treated with these.

*Possible interaction*: with other plasma protein-bound drugs, i.e. anticoagulants.

*Side effects*: mainly nausea, vomiting and bleeding usually confined to puncture site but can occur elsewhere including intracerebral haemorrhage. Severe bleeding necessitates halting of treatment and possible administration of drugs to counter the fibrinolytic. Hence close monitoring is essential during treatment.

*Manufacturer*: Boehringer Ingelheim.

## ACTINAC

*Description*: an antibacterial steroid (corticosteroid) preparation with skin softening properties, available as a powder with solvent to be made up as a lotion. Contains the broad spectrum antibiotic chloramphenicol (4%), hydrocortisone acetate (4%) and also sulphur precipitate, allantoin and butoxyethyl nicotinate.

*Used for*: acne.

*Dosage*: apply to affected skin morning and night for 4 days then at night only for up to 3 weeks, continuing for 3 days after spots have disappeared.

*Special care*: pregnant women, avoid contact with jewellery.

*Side effects*: possible erythema, which may be severe.

*Manufacturer*: Peckforton.

## ACUPAN

*Description*: an analgesic non-narcotic drug available in the form of white tablets or as a solution for injection. Contains 30mg nefopam hydrochloride, tablets being marked APN. (Injection contains 20mg nefopam hydrochloride per ml in each ampoule.)

*Used for*: relief of moderate and severe pain, e.g. following surgery, muscle and joint pain, dental cancer.

*Dosage*: tablets 3 times per day, adults only, total dose in the order of 30 to 90mg. Injection, one 20mg dose intramuscularly 3 times a day.

*Special care*: elderly patients (1 tablet, 3 times a day initially), pregnant women, patients with kidney or liver disorders or suffering from urine retention.

*Avoid use*: children, history of convulsions or heart attack (myocardial infarction) and also glaucoma.

*Possible interaction*: drugs including sympathomimetics, tricyclics, anticholinergics and MAOIs (antidepressants).

*Side effects*: nervousness, irritability, dry mouth, dizziness and nausea, headaches. Occasionally, insomnia, irregular heartbeat and sweating. Urine may be tinged pink.

*Manufacturer*: 3M Health Care.

## ACUPHASE *SEE*: CLOPIXOL.

## ACWY VAX

*Description*: a preparation of vaccine for meningitis containing in excess of 50µg of polysaccharides of each of the meningococcal serogroups A, C, W135 and Y per 0.5ml of solution. Supplied in vials as freeze-dried powder with diluent.

*Used for*: immunisation against the above listed types of meningococcal meningitis. Especially for close contacts of an affected person or those living in or visiting a country where disease is prevalent. Also, when certain specialised conditions apply.

*Dosage*: people over 2 years of age, 0.5ml given by deep subcutaneous injection.

*Special care*: does not give protection to younger children.

*Avoid use*: fever and infection.

*Side effects*: Soreness and redness at injection site, localised reactions.

*Manufacturer*: GlaxoSmithKline.

## ADALAT

*Description*: a calcium antagonist and vasodilator, available as liquid-filled orange capsules, containing the active ingredient nifedipine (5mg and 10mg). Also available as sustained-release tablets and as a preparation for injection.

*Used for*: angina and Raynaud's phenomenon.

*Dosage*: 10mg 3 times a day (5mg in elderly patients) in first instance, depending upon response, up to 60mg a day thereafter. Capsules taken with or immediately after food.

*Special care*: patients with significant left ventricle disorders or congestive heart failure, low blood pressure, kidney and liver disease.

*Avoid use*: if pain worsens during treatment, pregnant and nursing mothers, children, patients with very low blood pressure.

*Possible interaction*: antihypertensive drugs; quinidine and cimetidine.

*Side effects*: dizziness, flushing, nausea, palpitations, sweating, headaches, fluid retention, digestive upset, increased frequency of urination, drowsiness and insomnia. Rarely jaundice and swelling of gums.

*Manufacturer*: Bayer. Nifedipine capsules are also produced by other manufacturers.

## ADIZEM

*Description*: a calcium antagonist and vasodilator containing the active ingredient diltiazem hydrochloride. Available as tablets in 2 forms: **ADIZEM-SR**—white 90mg; brown 120mg; white/brown 180mg. Also as 120mg white tablets (DL/120). All continuous-release capsules. **ADIZEM XL**—pink/blue 120mg; pink/blue 180mg; red/blue 240mg; maroon/blue 300mg. All continuous-release capsules marked with strength.

*Used for*: angina and hypertension.

*Dosage*: 60mg 3 times a day increasing if required to a maximum of 480mg. Elderly, twice a day in first instance.

*Special care*: patients with heart block, reduced function in left ventricle of heart, bradycardia, diabetes.

*Avoid use*: in children, pregnant and nursing mothers, severe heart block or bradycardia, impairment of kidney and liver function.

*Possible interaction*: digoxin, ß-blockers, antihypertensive drugs, cardiac depressants, diazepam, ciclosporin, cimetidine, theophylline and cartamazepine.

*Side effects*: swelling of ankles, nausea, headache, bradycardia, rash, first degree heart block.

*Manufacturer*: Napp.

## AEROBEC AUTOHALER

*Description*: a corticosteroid preparation for inhalation containing beclometasone dipropionate. Available in two strengths, 50μg or 100μg per metered dose, delivered by breath-actuated, aerosol inhalation.

*Also*, **AEROBEC FORTE AUTOHALER** containing 250μg beclometasone dipropionate per metered dose, delivered by breath-actuated, aerosol inhalation.

*Used for*: obstructive airways disease which is chronic and reversible.

*Dosage*: Aerobec, Adults: 100μg inhaled 3 to 4 times each day or 200μg twice daily. If condition severe, 600 to 800μg may be inhaled each day in divided doses with absolute maximum of 1mg. Children: 50 to 100μg inhaled between 2 and 4 times daily. Aerobec Forte, Adults only: 250μg inhaled 4 times daily or 500μg twice each day. If necessary, dose can be increased to 500μg 4 times each day.

*Special care*: pregnancy, patients who have been taking other steroid drugs, pulmonary tuberculosis, both active and past infection.
*Side effects*: throat irritation and hoarseness, Candida (thrush-type) infections of throat and mouth.
*Manufacturer*: 3M Health Care.

## AERODIOL

*Description*: a hormonal, oestrogen preparation in a nasal spray comprising 150μg oestradiol hemihydrate per spray.
*Used for*: hormone replacement therapy in post-menopausal women.
*Dosage*: Women: start with 1 spray in each nostril (given one after the other) once daily; if necessary, increase to 3 to 4 sprays total dose, divided between morning and evening or decrease to 1 spray, according to response. Take for 3 to 4 cycles (if present), to gauge response before adjusting. For maintenance, use lowest effective dose and use continuously (or cyclically, if applicable). Women who have not had a hysterectomy require progestogen for at least 12 days of assumed 28 day cycles.
*Special care*: women who are judged to be at increased risk of thromboembolism, patients undergoing surgery, women immobilised due to accident or illness, trauma or injury. Also, ongoing, mild liver disorders (checks required on liver function every 2 to 3 months). Women with any of the following require careful monitoring: high blood pressure, uterine fibroids, nodules in breast, fibrocystic disease, multiple sclerosis, impaired kidney

function, porphyria, epilepsy, migraine, cholelithiasis, diabetes, elevated blood calcium levels, tetany, asthma, otosclerosis. Women should be encouraged to self-examine breasts and to have breast screening and cervical smear tests.

*Avoid use*: pregnancy, breastfeeding, previous breast or other cancer, especially if hormone-dependant, family history of breast cancer, thromboembolic disorders, serious liver, kidney or heart disease, Rotor syndrome or Dubin–Johnson syndrome.

*Possible interaction*: drugs that induce liver enzymes.

*Side effects*: gastrointestinal upset, sickness and nausea, tender and enlarged breasts, weight gain, skin itching and redness, dizziness and headache, rise in blood pressure, decrease in glucose tolerance, deterioration in existing varicose veins, cholestatic jaundice, impaired liver function. Increased risk of thromboembolic episode, breast cancer. In the event of any of the following, drug should be discontinued: planned surgery, thromboembolic episode or thrombophlebitis, severe headaches or migraine, disturbance of vision, serious rise in blood pressure, hepatitis, jaundice, severe itching of whole body, seizures, pregnancy.

*Manufacturer*: Servier.

## AGRIPPAL

*Description*: a vaccine preparation comprising inactivated surface antigens of three strains of influenza virus: A/New Caledonia/20/99(H1N1)-like strain, A/Moscow/10/

99(H1N2)-like strain, B/Hong Kong/330/2001-like strain. Preparation comprises 15µg of each strain per 0.5ml, available as suspension in ready to use syringes.

*Used for*: immunisation against above strains of influenza.

*Dosage*: Adults: 0.5ml; children aged 6months to 3 years: 0.25ml or 0.5ml; 3 years and above, 0.5ml. If child not previously vaccinated or infected, dose is repeated after at least one month has passed. All injections are either deep subcutaneous or intramuscular.

*Special care*: pregnancy.

*Avoid use*: infant less than 6 months old, feverish illness, known allergy to egg or chicken proteins.

*Side effects*: soreness at injection site, mild fever and malaise; rarely, neurological effects.

*Manufacturer*: Wyeth.

## AIROMIR

*Description*: a bronchodilator, salbutamol (as sulphate) delivered via an aerosol, 100µg per dose.

*Used for*: emphysema, bronchial asthma, chronic bronchitis. Prevention of exercise-induced asthma.

*Dosage*: in adults, 1 or 2 puffs for an acute attack, 2 puffs before exercise, maximum dosage 8 in 24 hours. Same for children except before exercise, 1 or 2 puffs.

*Special care*: hypertension, heart defects including angina, hyperthyroidism, pregnancy.

*Possible interaction*: sympathomimetics (bronchial muscle relaxant) ß-blockers.

*Side effects*: headache, hypokalaemia, tremor, peripheral vasodilatation.
*Manufacturer*: 3M Health Care.

## AKNEMIN

*Description*: an antibiotic drug, containing minocycline hydrochloride, available as 50mg red/fawn coloured capsules and 100mg red capsules.
*Used for*: acne.
*Dosage*: adults, twice daily dose of 50mg or 100mg. Tablets required for a minimum period of 6 weeks to 3 months with improvement not expected until after first month.
*Special care*: liver or kidney disorders.
*Avoid use*: pregnant and nursing mothers, children, kidney failure, SLE.
*Possible interaction*: alcohol, antacid stomach preparations, mineral supplements, anticoagulant drugs, penicillin.
*Side effects*: skin rashes, dizziness, blood abnormalities. Possible intracranial hypertension – drug should be discontinued.
*Manufacturer*: Crookes.

## ALDACTIDE

*Description*: a proprietary preparation containing a potassium-sparing diuretic (encourages potassium to be retained and not eliminated in kidney) combined with a thiazide (a drug which inhibits the reabsorption of chloride and sodium in the kidney). The preparation is available in two strengths. **ALDACTIDE 25** contains 25mg spironolactone and 25mg hydroflumethiazide in buff-coloured tablets marked Searle 101. **ALDACTIDE 50** (Gold Cross) contains 50mg of each drug.

*Used for*: congestive heart failure.

*Dosage*: *Aldactide 25*: adults, 4 tablets daily with food in first instance with a maximum of eight. *Aldactide 50*: two tablets daily with a maximum of four. In children: 1.5 to 3mg per kg of body weight given at intervals through the day.

*Special care*: the elderly, liver and kidney disorders, pregnant mothers, diabetic patients, gout, long-term use in young people. Blood tests and monitoring of electrolyte levels may be required.

*Avoid use*: nursing mothers, patients with liver or kidney failure, hypercalcaemia, hyperkalaemia, Addison's disease, sensitivity to sulfonamide drugs.

*Possible interaction*: potassium supplements, other potassium-sparing diuretic drugs, NSAIDs, anti-diabetic drugs, antihypertensive drugs, ACE inhibitors and cardiac glycosides.

*Side effects*: metabolic disorders, disturbance of electrolyte balance in blood, rash, drowsiness, sensitivity to light, gastro-intestinal upset, menstrual irregularities, deepening of voice.

*Manufacturer*: Pharmacia.

## ALDACTONE

*Description*: a diuretic, potassium-sparing preparation containing spironolactone. Tablets available: 25mg buff marked Searle 39, 50mg off-white (Searle 916), 100mg buff (Searle 314).

*Used for*: congestive heart failure, oedema caused by cirrhosis of the liver, malignancy or nephrotic syndrome, primary aldosteronism (over-production of the adrenal hormone, aldosterone).

*Dosage*: in adults with congestive heart failure, 100mg daily in first instance increasing to 400mg taken with food. Thereafter, 75 to 200mg per day. Children, 3mg per kg of body weight in first instance in several doses.

*Special care*: pregnant mothers, long-term use in young people patients with liver or kidney disorders. Blood electrolyte levels may need to be monitored.

*Avoid use*: nursing mothers, patients with kidney failure, Addison's disease, and hyperkalaemia.

*Side effects*: gastro-intestinal upset, rash, headache, disturbance of electrolyte levels, metabolic disturbance, breast enlargement, deepening of voice, menstrual irregularities, confusion, ataxia (unsteadiness).

*Manufacturer*: Pharmacia.

## ALDOMET

*Description*: a centrally acting (on central nervous system), antihypertensive preparation containing the drug methyldopa. It is available as tablets or in ampoules for injection. May be used in combination with a diuretic drug. Aldomet tablets are available in three strengths all marked Aldomet and coloured yellow: Aldomet 125mg code 135; Aldomet 250mg code 401, Aldomet 500mg code 516.

*Used for*: hypertension, especially useful for hypertension of pregnancy.

*Dosage*: in adults, 250mg 2 to 3 times a day in first instance with an eventual maximum of 3g, having gradually increased dose by increments at 2-day intervals. In children, 10mg per kg of body weight each day in 2 to 4 separate doses.

*Special care*: history of liver disease, kidney disorders, haemolytic anaemia, undergoing anaesthesia.

*Avoid use*: liver disease, a disease of the adrenal glands called phaeochromocytoma, patients with depression.

*Possible interaction*: sympathomimetics, other hypertensives, MAOIs, tricyclic antidepressants, lithium and phenothiazines.

*Side effects*: depression, sleepiness, headache, dry mouth, nasal congestion, gastro-intestinal upsets, bradycardia, jaundice, haemolytic anaemia, positive Coombs test.

*Manufacturer*: MSD.

## ALFUZOSIN *SEE*: XATRAL

## ALGINIC ACID *SEE*: GASTROCOTE, GAVISCON.

## ALIMEMAZINE *SEE*: VALLERGAN.

## ALKERAN

*Description*: a preparation of the alkylating, cytotoxic drug melphalan, for use by a physician skilled in cancer chemotherapy, available as white tablets containing 2mg of melphalan marked with A and gxEh3 and A. Also, **ALKERAN INJECTION**, available as a powder in ampoules with diluent for reconstitution and injection containing 50mg of melphalan.

For *Usages, Dosages, etc.* manufacturer's literature should be consulted.

*Manufacturer*: GlaxoSmithKline.

## ALLANTOIN *SEE*: ACTINAC.

## ALLEGRON

*Description*: a TCAD, nortriptyline, available in tablets of two strengths. It has less of a sedative effect than some other TCAD drugs. It is available as white scored tablets marked DISTA, containing 10mg nortriptyline hydrochloride, and orange scored tablets marked DISTA (25mg).

*Used for*: depressive illnesses and bedwetting in children.

*Dosage*: adults, 20 to 40mg each day in divided doses, increasing to 100mg if required. Maintenance, 30 to 75mg a day. Elderly persons; 10mg three times daily in first instance. Children (for bedwetting), seven to ten years, 10 to 20mg, 11 to 16 years, 25 to 50mg, given half an hour before bedtime.

*Special care*: patients with heart disease, elderly people (reduced doses), nursing mothers, those with diabetes, thyroid disease, liver disorders, tumours of the medulla of adrenal glands, epilepsy, glaucoma, urine retention, psychosis, suicidal tendencies. Withdrawal should be gradual. May reduce ability to perform skilled tasks such as driving.

*Avoid use*: pregnant mothers, heart block, heart attack, serious liver disorders.

*Possible interaction*: alcohol, MAOIs, barbiturate drugs, anticholinergic drugs, other antidepressant and antihypertensive drugs, adrenaline, noradrenaline, oestrogens, cimetidine.

*Side effects*: drowsiness, blurred vision, dry mouth, insomnia, urine retention, palpitations and shakiness, low blood pressure, weight changes, skin reactions, jaundice, blood changes, loss of libido.

*Manufacturer*: King.

## ALOMIDE

*Description*: a preparation containing lodoxamide trometha-mine with additives benzalkonium chloride and disodium edetate, available as 1% solution.

*Used for*: allergic conjunctivitis.

*Dosage*: 1 to 2 drops in each eye four times daily.

*Special care*: pregnant and nursing mothers.

*Avoid use*: those who wear soft contact lenses, children under four years of age.

*Side effects*: irritation, stinging, watering of eyes.

*Manufacturer*: Alcon.

## ALPHADERM

*Description*: a moderately strong steroid with a hydrating agent (to moisten the skin). Alphaderm combines 1% hydrocortisone, 10% urea in a slightly oily cream.

*Used for*: dermatitis and eczema.

*Dosage*: wash and dry affected skin and apply thinly twice a day.

*Special care*: short-term use only (especially in children or on face).

*Avoid use*: acne, scabies, tuberculosis, ringworm, untreated bacterial and fungal infections, viral skin diseases, leg ulcers, pregnant mothers.
*Side effects*: usually few but skin thinning, adrenal gland suppression, fluid retention possible.
*Manufacturer*: Alliance.

## ALPRAZOLAM *SEE*: XANAX.

## ALTACITE PLUS

*Description*: an antacid/anti-flatulence preparation in the form of a suspension containing 500mg of hydrotalcite and 125mg of activated dimeticone per 5ml.
*Used for*: acid inflammation of the stomach, over-production of stomach acid, flatulence, acid indigestion, peptic ulcer.
*Dosage*: adults and children over 12 years; 10ml taken 3 times a day, between meals and before going to bed. Children aged 8 to 12 years; 5ml taken 3 times a day in same way.
*Avoid use*: children aged under 8 years.
*Manufacturer*: Peckforton.

## ALTEPLASE *SEE*: ACTILYSE

## ALU-CAP

*Description*: a preparation which acts as an antacid and phosphate binder, containing 475mg of dried aluminium hydroxide gel in each red/green capsule. Capsules are marked 3M.

*Used for*: over production of stomach acid (hyperacidity) and to bind phosphate in kidney failure.

*Dosage*: adults, hyperacidity; 1 capsule 4 times each day and before going to bed. Adults, phosphate binding; 4 to 20 capsules each day in divided doses, taken with meals.

*Avoid use*: children, patients with low levels of phosphate in blood.

*Possible interaction*: tetracycline antibiotics.

*Manufacturer*: 3M Health Care.

## ALUMINIUM HYDROXIDE GEL (DRIED) *SEE*: ALU-CAP, GASTROCOTE, GAVISCON, KOLANTICON, MAALOX.

## ALUPENT

*Description*: a bronchodilator, containing the partially selective drug orciprenaline sulphate. It is available as off-white scored tablets marked A7 containing 20mg orciprenaline sulphate. Also as alupent sugar-free syrup (10mg/5ml of solution) and alupent aerosol containing 0.75mg per metered dose.

*Used for*: bronchial spasm due to asthma, chronic bronchitis and emphysema.

*Dosage*: tablets and syrup: adults, one tablet or 10mls four times a day. Children under 1 year, 2.5 to 5mls three times daily; 1–3 years, 2.5 to 5mls four times daily; 3–12 years, 5mls four times daily up to 10mls three times daily depending on age and symptoms. Aerosol: adults, 1–2 puffs which can be repeated after 30 minutes if required. Maximum dose 12 puffs in 24 hours. Children, 6 years and under, one puff, 6–12 years, one or two puffs. Must not be repeated within 30 minutes and maximum dose is four puffs in 24 hours.

*Special care*: patients with diabetes or hypertension. Patients should follow instructions carefully.

*Avoid use*: acute heart disease, hyperthyroidism or cardiac asthma.

*Possible interaction*: sympathomimetic drugs, tricyclic antidepressants, MAOIs.

*Side effects*: tachycardia, arrhythmia, fine tremor, headache and nervous tension, dilation of blood vessels.

*Manufacturer*: Boehringer Ingelheim.

## AMIKIN

*Description*: a broad spectrum antibiotic/aminoglycoside preparation, available as a suspension in vials for injection, containing 100mg or 500mg of amikacin as sulphate per 2ml.

*Used for*: serious infections caused by bacteria sensitive to amikacin. Generally for hospital use.

*Dosage*: adults and children; 15mg per kg of body weight; total quantity divided into two doses daily given by intramuscular or intravenous injection. Very severe infections may require higher dose of 500mg repeated every 8 hours. The maximum is 1.5g daily and can be continued for up to 10 days or to a top limit of 15g. New born infants; 10mg per kg of body weight, at start of treatment then 15mg per kg body weight, twice each day in divided doses.

*Special care*: kidney impairment, patient must be fully hydrated.

*Avoid use*: pregnancy.

*Possible interaction*: anaesthetics, drugs that block neuromuscular junction, furosemide, ethacrynic acid.

*Side effects*: ototoxicity (i.e. harmful effect on 8th cranial nerve affecting organs of balance and hearing), nephrotoxicity (toxic effects on kidneys).

*Manufacturer*: BMS.

## AMIL-CO

*Description*: a potent loop diuretic preparation with a rapid, short-acting mode of operation. A potassium-sparing, thiazide diuretic containing 5mg of hydrochloride and 50mg of hydrochlorothiazide (5/50 co-amilozide) in each pale orange coloured tablet. The tablets are scored and marked with logo and name.

*Used for*: congestive heart failure, high blood pressure, cirrhosis of the liver with ascites (abnormal fluid collection in abdominal cavity).

*Dosage*: adults; 1 to 2 tablets each day, either as single or divided dose. May be increased to a maximum of 4 tablets daily, in divided doses.

*Special care*: liver or kidney disease, gout, acidosis or diabetes.

*Avoid use*: children, pregnancy, breast feeding; patients with severe or progressive kidney disease or elevated blood potassium levels.

*Possible interaction*: other potassium-sparing diuretics,

potassium supplements, ACE inhibitors, lithium, antihypertensives, digitalis.
*Manufacturer*: IVAX.

## AMILORIDE *SEE*: AMIL CO, BURINEX A.

## AMIODARONE *SEE*: CORDARONE X.

## AMIODIPINE *SEE*: ISTIN.

## AMOXAPINE *SEE*: ASENDIS.

## AMOXIL

*Description*: a broad-spectrum antibiotic, penicillin preparation, available as capsules in two different strengths containing 250mg and 500mg amoxicillin (as trihydrate), respectively. The capsules are gold/maroon and each marked with strength and name. *Also*: **AMOXIL SYRUP SF**, available in two different strengths, containing 250mg and 500mg of amoxicillin (as trihydrate) per 5ml of sugar-free suspension. *Also*: **AMOXIL PAEDIATRIC SUSPENSION**, containing 125mg of amoxicillin (as trihydrate) per 1.25ml of liquid.
*Used for*: infections – ear, nose and throat, urinary tract, respiratory, soft tissue.
*Dosage*: adults and children aged over 10 years; 250mg to 500mg three times each day. Children aged less than 10 years; 125mg to 250mg three times each day. Infants aged under 6 months should receive paediatric suspension.

*Also*: **AMOXIL 3g SACHET SF**, containing 3g of amoxicillin (as trihydrate) in a sugar-free, sorbitol-based powder.

*Used for*: acute and severe and recurrent infections: urinary, respiratory, gonorrhoea, tooth abscess (in addition to surgical drainage). Also, prevention of bacterial endocarditis (inflammation and infection of the endocardium, the membrane lining the heart, cardiac veins and arteries and forming the cusps of the valves).

*Dosage*: adults and children over 10 years old; respiratory tract infections: 3g twice each day. Urinary infections: 3g with one further 3g dose after 10 to 12 hours. Gonorrhoea: single, 3g dose. Tooth abscess: 3g dose one hour before surgery followed by further 3g dose in 8 hours, if necessary. Prevention of bacterial endocarditis: 3g dose before dental surgery, followed by one further 3g dose after 6 hours, if necessary. Children; prevention of bacterial endocarditis: aged 5 years and under, 750mg; aged 5 to 10 years, 1.5g. All doses given one hour before dental surgery.

*Also*: **AMOXIL INJECTION**, available as powder in vials for reconstitution and injection, in three strengths, containing 250mg, 500mg and 1g of amoxicillin (as sodium salt).

*Used for*: severe bacterial infections.

*Dosage*: adults; either 1g given intravenously every 6 hours in very severe infections or 500mg given by intramuscular injection every 6 hours. Children; 50 to 100mg per kg of body weight each day in divided doses.

*Special care*: impaired kidney function, infectious mononucleosis.

*Possible interaction*: allopurinol, anticoagulant drugs.
*Side effects*: gastrointestinal upset, allergic reactions. Rarely, cholestatic jaundice, hepatitis, effects on blood and central nervous system.
*Manufacturer*: GlaxoSmithKline.

**AMOXICILLIN *SEE*: AMOXIL, AUGMENTIN, HELICLEAR.**

**AMPICILLIN *SEE*: PENBRITIN.**

**AMSACRINE *SEE*: AMSIDINE.**

**AMSIDINE**
*Description*: a cytotoxic, antibiotic, anti-cancer preparation containing amsacrine. This is available as a preparation for intravenous infusion for use by a physician skilled in cancer therapy. Amsidine concentrate contains 5mg amsacrine (as lactate) per ml when reconstituted.
*Used for*: acute myeloid leukaemia.
*Dosage*: as directed by physician. Usually no more than 450mg/m$^2$ of body surface area as a total cumulative dose.
*Special care*: patients with cardiac disorders, liver or kidney disease (reduced doses), elderly people, pregnant women. Caution in handling as irritant to tissues and skin; glass apparatus should be used for mixing. Cardiac monitoring and monitoring of electrolyte levels is essential during treatment.

*Side effects*: suppression of bone marrow function (myelosuppression), hair loss, mucositis. Rarely, tachycardia associated with ventricles of heart. Heart disease and potentially fatal heart failure.
*Manufacturer*: Goldshield.

## AMOBARBITAL *SEE*: AMYTAL

## AMYTAL[CD]

*Description*: a barbiturate preparation containing amobarbital, available as white tablets containing 50mg amobarbital.
*Used for*: severe intractable insomnia of a persistent nature for use by those patients already taking barbiturates.
*Dosage* : adults, 100–200mg at bedtime.
*Special care*: extremely dangerous, addictive drug with narrow margin of safety. Liable to abuse by overdose leading to coma and death or if combined with alcohol. Easily produces dependence and severe withdrawal symptoms. Drowsiness may persist next day affecting driving and performance of skilled tasks.
*Avoid use*: should be avoided if possible in all patients. Not to be used for children, young adults, pregnant and nursing mothers, elderly persons, those with drug or alcohol related problems, patients with liver, kidney or heart disease, porphyria, insomnia where the cause is pain.
*Possible interaction*: alcohol, central nervous system depressant drugs, griseofulvin, metronidazole, rifampicin,

phenytoin, chloramphenicol. Anticoagulant drugs of the coumarin type, steroid drugs including contraceptive pill.

*Side effects*: hangover with drowsiness, shakiness, dizziness, headache, anxiety, confusion, excitement, rash and allergic responses, gastro-intestinal upsets, urine retention, loss of sexual desire.

*Manufacturer*: Flynn.

## ANAFRANIL

*Description*: a TCAD containing clomipramine hydrochloride, available as capsules, syrup and in ampoules for injection. There are three strengths: yellow/caramel (10mg), orange/caramel (25mg), grey/caramel (50mg) all marked Geigy. Also **ANAFRANIL SR** sustained release pink capsules containing 75mg, marked Geigy and GD.

*Used for*: depression, phobic and obsessional states.

*Dosage*: adults, capsules for depression, 10mg each day gradually increasing to 30–150mg (maximum 250mg) in divided doses or as a single dose at bedtime. Obsession and phobia, 25mg at first increasing to 100–150mg daily. Elderly, 10mg each day at first increasing to a maximum of 75mg.

*Special care*: elderly (reduce dose), psychoses or suicidal tendencies. Persons with heart and circulatory disease, liver disorders, overactive thyroid gland (hyperthyroidism), epilepsy, diabetes, constipation, urine retention, glaucoma, tumour of the adrenal glands. Blood tests and monitoring of liver and heart function are advisable during therapy.

*Avoid use*: children, pregnancy, breastfeeding, patients with heart block, heart rhythm disorders, weak heart, mania, serious liver disease.

*Possible interaction*: MAOIs or within 14 days of their use, other antidepressant drugs, neuroleptics, anticholinergic drugs, alcohol, adrenaline, noradrenaline (or anaesthetics containing these), quinidine, carbamazepine, phenytoin, antihypertensive drugs, thyroid drugs, barbiturates, cimetidine, sympathomimetics, oestrogens.

*Side effects*: gastro-intestinal disturbances such as constipation, blurred vision, dry mouth, anxiety, ringing in ears (tinnitus), drowsiness, insomnia, urine retention, sweating, tremor, raised heartbeat rate, arrhythmias, conduction defects, palpitations, weight gain or loss. Also low blood pressure on rising upright, blood changes, allergic skin reactions, abnormal breast enlargement and milk production (gynaecomastia and galactorrhoea), alterations in blood sugar, jaundice, loss of libido and impotence may occur. Occasionally, symptoms of schizophrenia and mania may be activated, particularly in elderly persons.

*Manufacturer*: Novartis.

## ANHYDROL FORTE

*Description*: an antiperspirant solution containing 20% aluminium chloride hexahydrate in an alcohol base. It is available as a solution in a bottle with a roll-on applicator.

*Used for*: excessive sweating (hyperhidrosis) of armpits, hands and feet.

*Dosage*: apply at night to dry skin and wash off the following morning. Use less as condition improves.
*Special care*: avoid bathing immediately before use or use of depilatory creams and shaving of armpits within 12 hours of applying. Should only be used on feet in children.
*Avoid use*: contact with eyes, broken or inflamed skin. Contact with clothing and jewellery.
*Manufacturer*: Dermal.

## ANTABUSE

*Description*: a preparation containing the drug disulfiram, an enzyme (aldehyde dehydrogenase) inhibitor used in the treatment of alcoholism. It is available as white, scored tablets (200mg) marked DUMEX 110L.
*Used for*: adjunct in therapy for alcohol dependence.
*Dosage*: adults, 800mg as single dose on first day. Afterwards reducing to 200–100mg over period of five days. Should not be used for longer than six months.
*Special care*: liver or kidney disease, respiratory disease, diabetes mellitus, epilepsy. Careful counselling of patient essential before use as reaction of disulfiram with even a minute quantity of alcohol causes extremely unpleasant and possibly fatal consequences due to accumulation of acetaldehyde in body. With small amounts of alcohol reactions include severe throbbing headache, palpitations, nausea, vomiting, raised heartbeat, flushing of face. The quantity of alcohol in many medicines may be sufficient to precipitate this. Larger quantities of alcohol can cause hypotension, heart arrhythmias and collapse. No alcohol

should be consumed until one week after stopping the drug or for 24 hours prior to start of treatment.

*Avoid use*: patients with heart failure, coronary artery disease or high blood pressure. Children and pregnant women (first three months). Patients with severe mental disorders or suicidal tendencies.

*Possible interaction*: alcohol, some TCADs, paraldehyde, warfarin, barbiturate drugs, antiepileptic drugs, metronidazole (antibacterial drug).

*Side effects*: fatigue and drowsiness, vomiting and nausea, bad breath (halitosis), reduced libido, allergic skin reactions, liver damage. Rarely, mental disturbances (mania, paranoia, schizophrenia, depression).

*Manufacturer*: Alpharma.

## ANTAZOLINE *SEE*: OTRIVINE-ANTISTIN.

## ANTEPSIN

*Description*: a cytoprotectant (cell-surface protectant) preparation available in the form of tablets and suspension. The tablets are scored, white, oblong in shape and contain 1g sucralfate, marked Antepsin on one side and WY39 on reverse. **ANTEPSIN SUSPENSION** contains 1g/5ml of solution.

*Used for*: gastric and duodenal ulcers, chronic gastritis, prevention of haemorrhage from stress, ulceration in patients who are seriously ill.

*Dosage*: tablets, adults 2g twice a day in the morning and at bedtime or 1g four times a day one hour before meals.

Maximum dose 8g per day. Treatment period usually 4–6 weeks, sometimes up to 12 weeks. Prevention (prophylaxis) of stress ulceration, 1g suspension 6 times a day with a maximum of 8g daily.

*Special care*: patients with kidney failure, pregnancy and lactation.

*Avoid use*: children and patients with severe kidney failure

*Possible interaction*: antibacterial drugs (ciprofloxacin, ofloxacin, norfloxacin and tetracycline), warfarin, phenytoin, H2 antagonists, digoxin, ketoconazole – allow 2 hours to elapse before using antepsin. Enteral feeds – allow 1 hour to elapse before using antepsin.

*Side effects*: gastro-intestinal upsets—constipation, diarrhoea, indigestion, nausea, dry mouth, rash, back pain, dizziness, sleeplessness, drowsiness, vertigo are possible. Rarely, intestinal obstruction.

*Manufacturer*: Chugai.

## ANTURAN

*Description*: a preparation containing the active ingredient, sulfinpyrazone, which promotes the excretion of uric acid by preventing its reabsorption in the kidney tubules. Anturan is available in the form of yellow, sugar-coated tablets marked Geigy in 2 strengths, (100mg and 200mg).

*Used for*: hyperuricaemia (high blood levels of uric acid), chronic gout, recurrent gouty arthritis.

*Dosage*: adults, 100mg to 200mg with food per day at first increasing over a 2–3 week period to 600mg. After this the amount is reduced (once uric acid level has dropped) to a maintenance dose which may be as low as 200mg daily.

*Special care*: pregnant and breast-feeding mothers, kidney disease or heart failure. Plenty of fluids should be taken during treatment and blood and kidney function tests may be necessary

*Avoid use*: children. Patients with known allergies to anti-inflammatory drugs, severe liver or kidney disease, acute gout, history of peptic ulcers or acute peptic ulcer, blood disorders, porphyria.

*Possible interaction*: salicylates, aspirin, hypoglycaemic drugs, anticoagulants, sulfonamides, penicillins, phenytoin, theophylline.

*Side effects*: gastro-intestinal upset and bleeding, ulcers, acute gout, kidney stones, renal colic, liver and kidney disorders, rash, blood changes (treatment should stop).

*Manufacturer*: Novartis.

## ANUSOL HC

*Description*: an astringent antiseptic with soothing properties in the form of an ointment and suppositories. The ointment contains 1.25% benzyl benzoate, 0.87% bismuth oxide, 2.25% bismuth subgallate, 0.25% hydrocortisone acetate, 1.87% Peru balsam, 10.75% zinc oxide. The suppositories contain 33mg benzyl benzoate, 24mg bismuth oxide, 59mg bismuth subgallate, 10mg hydrocortisone acetate, 49mg Peru balsam and 296mg zinc oxide.

*Used for*: haemorrhoids, ano-rectal inflammation.

*Dosage*: adults, one application of ointment or one suppository night and morning and after bowel movement.
*Special care*: pregnant women. Not to be used for longer than 7 days.
*Avoid use*: children, patients with fungal or viral infections or suffering from tuberculosis.
*Side effects*: systemic (affecting whole body) corticosteroid effects.
*Manufacturer*: Pfizer Consumer.

## APRESOLINE

*Description*: a vasodilator available in the form of tablets of two strengths and as a powder for reconstitution for injection. It contains hydralazine hydrochloride. Yellow tablets (25mg) are sugar-coated and marked CIBA and GF, while the deep pink tablets are marked in the same way and contain 50mg. **APRESOLINE INJECTION** contains 20mg hydralazine hydrochloride as a powder in an ampoule for reconstitution.
*Used for*: moderate and severe chronic heart failure. Also used for moderate to severe hypertension.
*Dosage*: for hypertension in adults (along with ß-blocker and thiazide diuretic), 25mg twice a day at first increasing to a maximum of 200mg daily. For cardiac failure in adults (with diuretics and cardiac glycosides), 25mg 3–4 times each day increasing to 50–75mg 4 times a day every second day.
*Special care*: patients with coronary or cerebrovascular disease, liver disorders, severe kidney failure, nursing mothers. Withdrawal should be gradual.

*Avoid use*: children, first half of pregnancy, patients with certain heart disorders (aortic, mitral stenosis, tachycardia, idiopathic SLE, constructive pericarditis, dissecting aortic aneurysm, cor pulmonale).

*Possible interaction*: anaesthetics, TCADs, MAOIs, antihypertensive drugs, diazoxide, CNS depressants.

*Side effects*: hypotension, tachycardia, angina, headache, flushes, especially with daily dose exceeding 100mg. Protein in urine, blood in urine, kidney failure, urine retention. Possible though rare, liver damage, nerve disorders and blood changes.

*Manufacturer*: Sovereign.

## APRINOX

*Description*: a thiazide preparation which has diuretic properties and is available as white tablets of two strengths containing 2.5mg or 5mg of bendroflumethiazide.

*Used for*: hypertension, oedema such as occurs in mild to moderate heart failure.

*Dosage*: adults, for oedema, 5–10mg in morning or on alternate days at first and then 5–10mg once or twice per week for maintenance. For hypertension, 2.5–5mg once each day.

*Special care*: pregnancy and breast-feeding, elderly persons. Patients with liver or kidney disease, liver cirrhosis, gout, diabetes, SLE. Advisable to monitor fluid, electrolytes and glucose levels.

*Avoid use*: children. Patients with severe liver or kidney failure, hypercalcaemia, Addison's disease, allergy to sulfonamide drugs.

*Possible interaction*: alcohol, opioids, barbiturates, antidiabetic drugs, NSAIDs, corticosteroids, tubocurarine, carbenoxolone, cardiac glucosides, lithium.

*Side effects*: metabolic disturbance and upset of electrolyte balance, gastro-intestinal disturbance, blood changes, rash, dizziness, impotence, pancreatitis, anorexia.

*Manufacturer*: Sovereign.

## AREDIA

*Description*: a preparation of the biphosphonate drug disodium pamidronate available as a powder for reconstitution and intravenous infusion. Vials contain 15mg or 30mg.

*Used for*: hypercalcaemia caused by malignancy, metastases or lesions and bone pain secondary to breast cancer or multiple myeloma, Paget's disease of bone.

*Dosage*: adults, hypercalcaemia, depending upon levels of calcium in blood plasma, maximum dose of 90mg each treatment given by slow infusion at a rate not exceeding 30mg in two hours. Dose may be divided over 2–4 days. Lesions and bone pain: 90mg every 4 weeks or 3weeks (with chemotherapy) in breast cancer. Paget's disease: 30mg once each week for 6 weeks; or, 30mg in first week, 60mg in weeks 2, 4 and 6 to a maximum of 210mg. This can be increased, if necessary, to an absolute maximum of 360mg. The treatment regime can be repeated every 6 months until remission takes place and reinstigated in the event of relapse.

*Special care*: severe kidney disorders, may cause convulsions due to disturbance of electrolyte balance. Electrolytes balance, potassium and calcium levels should be monitored. If use of drug is prolonged, kidney function must be monitored. Pregnancy, breastfeeding.

*Avoid use*: children.

*Possible interaction*: other infusions containing biphosphonates, drugs for hypocalcaemia, plicamycin.

*Side effects*: diarrhoea, nausea, short-lived rise in body temperature, 'flu-like symptoms, muscle and bone pain, headache, hypocalcaemia, lowering of magnesium levels. Rarely, decrease in number of white blood cells (lymphocytes) in blood, anaemia, other blood effects.

*Manufacturer*: Novartis.

## ARTHROTEC 50

*Description*: an NSAID containing diclofenac sodium, a phenylacetic acid prostaglandin analogue. Arthrotec tablets contain 50mg diclofenac sodium, 200µg misoprostol and are marked with a symbol and Searle 1411.

*Also,* **ARTHROTEC 75**, containing 75mg of diclofenac sodium and 200µg of misoprostol in each white tablet, marked Searle 1421.

*Used for*: osteoarthritis, rheumatoid arthritis.

*Dosage*: adults, one 50mg tablet twice a day with food increasing to one three times a day if required. Or, one 75mg twice each day with food.

*Special care*: women of childbearing age should use effective contraception. Patients with gastric or duodenal ulcer, heart disease, coronary, cerebrovascular, peripheral vascular disease, kidney or liver disorders. Patients taking the drug for a long period should be monitored.

*Avoid use*: children, pregnant women or those planning pregnancy, breast-feeding. Patients with gastro-intestinal bleeding, those with allergy to aspirin or other anti-inflammatory drugs.

*Possible interaction*: NSAIDs, anticoagulants, quinolone, methotrexate, digoxin, lithium, steroids, diuretic drugs, oral hypoglycaemics.

*Side effects*: gastro-intestinal upset, erosion of gastro-intestinal tract, heavy menstrual bleeding and inter-menstrual bleeding, dizziness, headache, oedema, nausea, skin reactions.

*Manufacturer*: Pharmacia.

## ARYTHMOL

*Description*: a class I antiarrhythmic drug used to treat disturbances of heart rhythm. Arythmol contains propafenone hydrochloride and is available in tablets of two strengths (150 and 300mg) which are white, scored and film-coated.

*Used for*: treatment and prevention of ventricular arrhythmias.

*Dosage*: adults, 150mg 3 times daily in first instance, gradually increasing at 3-day intervals to 300mg twice a day. Maximum dose is 300mg 3 times a day.

*Special care*: patients with heart failure or who are fitted with pacemakers, those with liver or kidney disorders, elderly persons.

*Avoid use*: children, pregnant women, some particular forms of heart rhythm disturbance, patients with uncontrolled congestive heart failure, electrolyte balance disturbances, obstructive lung disease, severe hypotension, myasthenia gravis.

*Possible interaction*: other class I antiarrhythmic drugs, myocardial (heart muscle) depressant drugs, warfarin, digoxin, cimetidine rifampicin, propranolol, metoprolol, theophylline, ciclosporin, tricyclic and similar anti-depressants.

*Side effects*: gastro-intestinal upset including constipation, diarrhoea, vomiting, nausea, unpleasant bitter taste, fatigue, headache, allergic skin rashes, disturbances of heart rhythm, dizziness.

*Manufacturer*: Abbott.

## ASACOL

*Description*: a preparation of the salicylate drug, mesalazine, available as tablets and suppositories. Tablets (400mg strength) are oblong, red and resin-coated. Suppositories are available in two strengths containing 250mg and 500mg. Also, **ASACOL FOAM ENEMA** is available.

*Used for*: to induce and maintain remission in ulcerative colitis and to treat acute attacks of this condition.

*Dosage*: adults, tablets, acute attack, 6 daily in divided doses. For maintenance, 3–6 tablets daily in divided doses. Asacol suppositories, adults 750–1500mg daily in divided doses with last dose at night.

*Special care*: elderly persons, pregnant and nursing mothers, patients with kidney disease, elevated blood urea levels, proteinuria.

*Avoid use*: children, patients with severe kidney disease, known allergy to salicylates or kidney sensitivity to sulfasalazine.

*Possible interaction*: lactulose, substance which increases acidity of motions

*Side effects*: gastro-intestinal upset, headache. Rarely, kidney failure, nephritis, nephrotic syndrome, lung allergies, rash, inflammation of heart and pericardium or peripheral nerves, blood changes. Patients should report any adverse side effects to their doctor – further tests may be needed.

*Manufacturer*: Procter & Gamble.

## ASENDIS

*Description*: a TCAD preparation containing amoxapine, available in tablets of two strengths, both seven-sided, scored tablets: 50mg, orange, marked LL50; 100mg, blue, marked LL100.

*Used for*: depression.

*Dosage*: 100–150mg per day at first increasing to a maintenance dose in the region of 150–250mg. Maximum daily dose is 300mg. Elderly persons, 25mg twice a day at first increasing, after 5–7 days, to 50mg 3 times daily if required.

*Special care*: patients with psychoses or suicidal tendencies, elderly persons, pregnant and nursing mothers, people with cardiac disorders, epilepsy, hyperthyroidism, urine retention, closed angle glaucoma, liver disease, tumours of adrenal gland, diabetes.

*Avoid use*: children, patients with recent heart attack, heart arrhythmias, heart block, porphyria (rare blood disorder).

*Possible interaction*: alcohol, barbiturate drugs, local anaesthetics (containing adrenaline or noradrenaline), antihypertensive and sympathomimetic drugs, anticholinergic drugs, cimetidine, oestrogens.

*Side effects*: anticholinergic effects including urine retention, dry mouth, constipation, blurred vision, rapid heartbeat, palpitations, nervousness, insomnia, sweating, dizziness, fatigue, weight changes, jaundice, blood changes, allergic skin rashes, changes in libido, breast enlargement and impotence.

*Manufacturer*: Goldshield.

## ATARAX

*Description*: an antihistamine preparation containing hydroxyzine hydrochloride available as sugar-coated tablets of two strengths (10 and 25mg) coloured orange and green respectively and in the form of a syrup. **ATARAX SYRUP** contains 10mg hydroxyzine hydrochloride per 5ml.

*Used for*: anxiety (short-term treatment) and itching caused by allergy (chronic urticaria and dermatitis).

*Dosage*: anxiety, adults only, 50–100mg 4 times each day. Itching, adults, 25mg taken at night increasing to 25mg 3–4 times a day if required. Children, 6 months to 6 years, 5–15mg daily increasing to 50mg in divided doses if required; 6 years and over, 15–25mg daily increasing to 50–100mg in divided doses if required.

*Special care*: patients with kidney disease. Patients must be warned that judgement and dexterity is impaired. Children should be given reduced doses for itching only.

*Avoid use*: pregnant women.

*Possible interaction*: central nervous system depressants, alcohol.

*Side effects*: drowsiness, anticholinergic effects, if high doses are taken there may be involuntary muscle movements.

*Manufacturer*: Pfizer.

## ATENOLOL *SEE*: BETA-ADALAT, TENORMIN.

## ATIVAN

*Description*: an anxiolytic benzodiazepine, lorazepam, which is for short-term use only as it carries a risk of dependency. **ATIVAN INJECTION** contains 4mg lorazepam per ml in ampoules.

*Used for*: anxiety, status epilepticus (a condition where a person with epilepsy suffers a series of fits in close succession and is deprived of oxygen), a sedative premedication prior to full anaesthesia.

*Dosage*: tablets, adults, for anxiety, 0.025 to 0.03mg per kg of body weight by means of intramuscular or intravenous injection. Not for children. For status epilepticus, adults, 4mg by intravenous injection, children half the adult dose. For premedication, adults, 0.05mg per kg of body weight intravenously about 30–45 minutes before operation. Not for children.

*Special care*: elderly, liver or kidney disorders, acute narrow angle glaucoma, lung disease. Short-term use only, withdraw gradually. Patients should be warned that dexterity and judgement may be adversely affected. Should not be used as sole treatment for depression.

*Avoid use*: pregnancy, labour, breastfeeding, acute lung diseases, depression of breathing, those with chronic psychoses, obsessional states and phobias.

*Possible interaction*: CNS depressant drugs, alcohol, anticonvulsants, narcotic painkillers, scopolamine, rifampicin, drugs that inhibit cytochromeP450, cimetidine.

*Side effects*: light-headedness, drowsiness, vertigo, confusion, muscular weakness, impaired ability, unsteadiness in walking, gastro-intestinal upset, disturbance of vision, rash, retention of urine, changes in libido, low blood pressure. Rarely, blood changes and jaundice. Risk of dependence especially with high doses.

*Manufacturer*: Wyeth.

## ATORVASTATIN *SEE*: LIPITOR.

## ATROPINE SULPHATE *SEE*: ISOPTO ATROPINE, LOMOTIL.

## ATROVENT

*Description*: an anticholinergic containing ipratropium

bromide available in various forms: aerosol inhalation, 20μg per dose delivered by metered dose inhaler; **ATROVENT AUTOHALER**, 20μg per dose delivered by breath-actuated metered dose aerosol; **ATROVENT FORTE**, 40μg per dose delivered by metered dose inhaler; **ATROVENT SOLUTION**, 250μg per ml, in preservative-free isotonic solution in unit dose vials for use with nebulizer. **ATROVENT AEROCAPS**, containing 40μg ipratropium bromide in capsules of two shades of green.

*Used for*: severe obstruction of airways, especially that caused by chronic bronchitis.

*Dosage*: adults, inhaler, 1–2 puffs three or four times a day. Children under 6 years, one puff, 6–12 years, 1–2 puffs, both three times a day. Adults, Atrovent Forte, 1 or 2 puffs three to four times daily; children 6–12 years, 1 puff three times daily. Adults, Atrovent solution, 0.4–2ml nebulized up to four times each day. Children over 3 years, 0.4–2ml nebulized up to three times each day. Aerocaps, adults; 1 or 2 inhaled 3 or 4 times each day. Not for use in children.

*Special care*: pregnancy, patients with enlarged prostate gland (prostate hypertrophy), glaucoma.

*Side effects*: urine retention, constipation, dry mouth, headache, raised heartbeat, nausea.

*Manufacturer*: Boehringer Ingelheim.

## AUDICORT

*Description*: a combined antibacterial, antifungal and anti-inflammatory (corticosteroid) preparation available in the form of ear drops. Audicort contains 1mg triamcinolone

acetate and neomycin undecenoate (antibiotic) (equivalent to 3.5mg neomycin base).
*Used for*: chronic and acute inflammation and/or bacterial infection of the outer ear.
*Dosage*: adults, 2–5 drops three or four times each day.
*Special care*: pregnant and nursing mothers.
*Avoid use*: children, patients with perforated ear drum.
*Side effects*: localized irritation, additional infection.
*Manufacturer*: Goldshield.

## AUGMENTIN

*Description*: a broad-spectrum, penicillin-like antibiotic, amoxicillin as the trihydrate, with clavulanic acid as the potassium salt. The latter makes the antibiotic effective against a wider range of infections by combating certain enzymes produced by some bacteria. Available as oval, white film coated tablets, Augmentin 375mg (250mg/125mg) and 625mg (500mg/125mg), all marked AUGMENTIN. Also, **AUGMENTIN DISPERSABLE** (250mg/125mg), white tablets marked Augmentin. Also **AUGMENTIN SUSPENSION 125/31 SF** (sugar-free) contains 125mg amoxicillin as trihydrate, 31mg clavulanic acid as potassium salt, per 5ml when reconstituted with water. Similarly, **AUGMENTIN SUSPENSION 250/62 SF** (250/62mg). **AUGMENTIN INTRAVENOUS** is a powder for intravenous injection available in 2 strengths containing amoxicillin as sodium salt and clavulanic acid as potassium salt (500/100mg, and 1g/200mg). **AUGMENTIN DUO 400/57**, containing 400mg amoxicillin as trihydrate and 57mg clavulanic acid as potassium salt per 5ml of reconstituted suspension.

*Used for*: respiratory tract and ear, nose and throat infections, skin and soft tissue infections, urinary tract infections.

*Dosage*: adults, tablets, 375mg three times a day (severe infections 625mg) for 14 days. Children, use suspension, under 6 years use lower strength 125/31. Under one year 25mg per kg body weight each day; 1–6 years, 5ml three times a day for 14 days. 6–12 years use 250/62 suspension, 5ml 3 times each day for 14 days. Intravenous injection: adults, 1.2g or by intermittent infusion 6 to 8-hourly for 14 days. Children, under 3 months, 30mg per kg of body weight every 12 hours in newborns increasing to every 8 hours in older infants. 3 months–12 years, 30mg per kg of body weight every 8 or 6 hours. By intravenous or intermittent infusion for up to 14 days. Augmentin Duo: children aged 2 months to 2 years; 25/3.6 to 45/6.4mg per kg of body weight each day in two divided doses. 2 years to 6 years; 2.5 to 5ml twice each day. 7 years to 12 years; 5 to 10ml twice each day. All doses should be taken just before eating a meal.

*Special care*: pregnant and breast-feeding mothers, patients with liver and kidney disease, glandular fever. Review after 14 days.

*Avoid use*: allergy to penicillin.

*Possible interaction*: allopurinol, anticoagulants.

*Side effects*: gastro-intestinal upset, allergic responses, rarely cholestatic jaundice, hepatitis, blood abnormalities, effects on central nervous system, phlebitis at site of injection.

*Manufacturer*: GlaxoSmithKline.

## AUREOCORT

*Description*: a combined antibacterial and steroid preparation available in the form of cream or ointment, containing 0.1% of the corticosteroid triamcinolone acetonide and 3% of the tetracycline antibiotic, chlortetracycline hydrochloride.

*Used for*: inflammation and irritation of the skin where infection is present also.

*Dosage*: apply sparingly to affected skin two or three times daily.

*Special care*: limit use to a short time period. In children and on face, treatment should not exceed 5 days.

*Avoid use*: on extensive areas of skin or for long time periods or for prevention. Acne (including rosacea), urticaria, scabies, leg ulcers, viral skin infections, tuberculosis, ringworm.

*Side effects*: thinning of skin and skin changes, adrenal gland suppression, fluid retention.

*Manufacturer*: Lederele.

## AXID

*Description*: a preparation containing nizatidine (an H2 blocker) available in the form of capsules: pale, yellow/dark yellow, coded 3144 (150mg) and yellow/brown coded 3145 (300mg). **AXID INJECTION** contains 25mg nizatidine per ml.

*Used for*: duodenal and benign gastric ulcers and their prevention. Gastro-oesophageal reflux disease.
*Dosage*: adults, for duodenal and gastric ulcers, 300mg taken in the evening or 150mg morning and evening for 4–8 weeks. Prevention, 150mg in evening for up to one year. Adults, for gastro-oesophageal reflux disease, 150mg–300mg twice a day for up to 12 weeks. Axid injection, adults, dilute before use, 100mg by slow intravenous injection three times each day or 10mg per hour by intravenous infusion. Maximum 480mg per day.
*Special care*: patients with liver or kidney disease, pregnant or breast-feeding mothers.
*Avoid use*: children.
*Possible interaction*: salicylates.
*Side effects*: sweating, sleepiness, itchiness, headache, muscle and joint pain, jaundice, raised levels of liver enzymes, hepatitis, anaemia, pain at site of injection. Rarely, allergic responses.
*Manufacturer*: Lilly.

## AXSAIN

*Description*: a topical counter-irritant analgesic preparation available as a cream containing 0.075% capsaicin.
*Used for*: post-herpetic neuralgia, diabetic neuropathy.
*Dosage*: adults only, massage in 3 to 4 times daily once lesions have healed.
*Avoid use*: children, on broken, irritated skin.
*Side effects*: local skin irritation.
*Manufacturer*: Elan.

## AZACTAM

*Description*: a powder for injection and infusion, containing 500mg aztreonam available as 1g or 2g powder in vials.

*Used for*: serious infections caused by Gram-negative bacteria, including those of the lower respiratory tract and lung infections in cystic fibrosis sufferers. Also, soft tissue, skin, joint, bone, gynaecological and abdominal infections. Urinary tract infections and gonorrhoea, meningitis (where *H. influenzae* or *N. Meningitidis* is the causal organism), septicaemia and bacteraemia (bacteria in blood indicating infection).

*Dosage*: adults, 1g by intramuscular or intravenous injection every eight hours or 2g intravenously every 12 hours. If infection is severe, 2g six to eight hourly intravenously. Maximum daily dose is 8g. For urinary tract infections, 0.5–1g intramuscularly or intravenously every eight to twelve hours. For cystitis, 1g intramuscularly as a single dose. Children, one week to two years, 30mg per kg of body weight every six to eight hours. Severe infections in children over two years, 50mg per kg of body weight every six to eight hours. Maximum dose is 8g each day.

*Special care*: patients with allergy to penicillin or cephalosporin. Persons with kidney or liver disease. Breastfeeding mothers.

*Avoid use*: children under one year, pregnancy.

*Side effects*: gastro-intestinal upset, vomiting and diarrhoea, local skin inflammation at injection site. Rarely, blood and liver reactions.

*Manufacturer*: BMS.

## AZAPROPAZONE *SEE*: RHEUMOX.

## AZELASTINE *SEE*: OPTILAST, RHINOLAST.

## AZOPT

*Description*: a carbonic anhydrase 11 inhibitor used in the treatment of glaucoma. Contains 10mg of brinzolamide per ml, as eye drops.

*Used for*: open angle glaucoma, high blood pressure within the eye. As sole therapy when Beta blockers cannot be used or have not worked or in addition to Beta blockers.

*Dosage*: adults; 1 drop directly into eye two or three times each day.

*Special care*: pregnancy, dry eye conditions (patient must be monitored), people who wear contact lenses, other forms of glaucoma.

*Avoid use*: children, breastfeeding, liver or serious kidney disease, sensitivity to sulfonamides, hyperchloraemic acidosis.

*Possible interaction*: CYP3A4 inhibitors, carbonic anhydrase inhibitors. Wait quarter of an hour before inserting contact lenses. Do not use other eye drops for at least 5 minutes.

*Side effects*: headache, short-lived discomfort in eye and disturbance of sight, aversion of taste. Any adverse side effects should be reported to the CSM.

*Manufacturer*: Alcon.

## AZTREONAM *SEE*: AZACTAM.

# B

## BACITRACIN *SEE*: CICATRIN, POLYFAX.

## BACTROBAN

*Description*: a broad-spectrum antibiotic preparation containing 2% mupirocin in the form of an ointment. **BACTROBAN NASAL** is an ointment containing 2% mupirocin in a soft white paraffin base.*Also*: **BACTROBAN CREAM** containing 2% mupirocin.

*Used for*: bacterial skin infections. Nasal ointment, infections of the nose and nostrils caused by staphylococci bacteria. Cream used for secondary infections of wounds and lesions.

*Dosage*: ointment, apply to skin 3 times a day for up to 10 days. Nasal ointment, apply to the inner surface of nostrils 2 or 3 times daily. Cream, applied as for ointment.

*Special care*: patients with kidney disorders (ointment), avoid eyes.

*Avoid use*: ointment: infants aged less than 1 year.

*Side effects*: may sting on application. Cream: nausea, headache, diarrhoea.

*Manufacturer*: GlaxoSmithKline.

## BAMBEC

*Description*: a preparation containing bambuterol hydrochloride which is a selective ß2-agonist used in the treatment of asthma. Bambec is available as tablets of 2 strengths containing 10mg (marked A/BM) and 20mg (marked A/BA). Tablets are oval, white and scored.

*Used for*: asthma (bronchospasm) and reversible airways obstruction.

*Dosage*: 10mg as one dose taken at night increasing to 20mg once a day if necessary. If the patient has been used to treatment with a ß2–agonist, then 20mg may be taken from the start.

*Special care*: pregnant women and breast-feeding mothers, diabetics, moderate or severe kidney disorders, heart disorders, thyrotoxicosis. In cases of severe asthma, potassium levels in blood should be monitored.

*Avoid use*: children.

*Possible interaction*: Other ß-blockers, suxamethonium.

*Side effects*: headache, palpitations, cramps, tremor, hypokalaemia, skin reactions.

*Manufacturer*: AstraZeneca.

## BAMBUTEROL *SEE* BAMBEC.

## BARATOL

*Description*: an antihypertensive, alpha-adrenoceptor blocking drug, indoramin hydrochloride, available as blue tablets, 25mg strength, marked MPL020 and 25 which are film-coated and scored.

*Used for*: hypertension (high blood pressure).

*Dosage*: adults, 25mg twice each day at start increasing by 25mg or 50mg each fortnight. Maximum dose is 200mg per day in 2 or 3 divided doses.

*Special care*: elderly people, patients with liver or kidney disorders, Parkinson's disease, epilepsy, history of depression. Patients with incipient heart failure should be treated with digoxin and diuretics. Performance of skilled tasks such as driving may be impaired.

*Avoid use*: children, cardiac failure.

*Possible interaction*: alcohol, antihypertensive drugs (dose requires adjustment), MAOIs.

*Side effects*: drowsiness, dizziness, depression, dry mouth, blocked nose, weight gain, failure to ejaculate.

*Manufacturer*: Shire.

## BAXAN

*Description*: a cephalosporin antibiotic preparation available as tablets and as powder for reconstitution with water, in 3 strengths. Baxan white capsules contain 500mg cefadroxil (as monohydrate) and are marked 7244. **BAXAN SUSPENSION** contains either 125mg, 250mg or 500mg per 5ml when reconstituted with water, available as powder to make 60ml.

*Used for*: various infections of skin, urinary and respiratory tracts, ear and soft tissues.

*Dosage*: adults, 500mg–1g twice each day (1 to 2 tablets); children under 1 year, 25mg per kg of body weight in divided doses; 1 to 6 years, 250mg twice each day; 6 years and over, 500mg twice each day.

*Special care*: pregnancy, breastfeeding, patients with penicillin allergy or kidney disease.

*Side effects*: gastro-intestinal upset, allergic responses.
*Manufacturer*: BMS.

## BECLAZONE EASI-BREATHE

*Description*: a corticosteroid preparation containing either 50 or 100μg beclometasone dipropionate per dose, delivered by breath activated metered dose aerosol. *Also,* **BECLAZONE INHALER**, available in three strengths, containing 50, 100 or 200μg beclometasone dipropionate delivered by breath-activated metered dose inhaler. *Also*, **BECLAZONE 250 INHALER**, containing 250μg beclometasone dipropionate per breath-activated metered dose. *Also,* **BECLAZONE 250 EASI-BREATHE** containing 250μg beclometasone dipropionate delivered by breath-activated inhaler.

*Used for*: chronic reversible obstructive airways disease (asthma).

*Dosage*: Beclazone Easi-Breathe, Beclazone Inhaler; adults: 100μg three to four each day or 200μg twice each day. Severe asthma, 600 to 800μg at start, reducing dosage as condition responds. Children: 100 to 200μg twice each day or 50 to 100μg two to four times each day according to need. Beclazone 250 Inhaler, Beclazone 250 Easi-Breathe; adults: 500μg twice each day or 250μg four times each day. The maximum daily dose is 2000μg. These preparations are not recommended for children.

*Special care*: pulmonary tuberculosis, pregnant women, patients who have been taking systemic steroid drugs.

*Side effects*: hoarseness, fungal infections of throat and mouth.
*Manufacturer*: IVAX.

## BECLOFORTE

*Description*: a corticosteroid preparation for inhalation containing 250µg beclometasone dipropionate per dose delivered by metered dose aerosol. *Also*, **BECLOFORTE DISKHALER** consisting of blisters containing 400µg beclometasone dipropionate per dose delivered by breath-actuated inhaler.
*Used for*: patients with chronic and severe asthma, emphysema or chronic bronchitis who require high doses of beclometasone.
*Dosage*: adults only, 500µg twice each day or 250µg 4 times a day. May be increased to 500µg 3 or 4 times each day if necessary. Diskhaler, adults, 1 blister twice each day increasing to 2 blisters twice each day if condition is severe.
*Special care*: pregnancy, breastfeeding, patients with active or quiescent pulmonary tuberculosis, those transferring from systemic steroids. Risk of systemic effects such as suppression of adrenal glands if high doses are used for a long period.
*Avoid use*: children.
*Side effects*: hoarseness, fungal infections of throat and mouth, paradoxical bronchospasm, allergic reactions.
*Manufacturer*: A & H.

## BECLOMETASONE *SEE*: AEROBEC, BECLAZONE, BECLOFORTE, BECODISKS, BECOTIDE.

## BECODISKS

*Description*: a corticosteroid preparation available as a dry powder for inhalation with Diskhaler. Beige disks contain 100µg beclometasone dipropionate; brown disks contain 200µg; dark brown disks contain 400µg.

*Used for*: prevention of bronchial asthma.

*Dosage*: adults, 400µg twice each day or 200µg 3 to 4 times each day. Children, 100µg 2 to 4 times each day or 200µg twice each day.

*Special care*: pregnant or breastfeeding women, patients with active or quiescent pulmonary tuberculosis, those transferring from systemic steroids. Risk of suppression of adrenal glands and other systemic effects with prolonged use. Height of children should be monitored if use is prolonged.

*Side effects*: hoarseness, fungal infections of throat and mouth, paradoxical bronchospasm.

*Manufacturer*: A & H.

## BECOTIDE

*Description*: a corticosteroid preparation, beclometasone dipropionate, available in the form of an aerosol of different strengths for inhalation. Becotide-50 (50µg per metered inhalation), Becotide-100 (100µg) and Becotide-200 (200µg).

*Used for*: prevention of bronchial asthma.

*Dosage*: adults, 400μg each day in 2, 3 or 4 divided doses. If asthma is severe, 600–800μg may be required in first instance in daily divided doses. This should be reduced as condition improves. Children, 100μg twice each day increasing to 400μg in two to four divided doses, if required and according to response.

*Special care*: pregnant or breastfeeding women, patients with active or quiescent pulmonary tuberculosis, those transferring from systemic steroids. Risk of suppression of adrenal glands and other systemic effects with high doses and prolonged use. Height of children should be monitored with long term usage.

*Side effects*: hoarseness, paradoxical bronchospasm, fungal infections of throat and mouth.

*Manufacturer*: A & H.

## BECOTIDE ROTACAPS

*Description*: a corticosteroid preparation, beclometasone dipropionate, available as a dry powder in capsules for inhalation: buff/clear (100μg), brown/clear (200μg), dark brown/clear (400μg), all marked with name and strength and each is a single dose for use with a Rotahaler.

*Used for*: prevention of bronchial asthma.

*Dosage*: adults, 400μg twice each day or 200μg 3 or 4 times each day. Children, 100μg 2 to 4 times each day or 200μg twice each day.

*Special care*: pregnant or breastfeeding women, patients with active or quiescent pulmonary tuberculosis, those transferring from systemic steroids. Risk of adrenal gland suppression and other systemic effects with prolonged usage or high doses. Height of children should be monitored if treatment is long-term.

*Side effects*: hoarseness, paradoxical bronchospasm, fungal infections of throat and mouth.

*Manufacturer*: A & H.

## BEGRIVAC

*Description*: a preparation of vaccine (inactivated split virion) against various strains of influenza, available as a suspension in pre-filled syringes. The strains included are A/New Caledonia 20/99(H1N1)-like strain, A/Moscow/10/99(H3N2)-like strain and B/Hong Kong/330/2001-loke strain with 15μg of each for every 0.5ml suspension.

*Used for*: immunisation against influenza.

*Dosage*: adults and children over 3 years; 0.5ml given by intra-muscular or deep sub-cutaneous injection. Infants aged 6 months to 3 years, 0.25ml or 0.5ml – a second dose may be needed after 4 weeks in a child not previously vaccinated or infected.

*Special care*: pregnant women.

*Avoid use*: fever, persons with known allergy to eggs or chicken protein.

*Side effects*: soreness at injection site, headache, malaise, fever. Rarely, neurological effects.

*Manufacturer*: Wyeth.

## BENDROFLUMETHIAZIDE *SEE*: APRINOX, CORGARETIC.

## BENZALKONIUM CHLORIDE *SEE* BRADOSOL.

## TRIHEXYPHENIDYL *SEE* BROFLEX.

## BENZATROPINE MESYLATE *SEE* COGENTIN.

## BENZYL BENZOATE *SEE*, ANUSOL HC.

## BETA-ADALAT

*Description*: a cardio-selective ß-blocker/Class II calcium antagonist containing atenolol and nifedipine available as red-brown capsules marked with the Bayer cross and name and containing 50mg atenolol and 20mg nifedipine.

*Used for*: hypertension, angina (where therapy with a calcium-channel blocker or beta-blocker alone proves to be ineffective).

*Dosage*: for hypertension, 1 capsule each day increasing to 2 per each 24 hour period, if required. Elderly persons, 1 capsule. Angina, 1 capsule twice each day (two in each 24 hour period).

*Special care*: elderly persons, weak heart, liver or kidney disease, diabetes, anaesthesia.

*Avoid use*: children, pregnancy, breast-feeding, heart block, heart shock or heart failure, asthma, wheezing.

*Possible interaction*: cardiac depressant drugs, cimetidine, quinidine, digoxin, rifampicin, grapefruit juice.

*Side effects*: headache, dizziness, flushing, dryness of eyes, skin rashes, oedema, swelling of gums, breast enlargement.

Rarely, allergic jaundice, mood swings, heart pain (withdraw drug), heart attack.
*Manufacturer*: Bayer.

## BETA-CARDONE

*Description*: a non-cardioselective ß-blocker, sotalol hydrochloride, available as tablets in 3 strengths: green-scored tablets marked Evans/BC4 (40mg); pink-scored tablets marked Evans/BC8 (80mg) and white-scored tablets marked Evans/BC20 (200mg).
*Used for*: ventricular heart arrhythmias and their prevention.
*Dosage*: adults only; initially, 80mg each day either as single or divided dose. Increase at 2 to 3 day intervals to 160 to 320mg each day in two divided doses.
*Special care*: patients with diabetes, liver or kidney disorders, poor cerebral circulation, history of bronchospasm, those undergoing general anaesthesia (drug may need to be stopped). Pregnant women and nursing mothers. Patients with weak hearts may need to be treated with digitalis and diuretic drugs.
*Avoid use*: children, patients with asthma or history of bronchospasm, those with heart block, heart attack, heart shock and various other cardiac disorders. Drug should be stopped gradually.
*Possible interaction*: verapamil, clonidine withdrawal, hyperglycaemics, class I anti-arrhythmic drugs, some anaesthetics, reserpine, sympathomimetics, antidepressants, ergotamine, ergot alkaloids, indometacin,

cimetidine, diltiazem, class II calcium antagonists, CNS depressants, theophylline, warfarin, ibuprofen.

*Side effects*: slow heartbeat, disruption of sleep, cold hands and feet, fatigue in exercise, hair loss, gastro-intestinal upset, wheezing, heart failure, skin rash, dry eyes (withdraw drug gradually).

*Manufacturer*: Celltech.

## BETA-PROGRANE

*Description*: a non-cardioselective ß-blocker available as white, sustained-release capsules containing 160mg of propranolol hydrochloride. *Also*, **HALF-BETA PROGRANE**, available as white/clear, sustained-release capsules, containing 80mg of propranolol hydrochloride.

*Used for*: angina, hypertension, additional therapy in thyrotoxicosis, prevention of migraine.

*Dosage*: adults only; angina: 80 to 160mg each day to a maximum dose of 240mg. Hypertension: 160mg each day increasing gradually, if required, by 80mg daily to a maximum dose of 320mg. Thyrotoxicosis and prevention of migraine: 80mg or 160mg each day with a maximum dose of 240mg.

*Special care*: patients with diabetes, liver or kidney disorders, poor cerebral circulation, history of bronchospasm, those undergoing general anaesthesia (drug may need to be stopped). Pregnant women and nursing mothers. Patients with weak hearts may need to be treated with digitalis and diuretic drugs.

*Avoid use*: children, patients with asthma or history of

bronchospasm, those with heart block, heart attack, heart shock and various other cardiac disorders. Drug should be stopped gradually.

*Possible interaction*: verapamil, clonidine withdrawal, hyperglycaemics, class I anti-arrhythmic drugs, some anaesthetics, reserpine, sympathomimetics, antidepressants, ergotamine, ergot alkaloids, indometacin, cimetidine, diltiazem, class II calcium antagonists, CNS depressants, theophylline, warfarin, ibuprofen.

*Side effects*: slow heartbeat, disruption of sleep, cold hands and feet, fatigue in exercise, hair loss, gastro-intestinal upset, wheezing, heart failure, skin rash, dry eyes (withdraw drug gradually).

*Manufacturer*: Tillomed.

## BETAGAN

*Description*: a preparation which is a ß-blocker containing 0.5% levobunolol hydrochloride, available in the form of eye drops. *Also,* **BETAGAN UNIT DOSE** containing 0.5% levobunolol hydrochloride in solution, as single dose vials.

*Used for*: high blood pressure within the eye, open-angle glaucoma.

*Dosage*: adults only; 1 drop into affected eye once or twice each day.

*Special care*: breastfeeding women, diabetes, patients with respiratory disorders.

*Avoid use*: children, pregnant women, some forms of heart disease, asthma, previous obstructive pulmonary disease.

*Possible interaction*: other, (systemic) ß-blockers, reserpine.

*Side effects*: headache, local irritation in eye, dizziness, symptoms associated with systemic ß-blockers.

*Manufacturer*: Allergan.

## BETALOC

*Description*: a cardioselective ß-blocker, metoprolol tartrate, available as tablets of 2 strengths, as modified-release tablets and in ampoules for injection. Betaloc tablets are white, scored and contain 50mg (marked A/BB) or 100mg (marked A/ME). Also, **BETALOC-SA** modified-release tablets (Durules®), containing 200mg and marked A/MD. Also, **BETALOC INJECTION** containing 1mg per ml in 5ml ampoules.

*Used for*: heart arrhythmias, angina, maintenance therapy in heart attack, hypertension, additional therapy in thyrotoxicosis, prevention of migraine.

*Dosage*: all adults only; heart attack, 200mg each day in divided doses; heart arrhythmias, 50mg 2 or 3 times each day increasing to maximum daily dose of 300mg. Angina, 50–100mg twice or three times each day. Hypertension, 50mg twice each day at first increasing to 400mg if required. Thyrotoxicosis, 50mg 4 times each day; migraine prevention, 100mg–200mg each day in divided doses. Betaloc-SA; angina, hypertension: 1 tablet taken in the morning, increasing to 2, if needed; prevention of migraine: 1 tablet taken in the morning. Betaloc injection: early treatment after heart attack; 5mg every 2 minutes by intravenous injection to a maximum of 15mg. Fifteen minutes after final injection, patient is transferred to tablets – 50mg taken every 6 hours for 2 days.

*Special care*: pregnancy, breast-feeding, liver or kidney disease, diabetes, metabolic acidosis, poor cerebral blood supply, history of bronchospasm, those undergoing anaesthesia; patients with weak hearts should be treated with digitalis and diuretics. Drug should be stopped gradually.

*Avoid use*: children, patients with asthma, heart diseases including heart block, heart shock, slow heartbeat rate, heart failure.

*Possible interaction*: cardiac depressants, anaesthetics, reserpine, sedatives, class II calcium antagonists, antihypertensives, sympathomimetics, cimetidine, indometacin, ergotamine, class I antiarrhythmic drugs, verapamil, clonidine withdrawal, hypoglycaemics, rifampicin, warfarin, ibuprofen.

*Side effects*: sleep disturbance, cold feet and hands, slow heartbeat, fatigue on exercise, wheeziness, heart failure, gastro-intestinal disorders; dry eyes or skin rash (stop use gradually), hair loss, low blood pressure, thrombocytopenia (abnormal decline in blood platelets).

*Manufacturer*: AstraZeneca.

## BETNELAN

*Description*: a corticosteroid, glucocorticoid preparation, comprising 0.5mg of betamethasone in each scored, white tablet. Tablets are marked with name and EVANS.

*Used for*: allergies, serious asthma, inflammatory conditions, rheumatoid arthritis, collagen disorders.

*Dosage*: children and adults over 12 years; 0.5mg to 5mg each day, using minimum effective dose for maintenance. Children aged 1 to 7 years; one quarter to half the adult dose; aged 7 to 12 years; half to three-quarters the adult dose.

*Special Care*: elderly, pregnant or breastfeeding women, patients with tuberculosis, fungal, viral and other infections, amoebiasis. Patients should endeavour to avoid possible infection with chickenpox or herpes zoster virus; in the event of exposure or infection, special treatment is required. Also, many inflammatory gastrointestinal diseases, kidney and liver disorders, heart failure and heart disease, thyroid disorders, myasthenia gravis, thrombophlebitis, osteoporosis, secondary tumours, high blood pressure, glaucoma, cerebral malaria, previous steroid damage. Also, stress diabetes, epilepsy, psychotic disorders. Patients require close monitoring and drug use should be limited in time and dosage.

*Avoid use*: infants under 1 year, patients with systemic fungal infections, unless receiving particular treatment.

*Possible interaction*: amphotericin, acetazolamide, ciclosporin, azole anti-fungal drugs, methotrexate, live vaccines, carbenoxolone, salicylates, NSAIDs. Also, diuretics, anticholinesterases, rifampicin, hypoglycaemics, antihypertensives, cardiac glycosides, oestrogens, oral anticoagulants, rifampicin, phenytoin, carbamazepine, phenobarbital, rifabutin, ephedrine, primidone, aminoglutethimide.

*Side effects*: depending upon dose and duration of treatment, can include a range of systemic steroid effects: fluid retention, osteoporosis, cushingoid changes, suppression of growth in children, hyperglycaemia, electrolyte imbalances, thinning of skin and skin reactions, high blood pressure, mood changes, depression, gastrointestinal disturbances, muscle weakness, effects on bones, central nervous system effects, changes in sperm motility (ability to swim), reduction in wound healing, peptic ulcers.

*Manufacturer*: Celltech.

## BETIM

*Description*: a non-cardioselective ß-blocker available as white, scored tablets containing 10mg timolol maleate and marked with 102 and symbol.

*Used for*: prevention of second heart attack following initial episode, angina, hypertension, prevention of migraine.

*Dosage*: adults, prevention of secondary heart attack, 5mg twice each day for first 2 days, thereafter 10mg twice each day. Angina, 10mg twice each day at first, adjusted according to response to a maximum of 60mg. Hypertension, 10mg a day at first in single or divided dose increasing by 10mg every 3 to 4 days to a maximum of 60mg. Usual maintenance dose is in the order of 10–30mg. Prevention of migraine, 10–20mg each day in 1 or 2 divided doses.

*Special care*: pregnancy, breast-feeding, liver or kidney disease, diabetes, those undergoing general anaesthesia, patients with weak hearts should receive digitalis and diuretics. Drug should be stopped gradually.

*Avoid use*: children, patients with asthma or history of breathing difficulties, those with various forms of heart disease including heart block, heart shock, slow heartbeat, heart failure.

*Possible interaction*: class I antiarrhythmics, cardiac depressant anaesthetics, ergotamine, sedatives, sympathomimetics, cimetidine, indometacin, reserpine, hypoglycaemic drugs, clonidine withdrawal, verapamil.

*Side effects*: sleep disturbance, cold feet and hands, slow heartbeat, fatigue in exercise, wheeziness, heart failure, gastro-intestinal upset, dry eyes or skin rash (stop drug gradually).

*Manufacturer*: ICN.

## BETNESOL

*Description*: a corticosteroid, glucocorticoid preparation containing 0.5mg of betamethasone, as sodium phosphate, in each scored, pink tablet. The tablets are marked with the name and EVANS. *Also,* **BETNESOL INJECTION** containing 4mg per ml of betamethasone as sodium phosphate, in ampoules.

*Used for*: tablets: allergies, serious asthma, inflammatory conditions, rheumatoid arthritis, collagen disorders. Betnesol injection: shock, anaphylactic reactions to drugs, lesions of soft tissue.

*Dosage*: tablets, adults and children over 12 years; 0.5 to 5mg each day, dissolved in water at first, reducing to minimum effective dose for maintenance. Children aged 1 to 7 years, $^1/_4$ to $^1/_2$ adult dose; aged 7 to 12 years, $^1/_2$ to $^3/_4$ adult dose.

Betnesol injection, adults and children over 12 years; 4 to 20mg by deep intramuscular or slow intravenous injection or infusion, 3 or 4 times in each 24 hour period. Children aged 0 to 1 year; 1mg; aged 1 to 5 years, 2mg; aged 6 to 12 years, 4mg, all given in same way as for adults and may be repeated 3 to 4 times in each 24 hour period.

*Special care*: elderly, pregnant or breastfeeding women, patients with tuberculosis, fungal, viral and other infections, amoebiasis. Patients should endeavour to avoid possible infection with chickenpox or herpes zoster virus; in the event of exposure or infection, special treatment is required. Also, many inflammatory gastrointestinal diseases, kidney and liver disorders, heart failure and heart disease, thyroid disorders, myasthenia gravis, thrombophlebitis, osteoporosis, secondary tumours, high blood pressure, glaucoma, cerebral malaria, previous steroid damage. Also, stress diabetes, epilepsy, psychotic disorders. Patients require close monitoring and drug use should be limited in time and dosage.

*Avoid use*: infants under 1 year, patients with systemic fungal infections, unless receiving particular treatment.

*Possible interaction*: amphotericin, acetazolamide, ciclosporin, azole anti-fungal drugs, methotrexate, live vaccines, carbenoxolone, salicylates, NSAIDs. Also, diuretics, anticholinesterases, rifampicin, hypoglycaemics, antihypertensives, cardiac glycosides, oestrogens, oral anticoagulants, rifampicin, phenytoin, carbamazepine, phenobarbital, rifabutin, ephedrine, primidone, aminoglutethimide.

*Side effects*: depending upon dose and duration of treatment, can include a range of systemic steroid effects: fluid retention, osteoporosis, cushingoid changes, suppression of growth in children, hyperglycaemia, electrolyte imbalances, thinning of skin and skin reactions, high blood pressure, mood changes, depression, gastrointestinal disturbances, muscle weakness, effects on bones, central nervous system effects, changes in sperm motility (ability to swim), reduction in wound healing, peptic ulcers.
*Manufacturer*: Celltech.

## BETNOVATE

*Description*: a group of moderate to potent corticosteroid preparations containing betamethasone and available as ointment, cream or lotion. Betnovate cream and ointment both contain 0.1% betamethasone (as valerate); **BETNOVATE SCALP APPLICATION**, (0.1%) **BETNOVATE C** cream and ointment contains an antimicrobial drug (antifungal and antibacterial), 3% clioquinol and 0.1% betamethasone (as valerate); **BETNOVATE N** cream and ointment also contain an antimicrobial (antibacterial) drug, 0.5% neomycin sulphate and 0.1% betamethasone (as valerate). **BETNOVATE RD** cream and ointment are less potent containing 0.025% betamethasone (as valerate).
*Used for*: eczema, seborrhoeic and contact dermatitis, psoriasis, other skin disorders (lichen simplex and planus). For infected conditions, Betnovate C or N are used depending upon causal organism.

*Dosage*: adults, apply sparingly 2 or 3 times each day. More potent preparations may be used first with Betnovate RD then used for maintenance treatment. Children over 1 year same as adult dose.

*Special care*: should not be used extensively or for a prolonged period. Should be used for only 5 days on children or on face. Stop use gradually.

*Avoid use*: children under 1 year, continuous use especially by pregnant women, any conditions caused by ringworm, fungi, viruses, tuberculosis, acne, leg ulcers, scabies.

*Side effects*: thinning of skin, suppression of adrenal glands, hair growth, symptoms associated with Cushing's syndrome, e.g. reddening of skin on face and neck.

*Manufacturer*: GlaxoSmithKline.

## BETOPTIC

*Description*: a cardio-selective ß-blocker that reduces pressure within the eye. Contains 0.25% betaxolol as hydrochloride in suspension in single dose vials or in bottle. *Also,* **BETOPTIC SOLUTION** contains 0.5% betaxolol hydrochloride in the form of eye drops.

*Used for*: chronic open angle glaucoma and hypertension of eyes.

*Dosage*: 1 drop twice each day into eye.

*Special care*: patients with diabetes, thyrotoxicosis, blocked airways disease, those undergoing general anaesthetic.

*Avoid use*: children, patients with certain heart diseases including heart shock, cardiac failure, slow heart beat, those using soft contact lenses.

*Side effects*: passing slight discomfort, rarely staining or reddening of cornea and decreased sensitivity of cornea, keratitis.

*Manufacturer*: Alcon.

## BEZAFIBRATE *SEE* BEZALIP

## BEZALIP

*Description*: a preparation used to reduce high levels of fats (lipids) in the bloodstream, and available in the form of white, film-coated tablets marked BM/G6, containing 200mg bezafibrate. Bezalip-MONO are white, film-coated, modified-release tablets marked BM/D9 containing 400mg bezafibrate.

*Used for*: hyperlipidaemias (high blood levels of lipids, classified as type IIa, IIb, III, IV and V) which are resistant to changes in diet.

*Dosage*: adults, Bezalip-MONO, 1 tablet after food at night or in morning. Bezalip, 1 tablet 3 times each day with food.

*Special care*: patients with kidney disease; patients receiving dialysis require lesser dose.

*Avoid use*: children, patients with serious kidney, gall bladder or liver disease, nephrotic disease, light-sensitivity reactions to fibrates, pregnant and breast-feeding women.

*Possible interaction*: MAOIs, antidiabetic and anticoagulant drugs, statins, resins, ciclosporin.

*Side effects*: gastro-intestinal upset, rash, muscle pain, elevated levels of creatinine. Rarely, blood changes, hair

loss, gall stones, impotence, raised liver enzyme levels, cholestasis (disruption in the flow of bile).
*Manufacturer*: Roche.

## BICNU

*Description*: an alkylating cytotoxic drug used in the treatment of certain cancers and produced in the form of a powder for reconstitution and injection. Bicnu contains 100mg carmustine as a powder in a vial, with 3ml sterile ethanol for reconstitution.
*Used for*: leukaemia, lymphomas, myelomas, brain tumours.
*Dosage*: as directed by skilled cancer specialist.
*Special care*: patients should receive regular checks for blood count.
*Side effects*: vomiting and nausea, hair loss, bone marrow suppression (onset of which is delayed) necessitating regular blood checks, adverse effects on fertility. Possible kidney and liver damage may occur.
*Manufacturer*: BMS.

## BINOVUM

*Description*: a combined oestrogen/progesterone oral contraceptive preparation produced as a course of 21 tablets: 7 white tablets marked C over 535 contain 0.5mg (500μg) norethisterone and 35μg ethinylestradiol; 14 peach tablets, marked C over 135, contain 1mg norethisterone and 35μg ethinylestradiol.
*Used for*: oral contraception.
*Dosage*: 1 tablet each day starting with white tablets on first

day of period. There are 7 tablet-free days before the process is repeated.

*Special care*: hypertension, asthma, diabetes, varicose veins, multiple sclerosis, Raynaud's disease, kidney dialysis, chronic kidney disease, obesity, severe depression. Family history of heart disease, inflammatory bowel disease, Crohn's disease. Risk of arterial thrombosis especially in older women, those who smoke and those who are obese. Regular checks on blood pressure, breasts and pelvic organs should be carried out at intervals.

*Avoid use*: pregnancy, history of heart disease or thrombosis, hypertension, sickle cell anaemia, liver disease, cholestatic jaundice of pregnancy, abnormalities of liver function, porphyria, undiagnosed vaginal bleeding, some cancers, (hormone-dependent ones), infectious hepatitis, recent trophoblastic disease.

*Possible interaction*: barbiturates, tetracycline antibiotics, rifampicin, griseofulvin, carbamazepine, chloral hydrate, primidone, phenytoin, ethosuximide, glutethimide, dichloralphenazone.

*Side effects*: oedema and bloatedness, leg cramps, reduction in sexual desire, headaches, depression, weight gain, vaginal discharge, breakthrough bleeding, cervical erosion, nausea, chloasma (brownish patches on skin).

*Manufacturer*: Janssen-Cilag.

## BISMUTH OXIDE *SEE* ANUSOL HC.

## BISMUTH SUBGALLATE *SEE* ANUSOL HC.

## BISOPROLOL *SEE* EMCOR, MONOCOR.

## BONEFOS

*Description*: a preparation of the drug, sodium clodronate (a biphosphonate) which affects bone metabolism, preventing the increased rate of bone turnover associated with certain malignant conditions. Bonefos is available in the form of capsules, tablets and as a solution for intravenous infusion. Yellow capsules contain 400mg and the white, oval-shaped film-coated tablets contain 800mg. These are marked L134 and scored. The intravenous solution contains 60mg per ml in 5ml ampoules.

*Used for*: hypercalcaemia of malignancy. Bone pain and lesions associated with secondary bone growths as a result of multiple myeloma (malignant bone marrow disease) or breast cancer.

*Dosage*: adults, capsules or tablets, 1600mg each day either as one or two doses, taken 1 hour before or 1 hour after a meal. The maximum dose is 3200mg. Infusion, adults, 1500mg as single infusion over 4 hours or 300mg given by slow intravenous infusion for up to 7 days. Afterwards, capsules or tablets should be taken.

*Special care*: moderate kidney disorders. Ensure adequate fluid intake, monitor blood calcium levels and kidney function.

*Avoid use*: children, pregnancy, breast-feeding, severe kidney failure.

*Possible interaction*: other biphosphonates, NSAIDs, mineral supplements, antacid preparations.

*Side effects*: gastro-intestinal upset, disturbance of kidney function, parathyroid hormone, lactic acid dehydrogenase, creatinine, transaminase, alkaline phosphatase (enzymes) levels may be elevated for a time. Rarely, there may be hypocalcaemia which does not cause symptoms or skin reactions.

*Manufacturer*: Boehringer Ingelheim.

## BOTOX

*Description*: a bacterial (Clostridium) botulinum toxin, type A-haemagglutinin complex 100 units as powder in a vial.

*Used for*: relief of eyelid spasm, hemifacial spasm, idiopathic cervical dystonia (muscle tone impairment). Specialist treatment of equinus foot deformity (walking on tiptoe) because of spasticity in cerebral palsy cases.

*Dosage*: data sheet to be consulted before administration.

*Side effects*: all adverse reactions to be reported to the Committee on the Safety of Medicines.

*Manufacturer*: Allergan.

## BOTULINUM TOXIN *SEE* BOTOX.

## BRADOSOL

*Description*: an antiseptic preparation in the form of lozenges, each containing 0.5mg of benzalkonium chloride. *Also*, **BRADOSOL PLUS** lozenges, each containing 5mg of lidocaine hydrochloride and 0.5mg of domiphen bromide.

*Used for*: sore throat.

*Dosage*: Bradosol, adults and children over 5 years, 1 lozenge sucked slowly as needed. Bradosol Plus, adults only, 1 lozenge sucked slowly every 2 to 3 hours to a maximum of 8 in 24 hours. Can be taken for a maximum of 5 days.

*Avoid use*: Bradosol – children under 5 years. Bradosol Plus not recommended for children.

*Manufacturer*: Novartis Consumer.

## BREVIBLOC

*Description*: a cardio-selective ß-blocker available in the form of a solution for injection. Brevibloc contains either 10mg esmolol hydrochloride per ml in a 10ml vial or 250mg per ml (for dilution before use) in 10ml ampoules.

*Used for*: cardiac arrhythmias of various types, (sinus tachycardia; atrial flutter, atrial fibrillation), raised heartbeat rate and hypertension.

*Dosage*: 50–200µg per kg body weight per minute by intravenous infusion.

*Special care*: women in late pregnancy, breast-feeding, liver disease, kidney disease, angina, diabetes.

*Avoid use*: asthma, history of obstructive airways disease, heart failure, heart block, heart shock.

*Possible interaction*: other antiarrhythmic drugs.

*Manufacturer*: Baxter.

## BREVINOR

*Description*: a combined oestrogen/progestogen contraceptive preparation available as blue tablets, marked BX and

SEARLE contain 35μg ethinylestradiol and 0.5mg norethisterone.

*Used for*: contraception.

*Dosage*: 1 each day for 21 days starting on 5th day of period, then 7 tablet-free days.

*Special care*: women with asthma, hypertension, Raynaud's disease, haemolytic uraemic syndrome, diabetes, multiple sclerosis, chronic kidney disease, kidney dialysis, Sydenham's chorea, varicose veins, depression, epilepsy, history of cardiac failure, cholelithiasis, migraine, at risk of thrombosis, contact lenses, chloasma. Smoking, age and obesity increase the risk of thrombosis; there is a slightly increased risk of breast cancer. Blood pressure should be monitored and there may be a need for regular breast and pelvic examination.

*Avoid use*: pregnant women, patients with history of thrombosis or who may be at risk of this, heart disease, sickle cell anaemia, liver diseases, infectious hepatitis, history of cholestatic jaundice (caused by a failure of bile to reach the small intestine), porphyria, chorea, otosclerosis, haemolytic uraemic syndrome, hormone-dependent cancers, recent trophoblastic disease, undiagnosed vaginal bleeding.

*Possible interaction*: tetracycline antibiotics, ampicillin barbiturates, chloral hydrate, griseofulvin, rifampicin, carbamazepine, phenytoin, primidone, dichloralphenazone, ethosuximide, glutethimide, phenylbutazone, St John's Wort.

*Side effects*: oedema and bloatedness, leg cramps,

enlargement of breasts, loss of libido, headaches, nausea, depression, weight gain, breakthrough bleeding, cervical erosion, vaginal discharge, brownish patches on skin (chloasma). Discontinue immediately if any of the following occur: pregnancy, rise in blood pressure, disturbance of vision, new occurrence of severe or migraine-type headaches, signs or symptoms of thromboembolism or thrombophlebitis, serious depression, severe pains in upper abdomen, enlargement of liver, jaundice. Discontinue 6 weeks before planned surgery and do not retake until fully mobile.

*Manufacturer*: Pharmacia.

## BRICANYL

*Description*: a bronchodilator and a selective ß2-agonist (a selective beta receptor stimulant) and muscle relaxant containing terbutaline sulphate. Bricanyl is available as tablets, a syrup and as a variety of preparations suitable for use with different kinds of inhaler.

*Used for*: bronchospasm in asthma.

*Dosage*: Bricanyl white scored tablets, marked 5 and A/BT contain 5mg. Adult dose: 1 tablet twice each day or at 8-hour intervals. Children: 7 to 15 years, half adult dose. Young children under 7 should use syrup. Also, **BRICANYL SA** (sustained release) tablets, white, marked A/BD, contain 7.5mg. Adult dose: 1 twice each day. **BRICANYL Aerosol inhalation**, capsules contain 0.25mg per metered dose aerosol. Adults and children: 1 to 2 puffs as required, maximum dose 8 puffs in 24 hours.

**BRICANYL TURBOHALER** is a breath-actuated dry powder inhaler containing 0.5mg per metered dose. Adults and children, 1 inhalation as needed with a maximum of 4 in 24 hours. **BRICANYL SPACER INHALER** (with extended mouthpiece which is collapsible) contains 0.25mg per dose. Adults and children, 1 to 2 puffs as required with a maximum of 8 in 24 hours. **BRICANYL RESPULES** (for use with nebulizer) contain 5mg per 2ml solution as single dose units. Adults: 5–10mg 2, 3 or 4 times each day. Children over 25kg body weight: 5mg 2, 3 or 4 times daily. Both with nebulizer. **BRICANYL RESPIRATOR SOLUTION** (for use with power-operated nebulizer) contains 10mg per ml (diluted before use with sterile physiological saline). Adults, 5 to 10mg, children, 2–10mg diluted and used with nebulizer. **BRICANYL SYRUP** (sugar-free) contains 1.5mg per 5ml. Adults: 10–15ml; children under 3 years: 2.5ml; 3 to 7 years, 2.5–5ml, 7 to 15 years, 5–10ml. All at 8-hour intervals. **BRICANYL INJECTION** contains 0.5mg per ml in ampoules. Adults; 0.25–0.5mg by subcutaneous, intramuscular or slow intravenous injection up to 4 times each day. Children; 2 to 15 years, 10µg per kg of body weight, subcutaneously, intramuscularly or by slow intravenous injection. Maximum dose, 300µg.

*Special care*: pregnant or breastfeeding women, heart disorders, thyrotoxicosis, diabetes.

*Possible interaction*: sympathomimetics, hypokalaemic drugs (lowering potassium levels), ß-blockers.

*Side effects*: headache, nervous tension, trembling,

palpitations, muscle cramps, lowered potassium levels, nettle rash, skin effects, disturbance of sleep and behavioural upset in children.

*Manufacturer*: AstraZeneca.

## BROFLEX

*Description*: an antimuscarinic or anticholinergic preparation, produced in the form of a pink syrup containing 5mg trihexyphenidyl hydrochloride per 5ml.

*Used for*: Parkinsonism, including drug-induced.

*Dosage*: adults, 2mg each day at first increasing over a period of days by 1 or 2mg to a usual maintenance dose of 5–15mg, in 3 to 4 divided doses. Maximum daily dose is 20mg.

*Special care*: pregnant or breastfeeding women, high blood pressure, enlarged prostate gland, obstruction of gastro-intestinal tract, heart, liver or kidney disease. Withdraw drug slowly.

*Avoid use*: children, glaucoma.

*Possible interaction*: antidepressants, antihistamines, phenothiazines, amantadine, MAOIs, disopyramide.

*Side effects*: anti-cholinergic effects including gastro-intestinal disturbances, dry mouth, dizziness, blurred vision, sometimes nervousness, hypersensitivity, tachycardia (raised heart beat rate), urinary retention. In susceptible patients and/or with higher doses, psychiatric disturbances, mental confusion, excitability which may require treatment to be discontinued.

*Manufacturer*: Alliance.

## BROMPHENIRAMINE *SEE* DIMOTANE.

## BRUFEN

*Description*: an NSAID used as an analgesic to treat a variety of disorders and available as tablets, granules and syrup containing propionic acid – ibuprofen: magenta-coloured, oval, sugar-coated tablets are available in 3 strengths; coded BRUFEN (200mg); coded BRUFEN 400 (400mg) and coded BRUFEN 600 (600mg). **BRUFEN GRANULES** are effervescent, orange-flavoured granules in sachet containing 600mg. **BRUFEN SYRUP** contains 100mg per 5ml and **BRUFEN RETARD**, contain 800mg as white, oval film-coated sustained release tablets marked with name.

*Used for*: pain and inflammation in such conditions as rheumatic disorders, joint pain, juvenile arthritis, periarticular disorders, rheumatoid arthritis, seronegative arthritis, ankylosing spondylitis, osteoarthrosis, post-operative pain, period pain, soft tissue injuries.

*Dosage*: adults, tablets and granules, 1200–1800mg each day in divided doses (after food) with a maximum daily dose of 2400mg. A maintenance dose in the region of 600–1200mg may be sufficient. Adults, Brufen Retard, 2 tablets taken in the early evening or 3, in divided dose, if condition is very severe. Children, over 7kg body weight, Brufen tablets, 20mg/kg of body weight each day in divided doses. Junior rheumatoid arthritis, up to 40mg/kg of body weight each day in divided doses. Children, over 7 kg body weight, syrup, age 1 to 2 years, 2.5ml; age

3 to 7 years, 5ml; age 8 to 12 years, 10ml, all repeated up to 3 times each day.

*Special care*: pregnancy, nursing mothers, elderly persons, asthma, gastro-intestinal disorders, heart, liver or kidney disease, previous heart failure or high blood pressure. Patients on long-term therapy should receive monitoring of kidney function.

*Avoid use*: patients with known allergy to aspirin or anti-inflammatory drugs, those with peptic ulcer. Children under 7kg body weight.

*Possible interaction*: quinolones, anticoagulants, thiazide diuretics.

*Side effects*: gastro-intestinal upset and bleeding, rash, low levels of blood platelets (thrombocytopenia). All cases of aseptic meningitis should be reported to the Committee on the Safety of Medicines.

*Manufacturer*: Abbott.

## BUCCASTEM

*Description*: an anti-emetic and dopamine antagonist belonging to a group called the phenothiazines, available as pale yellow (buccal) tablets containing 3mg prochlorperazine maleate.

*Used for*: severe nausea, vomiting, vertigo due to labyrinthine disorders or Ménière's disease, migraine.

*Dosage*: 1 to 2 tablets twice each day, the tablet being placed high up between upper lip and gum and left to dissolve.

*Special care*: pregnancy, nursing mothers.

*Avoid use*: children under 14 years of age, patients with

Parkinson's disease, blood changes, narrow angle glaucoma, enlarged prostate gland, liver or kidney disease, epilepsy.

*Possible interaction*: alcohol, alpha-blockers, CNS depressants (sedatives).

*Side effects*: hypotension (low blood pressure), especially in elderly persons or dehydrated patients, anticholinergic effects, drowsiness, skin reactions, insomnia. Rarely extra-pyramidal symptoms may occur and Parkinsonism, especially in elderly patients.

*Manufacturer*: R&C.

## BUDENOSIDE *SEE* PULMICORT.

## BUMETANIDE *SEE* BURINEX, BURINEX A, BURINEX K.

## BURINEX

*Description*: a loop diuretic preparation, (acting on the part of the kidney tubules called loops of Henle), available in the form of tablets of two strengths containing bumetanide. White, scored tablets marked 133 and with lion logo contain 1mg, those marked with strength contain 5mg.

*Used for*: oedema caused by congestive heart failure, liver and kidney disease including nephrotic syndrome.

*Dosage*: adults, usually 1mg each day, according to response.

*Special care*: pregnancy, breast-feeding, diabetes, gout, liver or kidney disease, enlarged prostate gland, impaired micturition (urination). Potassium supplements may be needed.

*Avoid use*: children, patients in pre-comatose states as a result of liver cirrhosis.

*Possible interaction*: digitalis, lithium, antihypertensives, aminoglycosides.

*Side effects*: gastro-intestinal upset, cramps, skin rash, low blood potassium levels, enlarged breasts, thrombocytopenia.

*Manufacturer*: Leo.

## BURINEX A

*Description*: a combined loop and potassium-sparing diuretic preparation available as scored, cream, oval-shaped tablets, marked with lion and 149, containing 1mg bumetanide and 5mg amiloride hydrochloride.

*Used for*: patients requiring immediate diuresis, especially those in whom hypokalaemia may be a problem.

*Dosage*: adults, 1 to 2 tablets each day.

*Special care*: pregnancy, breast-feeding, diabetes, impaired micturition (urination), prostate gland enlargement, gout. Blood electrolyte levels should be monitored.

*Avoid use*: children, patients with severe imbalance of electrolyte levels (salts), severe kidney or liver disease, disorders of adrenal glands, hepatic pre-coma.

*Possible interaction*: antihypertensive drugs, digitalis, potassium supplements, potassium-sparing diuretics, lithium, ACE inhibitors, cephalosporins, aminoglycosides.

*Side effects*: gastro-intestinal upset, skin rash, cramps, thrombocytopenia.

*Manufacturer*: Leo.

## BURINEX K

*Description*: a combined loop diuretic, potassium supplement preparation available in the form of white, oval tablets, containing 0.5mg bumetanide, and 573mg potassium in a slow release wax core.

*Used for*: oedema accompanying congestive heart failure, kidney and liver disease in which a potassium supplement is needed.

*Dosage*: adults, 1 to 4 tablets each day.

*Special care*: pregnancy, breast-feeding, gout, diabetes, kidney or liver disorders, enlarged prostate gland, impaired micturition (urination). Patients receiving long-term treatment require monitoring of blood potassium levels.

*Avoid use*: children, patients with Addison's disease, hyperkalaemia, pre-comatose states in liver cirrhosis.

*Possible interaction*: aminoglycosides, digitalis, lithium, antihypertensives, potassium-sparing diuretics, ACE inhibitors, anti-arrhythmics, cephalosporins, sympathomimetic amines, NSAIDs, anti-diabetic drugs, lidocaine, TCADs, corticosteroids, mexiletine.

*Side effects*: gastro-intestinal upset, cramps, skin rash, enlarged breasts, thrombocytopenia, electrolyte imbalances, dizziness. Drug should be discontinued if obstruction or ulceration of small bowel occurs.

*Manufacturer*: Leo.

## BUSPAR

*Description*: an anxiolytic (anxiety-relieving) preparation, and an azaspirodecanedione. It is thought to be less open to abuse than the benzodiazepine drugs which are also used to relieve severe anxiety, and also to be less sedating in its effect. Buspar is produced in tablets of 2 strengths, containing 5mg or 10mg buspirone hydrochloride. The tablets are white, oval-shaped and marked with strength.

*Used for*: short-term relief of severe anxiety, i.e. that which is causing extreme distress and inability to function normally. This may be accompanied by depression.

*Dosage*: adults, 5mg 2 or 3 times each day at first, increasing every 2 or 3 days to a usual dose in the order of 15 to 30mg in divided dose. Maximum dose is 45mg daily.

*Special care*: if patient has been taking a benzodiazepine this should be slowly withdrawn before starting buspirone therapy. Special care in patients with liver or kidney disorders.

*Avoid use*: children, patients with severe kidney or liver disease, epilepsy, pregnant women, breast-feeding mothers.

*Possible interaction*: inhibitors of CYP3A4, verapamil, erythromycin, MAOIs, nefazodone, rifampicin, diltiazem, grapefruit juice.

*Side effects*: headache, nausea, nervous tension, dizziness, excitement. Rarely, confusion, fatigue, dry mouth, chest pain, tachycardia, sweating.

*Manufacturer*: BMS.

**BUSPIRONE *SEE* BUSPAR.**

**BUTOXYETHYL NICOTINATE *SEE* ACTINAC.**

# C

## CAFERGOT

*Description*: an analgesic preparation containing ergotamine which is available as white, sugar-coated tablets containing 1mg ergotamine tartrate and 100mg caffeine. **CAFERGOT SUPPOSITORIES** contain 2mg ergotamine tartrate and 100mg caffeine.

*Used for*: migraine.

*Dosage*: 1 or 2 tablets at start of attack with no more than 4 in 24 hours; should not be repeated within 4 days. Maximum dose, 8 tablets in one week. Suppositories, 1 at start of attack with maximum of 2 in 24 hours. Must not repeat within 4 days. Maximum dose, 4 suppositories in one week.

*Avoid use*: children, pregnancy, breast-feeding, liver or kidney disease, coronary, occlusive or peripheral vascular disease, sepsis, severe hypertension, Raynaud's disease. Should not be used to prevent migraine attack.

*Possible interaction*: ß-blockers, erythromycin, protease inhibitors.

*Side effects*: vomiting, nausea, abdominal pains, impairment of circulation (withdraw drug immediately), weakness in legs, pain affecting region in vicinity of heart. If pleural or retroperitoneal fibrosis occurs drug should be immediately stopped.

*Manufacturer*: Alliance.

## CALCIPARINE

*Description*: an anticoagulant available in the form of pre-filled syringes containing 25,000 units heparin calcium per use as subcutaneous injection only.

*Used for*: deep vein thrombosis, pulmonary embolism and prevention of these before surgery.

*Dosage*: 5000 units 2 hours before surgery then every 8 to 12 hours for 7 days.

*Special care*: pregnancy, kidney or liver disease. Blood platelet counts are required and therapy should be halted in patients who develop thrombocytopenia.

*Avoid use*: patients with allergy to heparin, those with haemophilia, haemorrhagic disorders, severe hypertension, peptic ulcer, cerebral aneurysm, recent eye surgery or concerning central nervous system, serious liver disease.

*Side effects*: haemorrhage, thrombocytopenia, allergic reactions. After prolonged use, osteoporosis and rarely, baldness may occur.

*Manufacturer*: Sanofi Synthelabo.

## CALCIUM HEPARIN *SEE*: CALCIPARINE.

## CALMURID HC

*Description*: a topical, moderately potent steroid with keratolytic and hydrating agents which have a softening and moistening effect on the skin. Available as a cream containing 1% hydrocortisone, 10% urea and 5% lactic acid.

*Used for*: dry eczemas and dermatoses.

*Dosage*: wash and dry affected skin, apply thinly twice a day at first and reduce frequency as condition improves.

*Special care*: limit use in children to 5 to 7 days, use extreme care with infants (napkin rash and infantile eczema). Also, use on face should be limited to 5 to 7 days. If stinging occurs, dilute to half-strength with water-based cream for 1 week before reverting to full strength preparation.

*Avoid use*: long-term use especially in pregnant women, patients with acne or skin conditions caused by tuberculosis, viral, fungal, bacterial infections which are untreated or ringworm, leg ulcers. Extensive or long term use should be avoided. Should not be used as long-term preventative treatment.

*Side effects*: not usually severe but thinning of skin, lines in skin (striae), blotchy red patches caused by distended blood vessels (capillaries) (telangiectasia), suppression of adrenal glands may occur.

*Manufacturer*: Galderma.

## CALPOL PAEDIATRIC

*Description*: a pain and fever relieving preparation available as a sugar-free suspension containing 120mg of paracetamol per 5ml of liquid. *Also*, **CALPOL SIX PLUS**, containing 250mg of paracetamol per 5ml of sugar-free suspension.

*Used for*: pain and fever relief.

*Dosage*: Children under 6 years, use Calpol Paediatric: infants aged 2 to 3 months, 2.5ml; 3months to 1 year, 2.5

to 5ml; 1 to 6 years, 5 to 10ml. Aged over 6 years, use Calpol Six Plus: aged 6 to 12 years, 5 to 10ml; aged over 12 years and adults, 10 to 20ml. All doses may be repeated up to 4 times each day.

*Special care*: impaired liver or kidney function.

*Avoid use*: infants aged under 2 months.

*Manufacturer*: Pfizer.

## CALSYNAR

*Description*: a manufactured form of a hormone, calcitonin, which is concerned with the regulation of calcium levels in the body. It is produced in ampoules for injection and contains 100 units salcatonin per ml in saline, (salcatonin is synthetic salmon calcitonin) or 200 iu/ml. Calcitonin lowers levels of calcium in blood plasma by inhibiting resorption of bone.

*Used for*: osteoporosis in post-menopausal women, Paget's disease, hypercalcaemia, in bone cancer, bone pain resulting from cancer.

*Dosage*: hypercalcaemia, initially, 400 units 6- to 8-hourly according to response, by subcutaneous or intramuscular injection to a maximum of 8 units per kg of body weight every 6 hours. Paget's disease of bone, 50 units 3 times each week to 100 units daily in single or divided doses, by subcutaneous or intramuscular injection. Post-menopausal osteoporosis, 100 units each day by subcutaneous or intramuscular injection along with 600mg calcium and 400 units vitamin D taken by mouth. Bone pain in cancer, 200 units every 6 hours or 400 units every 12 hours, for 48 hours by subcutaneous or intramuscular injection. Children should not receive therapy for more than a few weeks, as directed by physician.

*Special care*: history of allergy, perform scratch skin test. Pregnant women, breast-feeding mothers.

*Possible interaction*: cardiac glycosides.

*Side effects*: vomiting and nausea, tingling sensation in hands, flushing, allergic responses, unpleasant taste in mouth.

*Manufacturer*: R.P.R.

## CAMCOLIT

*Description*: an antidepressant preparation of lithium salts available as tablets of 2 strengths; as white, scored, film-coated tablets containing 250mg lithium carbonate (equivalent to 6.8mmol $Li^+$) marked CAMCOLIT. Also, as white, scored, modified release, film-coated tablets, containing 400mg lithium carbonate (10.8mmol $Li^+$), marked S and CAMCOLIT.

*Used for*: treatment and prevention of mania, recurrent bouts of depression, manic depression, aggressive and self-mutilating behaviour.

*Dosage*: adults, prevention, maintain serum levels of lithium in range of 0.4 to 8mmol per litre. Treatment: maintain serum levels of lithium in range of 0.6 to 1.0 mmol per litre, under direction of specialist physician.

*Special care*: treatment should be started in hospital with monitoring of plasma lithium concentrations at regular intervals. (Overdosage usually with plasma concentrations in excess of 1.5mmol $Li^+$ per litre can be fatal.) Adequate fluid and salt intake should be maintained. Monitor thyroid function. Pregnancy. Patients should be advised to report any intoxicating effects.

*Avoid use*: children, breast-feeding, heart or kidney disease, Addison's disease.

*Possible interaction*: NSAIDs, diuretics, haloperidol, phenytoin, metoclopramide, carbamazepine, flupentixol, methyldopa, tetracyclines, tricyclic and tetracyclic antidepressants.

*Side effects*: oedema, hypothyroidism, hyperparathyroidism, weight gain, gastro-intestinal upset, diarrhoea and nausea, trembling in hands, muscular weakness, heart and central nervous system disturbance, skin reactions, intense thirst, large volumes of dilute urine.

*Manufacturer*: Norgine.

## CANESTEN

*Description*: an antifungal/antibacterial preparation in the form of a cream, solution or spray (**CANESTEN SPRAY**), all containing 1% clotrimazole. Solution contains 1% clotrimazole in polyethylene glycol. *Also*, **CANESTEN POWDER** containing 1% clotrimazole.

*Used for*: fungal and Gram positive bacterial infections of the skin. Cream also used for balanitis and vulvitis and treatment of partner to prevent reinfection. Solution also used for fungal outer ear infections and inflammation.

*Dosage*: cream or solution, skin infections: apply thinly to affected skin twice or three times each day. Powder: dust on after applying cream, solution or spray and also apply to shoes and/or clothing. Ear infections: apply solution sparingly to affected area, 2 or 3 times each day. All treatments should be continued for two weeks after symptoms have cleared.

*Possible interaction*: barrier contraceptives, if cream is being used in genital area.

*Side effects*: slight burning or irritation, allergic reactions.

*Manufacturer*: Bayer.

## CAPOTEN

*Description*: an antihypertensive preparation, captopril, which is an ACE inhibitor, produced in tablets of 3 strengths: 12.5mg, 25mg and 50mg. All white, mottled and marked SQUIBB and 450, 452 or 482 repectively.

*Used for*: mild to moderate hypertension (with diuretics and digitalis), severe hypertension, where other methods have not been successful, congestive heart failure (with diuretics and digitalis), heart attack in which the left ventricle is at fault, diabetic nephropathy in insulin-dependent diabetes.

*Dosage*: adults, mild to moderate hypertension, 12.5mg twice each day at first with usual maintenance dose in the order of 25mg twice daily. Maximum dose is 50mg twice each day. Addition of a thiazide may be needed. Severe hypertension, 12.5mg twice each day at first, increasing to a maximum of 50mg 3 times each day if needed. Diabetic nephropathy, 75–100mg each day in divided doses. Heart failure, 6.25–12.5mg daily at first increasing to usual maintenance in the order of 25mg 2 or 3 times each day. Maximum dose is 150mg each day. N.B. therapy should be initiated in hospital under strict medical supervision with any diuretics being stopped or reduced before treatment begins. Post heart attack, 6.25mg daily at first beginning 3 days after attack increasing to 150mg daily in divided doses.

*Special care*: elderly persons, breastfeeding, severe congestive heart failure, kidney disease, reno-vascular hypertension, aortic stenosis, acute hypertensive crisis. Those with collagen vascular disease. White blood cell counts and checks on protein in urine and kidney function should be carried out before and during therapy. Contact manufacturer before use in children.

*Avoid use*: pregnancy, various heart disorders (aortic stenosis, outflow obstruction).

*Possible interaction*: NSAIDs, potassium supplements, potassium-sparing diuretics, immunosuppressants, vasodilators, antidiabetic drugs, allopurinol, probenecid, clonidine, procainamide, lithium.

*Manufacturer*: BMS.

## CAPOZIDE

*Description*: a combined thiazide diuretic with an ACE inhibitor, produced in the form of white, scored tablets marked SQUIBB containing 25mg hydrochlorothiazide and 50mg captopril. **CAPOZIDE LS** tablets are white, scored and contain 12.5mg hydrochlorothiazide and 25mg captopril and are marked SQUIBB 536.

*Used for*: mild to moderate hypertension in patients who are stable when taking the same proportions of captopril and hydrochlorothiazide individually.

*Dosage* : adults, 1 tablet daily with a possible maximum of 2. Capozide LS, 1 tablet each day.

*Special care*: breastfeeding, patients with kidney disease or receiving dialysis, liver disease, gout, collagen vascular disease, diabetes, undergoing anaesthesia or surgery. Kidney function, urinary protein and white blood cell count should be checked before and during treatment. Electrolyte levels must be monitored.

*Avoid use*: children, pregnant women, anuria (absence of urination).

*Possible interaction*: NSAIDs, potassium supplements, potassium-sparing diuretics, immunosuppressants, vasodilators, allopurinol, probenecid, clonidine, procainamide.

*Side effects*: blood dyscrasias (blood changes), low blood pressure, rash, proteinuria (protein in urine), loss of sensation of taste, sensitivity to light, pancreatitis, tiredness, thiazide side effects, rarely, a cough.

*Manufacturer*: BMS.

**CAPSAICIN *SEE*: AXSAIN.**

**CAPTOPRIL *SEE*: ACEZIDE, CAPOTEN, CAPOZIDE.**

## CARACE

*Description*: an ACE inhibitor produced in the form of blue, oval tablets marked MSD15 containing 2.5mg lisinopril; white, oval, scored tablets contain 5mg lisinopril; yellow, oval, scored tablets contain 10mg lisinopril; orange, oval, scored tablets contain 20mg lisinopril. All except 2.5mg tablets are marked with name and strength.

*Used for*: congestive heart failure (in conjunction with diuretics and possibly digitalis), essential and renovascular hypertension, acute heart attack in patients who are haemodynamically stable.

*Dosage*: adults, congestive heart failure, (reduce dose of any diuretic being taken before start of treatment) 2.5mg once each day at first increasing gradually to maintenance dose in the order of 5–20mg once daily, after 2 to 4 weeks. Hypertension, (discontinue any diuretic being taken 2 to 3 days before treatment starts); 2.5mg once a day increasing to a maintenance dose in the order of 10–20mg once daily. Maximum daily dose, 40mg. Following heart attack; 5mg straight away and then a further 5mg after 24 hours. Another 10mg after 48 hours and then 10mg once each day.

*Special care*: breast-feeding, patients with kidney disease, receiving dialysis, renovascular hypertension, severe congestive heart failure, undergoing anaesthesia. Kidney function should be monitored before and during treatment. Treatment should begin under hospital supervision for heart failure patients.

*Avoid use*: pregnancy, children, patients with various heart disorders (aortic stenosis, outflow obstruction), corpulmonale (a lung disorder), angioneurotic oedema as a result of previous ACE inhibitor treatment.

*Possible interaction*: potassium supplements, potassium-sparing diuretics, antihypertensives, neuroleptics, anti-diabetic drugs, tricyclic antidepressants.

*Side effects*: headache, dizziness, diarrhoea, nausea, tiredness, palpitations, low blood pressure, rash, angioedema, asthenia (weakness), cough.

*Manufacturer*: BMS.

## CARACE 10 PLUS

*Description*: an ACE inhibitor with a thiazide diuretic produced in the form of blue, hexagonal tablets marked 145 containing 10mg lisinopril and 12.5mg hydrochlorothiazide. **CARACE 20 PLUS** are yellow, hexagonal scored tablets, marked MSD 140, containing 20mg lisinopril and 12.5mg hydrochlorothiazide.

*Used for*: mild to moderate hypertension in patients who are stable when taking the same proportions of lisinopril and hydrochlorothiazide individually.

*Dosage*: adults, 1 Carace 10 Plus or Carace 20 Plus each day with a possible maximum of 2 tablets.

*Special care*: patients with liver or kidney disease receiving dialysis, heart and circulatory diseases, gout, hyperuricaemia (excess uric acid levels in blood), undergoing anaesthesia or surgery, with imbalances in salts (electrolytes) or fluid levels.

*Avoid use*: children, pregnancy, breast-feeding, anuria (absence of urination), angioneurotic oedema as a result of previous ACE inhibitor treatment, elevated potassium levels in blood, aortic stenosis.

*Possible interaction*: potassium supplements, hypoglycaemics, NSAIDs, lithium, tubocurarine.
*Side effects*: cough, headache, nausea, weariness, low blood pressure, gastrointestinal upset and diarrhoea, angioneurotic oedema, impotence, dizziness.
*Manufacturer*: BMS.

## CARBACHOL *SEE*: ISOPTO CARBACHOL.

## CARBALAX

*Description*: a laxative preparation available as suppositories containing 1.08g sodium bicarbonate and 1.30g of anhydrous sodium acid phosphate (equivalent to 1.69g of sodium acid phosphate).
*Used for*: constipation, anal dysfunction, before and after operations in radiology and sigmoidoscopy.
*Dosage*: adults, 1 suppository to achieve bowel movement.
*Avoid use*: children
*Manufacturer*: Forest

## CARBOMER *SEE*: GELTEARS.

## CARDENE

*Description*: a Class II calcium antagonist produced in the form of capsules: blue/white capsules contain 20mg nicardipine hydrochloride and pale blue/blue capsules containing 30mg.
*Used for*: prevention of chronic angina which is stable.
*Dosage*: adults; 20mg 3 times each day in first instance

increasing with 3-day intervals to a maintenance dose in the order of 30mg 3 times daily. Maximum daily dose, 120mg.

*Special care*: congestive heart failure, aftermath of stroke, liver or kidney disease, weak heart.

*Avoid use*: children, pregnancy, breast-feeding, aortic stenosis (a heart valve disease), within one month of heart attack, unstable angina, cardiogenic shock.

*Possible interaction*: cimetidine, digoxin, ciclosporin, rifampicin, grapefruit juice.

*Side effects*: headache, dizziness, nausea, palpitations, flushing and feeling of warmth; chest pain within half an hour of taking dose or on increasing dose, drug should be withdrawn.

*Manufacturer*: Yamanouchi.

## CARDENE SR

*Description*: a Class II calcium antagonist produced in the form of sustained-release capsules: white capsules marked SYNTEX 30 contain 30mg nicardipine hydrochloride; blue capsules marked SYNTEX 45 contain 45mg. *Also*, **CARDENE CAPSULES**, available in two strengths, white/blue containing 20mg of nicardipine hydrochloride and pale blue/blue containing 30mg. Each capsule is marked with strength, name and CO.

*Used for*: mild to moderate hypertension.

*Dosage*: adults; tablets, 30mg twice each day at first increasing to 45mg twice daily if required. Maximum dose is 60mg twice daily. (All doses at 12 hour intervals.)

Capsules, 20mg every 8 hours at first increasing, if necessary, allowing 3 day intervals to maintenance dose of 30mg, 8 hourly. Maximum is 120mg each day.

*Special care*: congestive heart failure, liver or kidney disease, weak heart, aftermath of stroke.

*Avoid use*: children, pregnant women, breast-feeding mothers, aortic stenosis (a heart valve disease), within one month of heart attack.

*Possible interaction*: cimetidine, digoxin, ciclosporin, rifampicin, grapefruit juice.

*Side effects*: headache, dizziness, nausea, palpitations, flushing and feeling of warmth, water retention in lower limbs; chest pain within half an hour of taking dose or on increasing dose, drug should be withdrawn.

*Manufacturer*: Yamanouchi.

## CARDICOR

*Description*: a cardioselective **ß**-blocker available as film-coated tablets in different strengths, containing bisoprolol fumarate. Round, white tablets contain 1.25mg or 2.5mg; off-white tablets contain 3.75mg; pale yellow tablets contain 5mg; yellow tablets contain 7.5mg; heart-shaped, orange tablets contain 10mg.

*Used for*: in conjunction with ACE inhibitors, diuretics and possibly cardiac glycosides; for chronic moderate to severe heart failure in which there is lowered, systolic ventricular function and where the condition is stable.

*Dosage*: starting dose, one 1.25mg tablet each day in the morning, swallowed whole, for 7 days. If well tolerated, dose increased by 1.25mg in second and consecutive weeks until a single daily, morning dose of 5mg is achieved. Continue for 4 weeks and then, dose can be similarly increased at weekly intervals, if required. Maximum daily dose is 10mg.

*Special care*: pregnancy, breastfeeding, liver or kidney disease, history of bronchospasm, diabetes, insufficient cerebrovascular circulation, weakness, atopy (inherited tendency to develop immediate allergic responses), anaesthesia (drug may need to be withdrawn before planned surgery), thyrotoxic crisis. Treatment should only be initiated under supervision of experienced physician and patient should be monitored for 4 hours after first dose. Drug should be stopped gradually.

*Avoid use*: children, various heart conditions (sinus bradycardia, 2nd or 3rd degree AV block, Prinzmetal's angina, right ventricular failure resulting from pulmonary hypertension, cardiogenic shock, significantly enlarged heart), severe peripheral arterial disease, metabolic acidosis, phaeochromocytoma which has not been treated.

*Possible interaction*: cardiac depressant anaesthetics, class II calcium antagonists, verapamil, diltiazem, class I antiarrhythmics, clonidine withdrawal, CNS depressants, hypoglycaemics, other antihypertensives, rifampicin, ibuprofen, sympathomimetics, reserpine, indometacin, ergot alkaloids warfarin, cimetidine, theophylline.

*Side effects*: bronchospasm, low blood pressure, cold hands and feet, slow heart beat, tiredness on exertion, sleep disturbance, heart failure, thrombocytopaenia (reduced platelets in blood), gastrointestinal upset, hair loss. If skin rash or unexplained dry eyes arise, gradually withdraw drug. Any adverse effects should be reported to the Committee on the Safety of Medicines (CSM).

*Manufacturer*: Merck.

## CARDURA XL

*Description*: a selective α1-blocker available as white, sustained-release tablets (with a hole) in two different strengths, containing 4mg and 8mg of doxazosin (as mesylate), respectively. *Also,* **CARDURA TABLETS**, pentagonal, white tablets contain 1mg doxazosin (as mesylate), marked PFIZER DXP1; oval, white tablets contain 2mg doxazosin (as mesylate), marked PFIZER DXP2.

*Used for*: high blood pressure, obstructed outflow of urine associated with benign enlargement of the prostate gland.

*Dosage*: adults, Cardura XL: at first, one 4mg tablet swallowed whole once each day, increasing if necessary to 8mg after one month of treatment. Cardura tablets: at first, single 1mg tablet once each day, increasing as required after 7 to 14 days to 2mg and then 4mg once daily. The maximum daily dose is 16mg.

*Special care*: pregnancy, liver disorders.

*Avoid use*: children, breastfeeding, history of gastrointestinal obstruction (applies only to Cardura XL).

*Possible interaction*: nausea, headache, weakness, dizziness, vertigo, tiredness, sleepiness, fluid retention, irritation of nasal passages (runny nose). More rarely, effects on blood, blurred vision, priapism, itching and skin rash, urinary incontinence, pain in abdomen, impotence, liver disorders, gastrointestinal upset, agitation, cholestasis, blood in urine, nose bleeds.

*Manufacturer*: Pfizer.

## CARISOMA

*Description*: a carbamate preparation which acts as a muscle relaxant and available as white tablets containing 125mg carisoprodol and white tablets marked with P in a hexagon contain 350mg carisoprodol.

*Used for*: muscle spasm resulting from bone and muscle disorders.

*Dosage*: adults: 350mg, elderly, 125mg, both 3 times each day.

*Special care*: history of drug abuse or alcoholism, liver or kidney disease. Long-term treatment should be avoided and the drug withdrawn gradually.

*Avoid use*: children, pregnancy, breast-feeding, acute intermittent porphyria.

*Possible interaction*: oral contraceptives, steroids, CNS depressants, tricyclics, griseofulvin, phenothiazines, rifampicin, phenytoin, anticoagulants.

*Side effects*: nausea, constipation, flushes, rash, weariness, drowsiness, headache.

*Manufacturer*: Forest.

## CARISOPRODOL *SEE*: CARISOMA.

## CARTEOLOL *SEE*: TEOPTIC.

## CARVEDILOL *SEE*: EUCARDIC.

## CATAPRES

*Description*: an antihypertensive preparation, clonidine hydrochloride, produced in the form of tablets of 2 strengths and in ampoules for injection. White scored tablets contain either 0.1mg marked with maker's symbol and O1C over O1C or 0.3mg marked with maker's symbol and 03C over O3C. Also, **CATAPRES INJECTION** contains 0.15mg per ml in ampoules.

*Used for*: hypertension, hypertensive crisis (injection).

*Dosage*: adults: tablets, 0.05 to 0.1mg 3 times each day, gradually increasing every second or third day. Injection, in accordance with specialist supervision.

*Special care*: breast-feeding, depression, peripheral vascular disease. Tablets should be stopped gradually especially if beta-blockers are being withdrawn.

*Avoid use*: children.

*Possible interaction*: other antihypertensives, tricyclics, CNS depressants, alpha-blockers.

*Side effects*: dry mouth, oedema, drowsiness, dizziness.

*Manufacturer*: Boehringer Ingelheim.

## CEFACLOR *SEE*: DISTACLOR.

## CEFADROXIL *SEE*: BAXAN.

## CEFOTAXIME *SEE*: CLAFORAN.

## CEFUROXIME SEE: ZINACEF.

## CEFUROXIME AXETIL *SEE*: ZINNAT.

## CELANCE

*Description*: a dopamine agonist, pergolide mesylate, produced as tablets: ivory, marked 4131 contain 0.05mg, green marked 4133 (0.25mg), and pink tablets, marked 4135 (1mg). All are rectangular, scored and marked LILLY.

*Used for*: sole therapy or additional therapy (to levodopa) in treatment of Parkinson's disease.

*Dosage* : additional therapy, 0.05mg each day at first in 3 divided doses increasing every third day by 0.1–0.15mg for a period of 12 days. Then the dose is increased by 0.25mg every third day until the best response is achieved. Maximum daily dose is 5mg. Levodopa dose should be carefully reduced. Sole therapy, at first, 0.05mg taken as evening dose on day one then 0.05mg taken at noon and evening on 2nd to 4th days. Afterwards, dose is gradually increased over 25 day period to 1.5mg each day in 3 divided doses, morning, noon and evening. Dose may then be further increased, if needed, by 0.25mg twice each week until optimal response is achieved.

*Special care*: pregnancy, breast-feeding, heart disease, heart arrhythmias, serosal inflammatory disorders associated with ergot derivatives, history of hallucinations. Patient should be monitored for signs of fibrosis. Drug should be gradually withdrawn.

*Avoid use*: children.

*Possible interaction*: anticoagulants, antihypertensives, other dopamine antagonists, drugs that affect protein binding.

*Side effects*: disturbances of heartbeat, movement disorder (dyskinesia), drowsiness, hypotension, inflammation of the nose, dyspepsia, nausea, dyspnoea (laboured breathing), diplopia, gastrointestinal upset, abdominal pain, abnormal liver tests and heart beat rate, rash, fever, serosal inflammatory disorders.

*Manufacturer*: Lilly.

## CELEBREX

*Description*: an NSAID available as capsules in two different strengths containing celecoxib. White capsules containing 100mg are marked with a pair of blue bands and 7767 and 100; white capsules containing 200mg are marked with paired gold bands and 7767 and 200.

*Used for*: rheumatoid arthritis, osteoarthritis.

*Dosage*: adults, rheumatoid arthritis, 200 to 400mg each day, divided into two doses; osteoarthritis, 100mg once each day or divided into two doses.

*Special care*: elderly persons aged over 65 years and black patients should be started on lower doses due to possible greater sensitivity. Oedema, risk of hypovolaemia (low blood volume), heart failure, malfunction of left ventricle of heart, liver or kidney disease, high blood pressure. Women of child-bearing age should use contraception.

*Avoid use*: children, pregnancy, breastfeeding, history of allergy to NSAIDs or sulfonamides, active gastrointestinal bleeding or ulceration, serious congestive heart failure, severe liver or kidney disorders, inflammatory disorders of the bowel.

*Possible interaction*: oral contraceptives, rifampicin, drugs metabolised by CYP2D6 or CYP2C19, carbamazepine, ACE inhibitors, fluconazole, diuretics, anticoagulants, barbiturates, antihypertensives, tacrolimus, methotrexate (monitor patient), ciclosporin, lithium.

*Side effects*: disorders of the upper respiratory tract, gastrointestinal upset, skin rashes, insomnia, fluid retention, dizziness. Any adverse effects should be reported to the Committee on the Safety of Medicines (CSM).

*Manufacturer*: Pharmacia.

## CELECOXIB *SEE*: CELEBREX.

## CELECTOL

*Description*: an antihypertensive which is a cardioselective beta1-blocker and partial beta2-agonist. It is produced in heart-shaped tablets of 2 strengths, yellow scored tablets (200mg celiprolol hydrochloride) and white tablets (400mg). The tablets are film-coated and marked with logo and strength.

*Used for*: mild to moderate hypertension.

*Dosage*: adults, 200mg once each day half an hour before food, maximum dose 400mg.

*Special care*: pregnancy, nursing mothers, anaesthesia or

planned surgery, diabetes, liver or kidney disease, metabolic acidosis. Patients with weak hearts should receive diuretic and digitalis. Patients with history of bronchospasm. Drug should be gradually withdrawn.

*Avoid use*: children, patients with forms of heart disease including heart block, heart failure, slow heart beat rate; sick sinus syndrome, peripheral arterial disease. Patients with obstructive airways disease (unless absolutely no alternative).

*Possible interaction*: sympathomimetics, central nervous system depressants, indometacin, antihypertensives, ergotamine, reserpine, cimetidine, cardiac depressant anaesthetics, hypoglycaemics, verapamil, Class I antiarrhythmics, clonidine withdrawal.

*Side effects*: gastro-intestinal disorders, fatigue with exercise, cold feet and hands, disruption of sleep, slow heartbeat rate. If dry eyes or skin rash occur, drug should be gradually withdrawn.

*Manufacturer*: Pantheon.

## CELEVAC

*Description*: a preparation which is a laxative and bulking agent, available as pink tablets containing 500mg methylcellulose.

*Used for*: constipation, diarrhoea, diseases of the diverticulum, ileostomy and colostomy control, obesity.

*Dosage*: adults, constipation, 3 to 6 tablets at night and in the morning taken with at least 300ml of water or other drink. Diarrhoea, etc., 3 to 6 tablets taken twice each day with as little fluid as possible – avoid drinks for 30 minutes before and after taking tablets. Obesity, 3 tablets taken 30 minutes before a meal with at least 30ml of a warm drink, or take when experiencing hunger pangs.

*Avoid use*: children, patients at risk of obstruction of the bowel and infective bowel disease.

*Manufacturer*: Shire.

## CELIPROLOL *SEE* CELECTOL.

## CEFALEXIN SEE: CEPOREX, KEFLEX.

## CEPOREX

*Description*: a cephalosporin antibiotic produced in the form of tablets, capsules and syrup. Pink, film-coated tablets, containing 250mg, 500mg cefalexin are marked with name and strength. **CEPOREX CAPSULES** coloured grey/caramel contain 250mg and 500mg and are marked with capsule name and strength. **CEPOREX SYRUP** (produced as granules for reconstitution), contains 125mg, 250mg and 500mg per 5ml when made up with water.

*Used for*: urinary tract infections, gonorrhoea, ear, nose and throat infections, respiratory tract, skin and soft tissue infections.

*Dosage*: adults, usual dose is 1g twice each day but 1g three times each day or 3g twice daily may be given in severe cases. For prevention of urinary tract infections, 125mg may be taken each night, continuing for several months, if needed. Children, under 12 months, 62.5mg–125mg twice each day; 1 to 6 years, 250–500mg each day; 7 to 12 years, 500mg to 1g twice each day. If infection is very severe, 100mg per kg of body weight may be given each day to a maximum daily dose of 4g.

*Special care*: patients with allergy to penicillins or kidney disease.

*Side effects*: allergic reactions, gastro-intestinal disorders, pseudomembranous colitis, skin rashes and other severe skin effects, neutropenia (deficiency in certain white blood cells), Stevens–Johnson syndrome.

*Manufacturer*: Galen.

## CERUMOL

*Description*: a cerumenolytic preparation (for softening ear wax) available as a solution containing 2% paradichlorobenzene, 5% chlorbutol and 57.3% arachis oil.

*Used for*: softening and removal of hardened ear wax.

*Dosage*: apply 5 drops into outer ear and leave for 10 to 30 minutes; ear may then be syringed with warm water to remove wax. Or, apply 5 drops for 3 consecutive days to dissolve wax – syringing may not then be required.

*Avoid use*: perforated ear drum, inflammation/infection of the outer ear, eczema or seborrhoeic dermatitis affecting the ear.

*Manufacturer*: L.A.B.

## CETRIZINE *SEE*: ZIRTEC.

**CETYLPYRIDINIUM CHLORIDE *SEE*: CALGEL**

**CHLORAMPHENICOL *SEE*: ACTINAC, CHLOROMYCETIN.**

**CHLORBUTOL *SEE*: CERUMOL.**

**CHLORDIAZEPOXIDE *SEE*: LIBRIUM.**

**CHLOROMYCETIN**

*Description*: a preparation which is a broad-spectrum antibiotic containing 1% chloramphenicol in the form of an ointment. *Also,* **CHLOROMYCETIN REDIDROPS**, containing 0.5% chloramphenicol in the form of eye drops.

*Used for*: conjunctivitis of bacterial origin.

*Dosage*: apply ointment, or two Redidrops, to eye (as advised by doctor) every three hours or more frequently, as directed by doctor, if required. Treatment should continue for a further 48 hours after symptoms have disappeared.

*Side effects*: Rarely, aplastic anaemia.

*Manufacturer*: Goldshield.

**CHLORPHENAMINE MALEATE *SEE*: PIRITON.**

**CHLORQUINADOL *SEE*: LOCOID C.**

**CHLORTETRACYCLINE *SEE*: AUREOCORT, DETECLO.**

## CICATRIN

*Description*: an aminoglycoside, antibacterial preparation available in the form of a cream and dusting powder. The cream and powder contain 3300 units neomycin sulphate, 250 units bacitracin zinc, 2mg l-cysteine, 10mg glycine and 1mg threonine per g.

*Used for*: minor bacterial skin infections.

*Dosage*: adults and children, cream and powder, apply up to 3 times each day to affected skin for a maximum period of 1 week. Infants (other than new-borns), apply a lesser dose.

*Special care*: on large areas of affected skin, kidney disorders.

*Avoid use*: new-born infants.

*Possible interaction*: neuromuscular blockers.

*Side effects*: allergic responses, ototoxicity (damage to organs of hearing and balance).

*Manufacturer*: GlaxoSmithKline.

## CIDOMYCIN

*Description*: an aminoglycoside antibiotic containing gentamicin as sulphate, produced for injection. Cidomycin injection contains 40mg gentamicin (as sulphate) per ml in ampoules and vials. **CIDOMYCIN PAEDIATRIC INJECTION** contains 10mg/ml in 2ml vials. **CIDOMYCIN INTRATHECAL INJECTION** contains 5mg/ml in ampoules.

*Used for*: Cidomycin, Cidomycin paediatric injection: serious infections sensitive to gentamicin; urinary tract infections. Cidomycin intrathecal injection, ventriculitis, bacterial meningitis.

*Dosage*: adults, Cidomycin, 5mg per kg of body weight by intramuscular or intravenous injection daily in 3 or 4 divided doses, for 1 week to 10 days. Children, use Cidomycin paediatric, up to 2 weeks of age, 3mg per kg of body weight at 12-hour intervals; over 2 weeks old, 2mg per kg of body weight at 8-hour intervals. Both intramuscularly or intravenously for a period of 7–10 days. Cidomycin intrathecal, according to manufacturer's instructions under supervision of specialist physician.

*Special care*: patients with kidney disease, myasthenia gravis; regular blood tests necessary as blood concentrations over 10 g/ml can cause damage to the organs of hearing and balance.

*Avoid use*: pregnant women.

*Possible interaction*: anaesthetics, neuromuscular blocking drugs, furosemide, ethacrynic acid.

*Side effects*: toxicity affecting organs of hearing and balance and kidneys.

*Manufacturer*: Hoechst.

## CIDOMYCIN EYE AND EAR DROPS

*Description*: an antibiotic preparation containing 0.3% gentamicin (as sulphate) in the form of ear and eye drops.

*Used for*: bacterial infections of the external ear and eye.

*Dosage*: ear drops, adults and children, 2 to 4 drops 3 or 4 times each day and at night. Eye drops, adults and children, 1 to 3 drops, 3 to 4 times each day.

*Avoid use*: ear infections where drum is perforated.

*Side effects*: risk of superinfection (another infection occurring during treatment).

*Manufacturer*: Hoechst.

## CILAZAPRIL *SEE*: VASCACE.

## CILEST

*Description*: a combined oestrogen/progestogen contraceptive preparation containing 35µg ethinylestradiol and 0.25mg norgestimate in the form of blue tablets marked C250.

*Used for*: oral contraception.

*Dosage*: 1 tablet each day for 21 days starting on first day of period, followed by 7 tablet-free days.

*Special care*: patients with asthma, diabetes, Raynaud's disease, ulcerative colitis, Crohn's disease, Sydenham's chorea, tetanus, varicose veins, hypertension, serious kidney disease, multiple sclerosis, haemolytic uraemic syndrome, serious depression. Also, uterine fibroids, endometriosis, contact lenses, history of heart failure, choliasis. The risk of thrombosis increases with age and if woman smokes or is obese. Slight increased chance of breast cancer. Pelvic organs, breasts and blood pressure should be checked regularly during the time oral contraceptives are being taken.

*Avoid use*: pregnancy, history of thrombosis, those with heart disease, heart valve disease and angina, some other circulatory conditions. Patient with sickle cell anaemia, infectious hepatitis, certain liver and kidney disorders, hormone-dependent cancers, undiagnosed vaginal bleeding. History of SLE and some other disorders that have previously occurred during pregnancy.

*Possible interaction*: tetracyclines, barbiturates, carbamazepine, primidone, griseofulvin, phenytoin, rifampicin, ampicillin, phenylbutazone, chloral hydrate, glutethimide, ethosuximide, dichloralphenazone, St John's Wort.

*Side effects*: nausea, headaches, bloatedness due to fluid retention, enlargement of breasts, cramps and leg pains, reduction in libido, depression, weight gain, bleeding, vaginal discharge, erosion of cervix.

*Manufacturer*: Janssen-Cilag.

## CILOXAN

*Description*: an antibiotic preparation available as eye drops containing 0.3% ciprofloxacin.

*Used for*: superficial bacterial eye infections and neighbouring tissues, ulcers on the cornea.

*Dosage*: adults and children aged over 1 year, conjunctivitis and eye infections, 1 to 2 drops 4 times each day; if severe, 1 to 2 drops every 2 hours through the day for 2 days, then normal dose. Corneal ulcers, first day, 2 drops every 15 minutes for 6 hours, followed by 2 drops every half hour for 18 hours; second day, 2 drops every 2 hours. 3rd to 14th day, 2 drops every 4 hours, continuing, if necessary, for a maximum period of 3 weeks.

*Special care*: pregnancy, breastfeeding.

*Avoid use*: children aged under 12 months, patients with soft contact lenses.
*Side effects*: short-lived irritation of eye, bitter taste in mouth, skin rashes (withdraw treatment).
*Manufacturer*: Alcon.

## CIMETIDINE *SEE*: DYSPAMET, TAGAMET.

## CINNARIZINE *SEE*: STUGERON.

## CIPRAMIL

*Description*: an antidepressant preparation which is a 5HT reuptake inhibitor. it selectively inhibits the reuptake of serotonin (a neurotransmitter), ensuring that this remains available for a longer period and facilitating beneficial serotonergic effects. Available as film-coated, white tablets in three different strengths containing citalopram as hydrobromide. White tablets contain 10mg, marked CL; white, oval tablets contain 20mg, marked CN; white, oval tablets contain 40mg, marked CR. *Also*, **CIPRAMIL DROPS,** containing 40mg of citalopram as hydrochloride per ml of solution (8 drops is equivalent to tablet of 20mg strength), for adding to water or fruit juice.
*Used for*: panic disorder which may be accompanied by agoraphobia, early stage depressive illness and as maintenance to prevent recurrence.
*Dosage*: adults, depressive illness, 20mg each day at start increasing to a maximum daily dose of 60mg, if needed; panic disorder, 10mg once each day at start, continuing

for 1 week and then increasing to 20mg daily, to a maximum of 60mg, if required. Elderly persons should receive same starting doses but with lower maximum of 40mg each day.

*Special care*: pregnancy, breastfeeding, liver or serious kidney disease, epilepsy which is unstable, patients at risk of bleeding disorders, diabetes, mania, ECT. Drug should be stopped gradually.

*Avoid use*: children.

*Possible interaction*: neuroleptics, tryptophan, 5HT agonists, lithium, MAOIs, St John's Wort.

*Side effects*: sleepiness, nausea, trembling, dry mouth, sweating.

*Manufacturer*: Lundbeck.

## CIPROFLOXACIN *SEE*: CILOXAN.

## CIPROXIN

*Description*: A 4-quinolone antibiotic, ciprofloxacin hydrochloride monohydrate, as tablets of 4 different strengths and as a suspension. White, film-coated tablets, marked with BAYER logo and CIP 100 contain 100mg; BAYER logo and CIP 250 contain 250mg; BAYER logo and CIP 500 (500mg); marked with BAYER logo and CIP 750 (750mg). **CIPROXIN SUSPENSION** contains 250mg ciprofloxacin per 5ml, available as granules with a non-aqueous diluent.

*Used for*: ear, nose, throat, respiratory tract infections. Skin, bone, joint, soft tissue and eye infections. Also, pelvic and gastro-intestinal infections, gonorrhoea and pneumonia caused by Gram-negative bacteria. Prevention of infection in endoscopy and surgery on upper gastro-intestinal tract, inhalation anthrax. In children, acute pulmonary flare-up of cystic fibrosis associated with infection by the organism, *P. aeruginosa.*

*Dosage*: adults, tablets, 100mg to 750mg twice each day for 5 to 10 days. For gonorrhoea, one 250mg dose. For prevention of infection, 750mg 1 hour to 1_ hours before operation. For gonorrhoea, 100mg by intravenous infusion. Uncomplicated cystitis in women, 100mg 2 times each day for 3 days. Inhalation anthrax, 500mg twice each day. Children, acute flare-up of cystic fibrosis, ages 5 to 17 years, 20mg per kg of body weight twice each day for 10 to 14 days; inhalation anthrax, 15mg per kg of body weight twice each day to a maximum of 1000mg total dose. Other exceptional conditions, 5 to 15mg per kg twice each day.

*Also,* **CIPROXIN INFUSION,** available in infusion bags or bottles as a solution containing 2mg of ciprofloxacin per ml.

*Used for*: some of severe conditions listed above where tablets are not appropriate.

*Dosage*: adults, 100 to 400mg by intravenous infusion over 30 minutes to 1 hour twice each day for 5 days to 1 week, depending upon severity of infection and response. Gonorrhoea, 100mg; inhalation anthrax, 400mg by intravenous infusion over 1 hour period, twice each day. Children aged 5 to 17 years, 10mg per kg of body weight by intravenous infusion over 1 hour, 3 times each day – for acute flare-up of cystic fibrosis. Inhalation anthrax, 10mg per kg of body weight by intravenous infusion twice each day to a maximum daily dose of 800mg. Other severe conditions, 4 to 8mg per kg of body weight by intravenous infusion twice each day.

*Special care*: severe kidney disorders (half doses), epilepsy or disorders of central nervous system, history of convulsions. Plenty of fluids should be drunk or patient well hydrated, operating machinery or driving, G-6-PD deficiency.

*Avoid use*: children aged under 5 years, all children and adolescents (except in exceptional circumstances outlined above), pregnancy, breast-feeding, tendon disorders.

*Possible interaction*: probenecid, premedicants, NSAIDs, opiates, theophylline (levels must be monitored or Ciproxin should not be used), ciclosporin (serum creatinine levels must be monitored), glibenclamide, iron, magnesium, calcium or aluminium salts, metoclopramide, corticosteroids, oral anticoagulants.

*Side effects*: headache, central nervous system effects, gastrointestinal disturbances, liver, kidney and blood changes, cardiovascular effects. Weakness, skin rash, allergic responses, pains in joints.

*Manufacturer*: Bayer.

## CLAFORAN

*Description*: a cephalosporin antibiotic preparation produced in the form of a powder for reconstitution and injection. Claforan contains 500mg, 1g or 2g of cefotaxime (as sodium salt), as powder in vials.

*Used for*: urinary tract and soft tissue infections, septicaemia, meningitis and respiratory tract infections.

*Dosage*: adults, mild to moderate conditions, 1g by intravenous or intramuscular injection at 12 hour intervals. For serious infections dose may need to be increased to up to 12g daily in 3 or 4 divided doses. The 2g dose should be given intravenously. Children, newborn babies, 50mg per kg of body weight daily in 2, 3 or 4 divided doses; older infants and children, 100 to 150mg per kg of body weight daily in 2, 3 or 4 divided doses.

*Special care*: pregnancy, breast-feeding, penicillin allergy and serious kidney failure. Monitor blood counts with prolonged treatment.

*Possible interaction*: aminoglycosides, probenecid, loop diuretics.

*Side effects*: gastro-intestinal upset, pain at injection site, allergic reactions, candidiasis, blood changes, haemolytic anaemia, rise in liver enzymes and blood urea. Positive Coomb's test, risk of effects on kidney function and encephalopathy if higher doses are used. Rarely, pseudomembranous colitis.

*Manufacturer*: Aventis Pharma.

**CLARITHROMYCIN *SEE*: HELICLEAR, HELIMET, KLARICID.**

## CLARITYN

*Description*: an antihistamine preparation produced in the form of a syrup containing 5mg loratadine per 5ml. of liquid.

*Used for*: relief of symptoms of allergic rhinitis, e.g. hay fever, urticaria.

*Dosage*: adults, 10ml syrup once each day. Children, 2 to 5 years, 5ml; 6 to 12 years, 10ml, both once each day.

*Avoid use*: children under 2 years of age, pregnancy, breast-feeding.

*Manufacturer*: Schering-Plough.

## CLAVULANIC ACID *SEE*: AUGMENTIN

## CLEXANE

*Description*: an anticoagulant preparation produced in pre-filled syringes for injection containing 20mg (low molecular weight heparin) enoxaparin per 0.2ml, or 40mg enoxaparin per 0.4ml, or 60mg per 0.6ml, or 80mg 0.8ml, or 100mg per ml. *Also*: **CLEXANE FORTE**, containing 150m of enoxaparin per ml in single dose, prepared syringes.

*Used for*: prevention of deep vein thrombosis especially associated with orthopaedic and general surgery and in people who are immobile and bed-ridden. Prevention of blood clot formation during haemodialysis; treatment of non-Q wave heart attack and angina which is unstable. Treatment of thromboembolic disease of the veins in which there is pulmonary embolism and/or deep vein thrombosis.

*Dosage*: adults, low to medium risk of thrombosis (in general surgery), 20mg 2 hours before operation by deep subcutaneous injection and then 20mg once each day for 7 to 10 days. High risk of thrombosis (orthopaedic surgery), 40mg 12 hours before operation by deep subcutaneous injection, and 40mg once a day for 7 to 10 days. Prevention in illness, 40mg once each day by deep, subcutaneous injection for at least 6 days, continuing until the patient is able to walk, but for a maximum period of 2 weeks, with alternating injection sites. Haemodialysis, 1mg per kg of body weight with a further dose of 0.5 to 1mg/kg if process lasts for longer than 4 hours. Treatment of venous thromboembolism, 1.5mg per kg of body weight each day for 5 days by subcutaneous injection, until the patient is able to take anticoagulation tablets by mouth. Treatment of angina which is unstable, 1mg per kg of body weight every 12 hours by subcutaneous injection for at least 2 days or until stabilised (usually, 2 to 8 days), with 100 to 325mg of aspirin taken by mouth.

*Special care*: pregnancy, breast-feeding, hypertension, history of liver disorders or ulcers, spinal anaesthesia or epidural, spinal puncture.

*Avoid use*: children, patients with peptic ulcer, serious bleeding disorders (e.g. haemophilia), those at risk of haemorrhage, thrombocytopenia, acute bacterial endocarditis, artificial heart valves, haemorrhagic CVA.

*Possible interaction*: aspirin, NSAIDs, dextran, anticoagulants taken by mouth, antiplatelet drugs, locoregional anaesthesia.

*Side effects*: effects on liver, thrombocytopenia, less commonly, bruising and haemorrhage. Hypoaldosteronism (low secretion of aldosterone, an adrenal gland hormone) causing elevated blood levels of potassium. Blood potassium levels should be monitored with longer term use of drug and in patients with diabetes, acidosis, chronic kidney failure or those who have been taking potassium-sparing drugs.

*Manufacturer*: R.P.R.

## CLIMAGEST

*Description*: a combined oestrogen, progestogen hormonal preparation, produced in the form of tablets. Climagest 1mg consists of 16 blue-grey tablets containing 1mg oestradiol valerate, coded OC/CG, and 12 white tablets, containing 1mg oestradiol valerate and 1mg norethisterone, coded OE/CG. Also, **CLIMAGEST 2MG** consists of 16 blue tablets containing 2mg oestradiol valerate, coded OD/CG, and 12 pale yellow tablets containing 2mg oestradiol valerate and 1mg norethisterone, coded OF/CG.

*Used for*: relief of menopausal symptoms.

*Dosage*: women, 1 tablet daily starting with oestradiol valerate on first day of period (if present), and finishing with the 12 tablets containing norethisterone.

*Special care*: patients considered to be at risk of thrombosis, those with diabetes, epilepsy, hypertension, multiple sclerosis, migraine, fibroids in uterus,fibrocystic disease, breast nodules, otosclerosis, tetany, liver disease(monitor liver function), porphyria, kidney disorder, cholelithiasis. All this group should be monitored closely. Regular examination of breasts and pelvic organs should be carried out and blood pressure checked. Persistent breakthrough bleeding. Women should self-examine breasts, attend for mammography (if applicable) and have cervical smear tests.

*Avoid use*: pregnancy, breast-feeding, hormone-dependent cancers, breast or uterus cancer, endometriosis, undiagnosed vaginal bleeding. Serious heart, kidney or liver disease, thrombophlebitis and thromboembolic diseases. Patients suffering from Dublin–Johnson syndrome or Rotor syndrome.

*Possible interaction*: drugs which induce liver enzymes.

*Side effects*: weight gain, enlargement and tenderness of breasts, fluid retention, cramps, gastro-intestinal upset, nausea and vomiting, headaches, breakthrough bleeding, dizziness. Cholestatic jaundice, effects on liver function, migraine, nose bleeds, worsening of varicose veins, lowered glucose tolerance, itching and reddening of skin (usually short-lived). Withdraw if migraines or other severe headaches occur for first time, or serious vision disturbances, signs of thromboembolic disorders, seizures, jaundice, hepatitis, serious, whole body itching, pregnancy. Stop 6 weeks before planned surgery or prolonged immobilisation.

*Manufacturer*: Novartis.

## CLIMAVAL

*Description*: a hormonal oestrogen preparation produced in tablets of 2 strengths. Climaval 1mg are grey/blue tablets containing 1mg oestradiol valerate marked OC/CG; Climaval 2mg are blue tablets containing 2mg oestradiol valerate and marked OD/CG.

*Used for*: treatment of menopausal symptoms in women who have had a hysterectomy.

*Dosage*: 1 tablet each day either 1mg or 2mg according to response. May be taken continuously for up to 2 years.

*Special care*: patients considered to be at risk of thrombosis, those with diabetes, epilepsy, hypertension, multiple sclerosis, migraine, fibroids in uterus,fibrocystic disease, breast nodules, osteosclerosis, tetany, liver disease(monitor liver function), porphyria, kidney disorder, cholelithiasis. All this group should be monitored closely. Regular examination of breasts and pelvic organs should be carried out and blood pressure checked. Persistent breakthrough bleeding. Women should self-examine breasts, attend for mammography (if applicable) and have cervical smear tests.

*Avoid use*: pregnancy, breast-feeding, hormone-dependent cancers, breast or uterus cancer, endometriosis, undiagnosed vaginal bleeding. Serious heart, kidney or liver disease, thrombophlebitis and thromboembolic diseases. Patients suffering from Dublin–Johnson syndrome or Rotor syndrome.

*Possible interaction*: drugs which induce liver enzymes.

*Side effects*: weight gain, enlargement and tenderness of

breasts, fluid retention, cramps, gastro-intestinal upset, nausea and vomiting, headaches, breakthrough bleeding, dizziness. Cholestatic jaundice, effects on liver function, migraine, nose bleeds, worsening of varicose veins, lowered glucose tolerance, itching and reddening of skin (usually short-lived). Withdraw if migraines or other severe headaches occur for first time, or serious vision disturbances, signs of thromboembolic disorders, seizures, jaundice, hepatitis, serious, whole body itching, pregnancy. Stop 6 weeks before planned surgery or prolonged immobilisation.

*Manufacturer*: Novartis.

## CLIMESSE

*Description*: a combined, hormonal, oestrogen/progestogen preparation comprising pink tablets containing 2mg of oestradiol valerate and 0.7mg of norethisterone marked OG/CG.

*Used for*: menopausal symptoms and prevention of osteoporosis following the menopause.

*Dosage*: women, starting at least one year after final period, 1 tablet every day, taken continuously.

*Special care*: patients considered to be at risk of thrombosis, those with diabetes, epilepsy, hypertension, multiple sclerosis, migraine, fibroids in uterus, fibrocystic disease, breast nodules, otosclerosis, tetany, liver disease (monitor liver function), porphyria, kidney disorder, cholelithiasis. All this group should be monitored closely. Regular examination of breasts and pelvic organs should be carried out and blood pressure checked. Persistent breakthrough bleeding. Women should self-examine breasts, attend for mammography (if applicable) and have cervical smear tests.

*Avoid use*: pregnancy, breast-feeding, hormone-dependent cancers, breast or uterus cancer, endometriosis, undiagnosed vaginal bleeding. Serious heart, kidney or liver disease, thrombophlebitis and thromboembolic diseases. Patients suffering from Dublin–Johnson syndrome or Rotor syndrome.

*Possible interaction*: drugs which induce liver enzymes.

*Side effects*: weight gain, enlargement and tenderness of breasts, fluid retention, cramps, gastro-intestinal upset, nausea and vomiting, headaches, breakthrough bleeding, dizziness. Cholestatic jaundice, effects on liver function, migraine, nose bleeds, worsening of varicose veins, lowered glucose tolerance, itching and reddening of skin (usually short-lived). Withdraw if migraines or other severe headaches occur for first time, or serious vision disturbances, signs of thromboembolic disorders, seizures, jaundice, hepatitis, serious, whole body itching, pregnancy. Stop 6 weeks before planned surgery or prolonged immobilisation.

*Manufacturer*: Novartis.

## CLINDAMYCIN *SEE*: DALACIN C, DALACIN T.

## CLINORIL

*Description*: a proprietary analgesic NSAID (indene),

produced in the form of hexagonal, yellow, scored tablets containing 100mg or 200mg sulindac and marked MSD 943 and MSD 942 respectively.

*Used for*: inflammation and pain in rheumatic diseases including gouty arthritis, rheumatoid arthritis, periarticular diseases, ankylosing spondylitis and osteoarthritis.

*Dosage*: adults, 200mg twice each day with food or drink.

*Special care*: elderly persons, diabetes, history of lithiasis (gallstones, kidney stones, stones in lower urinary tract), sepsis, patients with heart failure, liver or kidney disease (monitor function), history of gastro-intestinal haemorrhage or ulcers. Also, coagulation disorders (monitor), those at risk of fluid retention. Eye disorders should be investigated and plenty of fluids should be taken.

*Avoid use*: children, pregnancy, breast-feeding, allergy to aspirin or anti-inflammatory drugs, those with gastro-intestinal bleeding or peptic ulcer.

*Possible interaction*: aspirin, anticoagulants, diflunisal, hypoglycaemic drugs, methotrexate, dimethyl sulfoxide, ciclosporin, other NSAIDs, drugs toxic to the kidneys.

*Side effects*: allergic responses including liver failure and fever (stop drug immediately). Disturbance of vision, central nervous system effects, heart arrhythmias, changes in blood, kidney stones and disturbance of kidney function, pancreatitis, hyperglycaemia, gastro-intestinal bleeding and upset. Also rash, dizziness, glossitis (inflammation of tongue), tinnitus, muscle weakness, effects on urine including discolouration, proteinuria (protein in urine), crystals in urine (crystalluria), oedema, Stevens–Johnson syndrome.

*Manufacturer*: M.S.D.

## CLIOQUINOL *SEE*: BETNOVATE-C, SYNALAR C.

## CLOBETASOL *SEE*: DERMOVATE.

## CLOBETASONE BUTYRATE *SEE*: EUMOVATE, TRIMOVATE.

## CLOMID

*Description*: an anti-oestrogen hormonal preparation produced in the form of scored, beige coloured tablets, containing 50mg clomifene citrate, and marked with a circle containing the letter M.

*Used for*: treatment of sterility in women due to failure of ovulation.

*Dosage*: women, 1 tablet each day for 5 days starting on the fifth day of menstruation, if achievable. Treatment may continue for a maximum of 3 monthly cycles.

*Special care*: ensure patient is not pregnant before and during the course of treatment.

*Avoid use*: women with large ovarian cyst, cancer of the womb, undiagnosed uterine bleeding, liver disease.

*Side effects*: hot flushes, thinning of hair, enlargement of ovaries, abdominal discomfort, blurring of vision (withdraw drug).

*Manufacturer*: Aventis.

## CLOMIFENE *SEE*: CLOMID.

## CLOMIPRAMINE *SEE*: ANAFRANIL.

## CLOPAMIDE *SEE*: VISKALDIX.

## CLOPIXOL

*Description*: an antipsychotic drug and thioxanthene produced as tablets and as solutions for injection. Tablets in various strengths and all are film-coated; red tablets contain 2mg zuclopenthixol hydrochloride; light brown tablets contain 10mg; brown tablets contain 25mg. **CLOPIXOL INJECTION** contains 200mg per ml (as oily injection) contained in ampoules and vials. **CLOPIXOL CONCENTRATED INJECTION** contains 500mg per ml (as oily injection) contained in ampoules. **CLOPIXOL ACUPHASE** contains 50mg per ml (as oily injection) contained in ampoules.

*Used for*: psychoses, particularly schizophrenia and especially when accompanied by aggression and agitated behaviour. Clopixol acuphase is used for initial treatment of acute psychotic states.

*Dosage*: adults, tablets, 20–30mg each day in divided doses in first instance. Usual maintenance dose is in the order of 25–50mg each day with a maximum daily dose of 150mg. Clopixol injection and concentrated injection, 200–500mg every 1 to 4 weeks by deep intramuscular injection with a maximum weekly dose of 600mg. Clopixol acuphase (for immediate treatment of acute psychoses),

50–150mg by deep intramuscular injection repeated after 1, 2 or 3 days if required. Maximum total dose is 400mg and number of injections must not exceed 4. Maintenance should be by means of tablets or other Clopixol injections.

*Special care*: elderly, pregnancy, breast-feeding, severe heart, circulatory, liver or kidney disease, known intolerance to neuroleptic drugs taken by mouth.

*Avoid use*: children, coma, Parkinsonism, acute intoxication states – alcohol, barbiturate or opiate-induced.

*Possible interaction*: alcohol, antidiabetic drugs, levodopa, anticonvulsant drugs, analgesics, CNS depressants, antihypertensive drugs, anticoagulants.

*Side effects*: Parkinsonism-like effects, spasms in muscles and involuntary, repetitive movements, rapid heartbeat rate, vision disturbance, tremor. Also hypotension, changes in weight, difficulty in passing urine, constipation, dry mouth and stuffiness in nose, impotence, enlargement of breasts, abnormal milk production, hypothermia (especially in elderly persons). There may be blood and skin effects, weariness and lethargy, fits and jaundice. Drug should be withdrawn if neuroleptic malignant syndrome arises.

*Manufacturer*: Lundbeck.

## CLORAZEPATE POTASSIUM *SEE*: TRANXENE.

## CLOSTET

*Description*: a preparation of tetanus toxoid vaccine

(comprising at least 40iu per 0.5ml) adsorbed onto aluminium hydroxide and contained in pre-filled (0.5ml) syringes.

*Used for*: immunization against tetanus and for "booster" injections to reinforce immunity.

*Dosage*: adults, a course of 0.5ml by subcutaneous or intramuscular injection given a total of 3 times at 4 week intervals. After 10 years, a "booster" reinforcing dose of 0.5ml may be given by subcutaneous or intramuscular injection. If an injury is received which might give rise to tetanus, a booster reinforcing dose should be given to patients previously immunized. Those who have not, should be given a first dose of the primary course and an injection of antitetanus immunoglobin at a different site. Children normally receive a combined triple vaccine consisting of adsorbed tetanus, diphtheria and pertussis (whooping cough) vaccine, and can later receive booster reinforcing doses against tetanus. Vaccine (either primary course or reinforcing dose) may be given as protective treatment in the event of a wound, if patient's state of immunisation is in doubt or if considered advisable.

*Special care*: allergic reactions especially in persons receiving vaccine within 1 year of receiving a previous booster dose. Normally, 10 years should have elapsed before a reinforcing dose is given.

*Avoid use*: patients with serious infections unless there is a wound likely to be prone to tetanus.

*Side effects*: malaise, fever, slight soreness and local reactions.

*Manufacturer*: Evans Vaccines.

## CLOTRIMAZOLE *SEE*: CANESTEN.

## CO-AMILOZIDE *SEE*: AMIL-CO.

## CO-AMOXICLAV *SEE*: AUGMENTIN.

## CO-BETALOC

*Description*: an antihypertensive preparation combined with a cardioselective ß-blocker with a thiazide diuretic, available as white scored tablets, marked A/MH, contain 100mg metoprolol tartrate and 12.5mg hydrochlorothiazide. Also **CO-BETALOC SA** are yellow, film-coated tablets, marked A/MC, containing 200mg metoprolol tartrate and 25mg hydrochlorothiazide and having a sustained-release core.

*Used for*: mild to moderate hypertension.

*Dosage*: adults, 1 to 3 tablets each day in single or divided doses, or 1 Co-Betaloc SA tablet daily.

*Special care*: pregnancy, breast-feeding, diabetes, history of bronchospasm, wheezing, asthma etc., kidney or liver disorders, metabolic acidosis, thyrotoxic crisis, insufficient blood supply to brain, weakness, undergoing general anaesthesia, (may need to be withdrawn before planned surgery). Monitor electrolyte levels. Patients with weak hearts may need treatment with digitalis and diuretics. Withdraw drug gradually. Potassium supplements may be required.

*Avoid use*: children, sinus bradycardia, Prinzmetal's angina, heart block, heart shock, uncompensated heart failure, severe peripheral arterial disease, sick sinus syndrome, hypotension, failure of right ventricle of heart secondary to high blood pressure, severe kidney failure, anuria, metabolic acidosis, untreated phaeochromocytoma.

*Possible interaction*: sympathomimetics, warfarin, cardiac depressant anaesthetics, clonidine withdrawal, theophylline, hypoglycaemics, class I antiarrhythmic drugs, diltiazem, other antihypertensives, class II calcium antagonists, verapamil, ergot alkaloids, reserpine, ibuprofen, indometacin, rifampicin, cimetidine, CNS depressants, sympathomimetics. Also, potassium-sparing diuretics, potassium supplements, NSAIDs, amantadine lithium, digitalis, allopurinol.

*Side effects*: slow heart beat, heart failure, gastrointestinal upset, tiredness with exercise, cold hands and feet, low blood pressure, baldness, sleep disturbances, bronchospasm, blood changes. Also, sensitivity to light, enlargement of breasts, gout. If unexplained dry eyes or skin rashes occur, drug may need to be stopped gradually.

*Manufacturer*: Pharmacia.

**CO-DANTHRAMER *SEE*: CODALAX.**

**CO-DANTHRUSATE *SEE*: NORMAX.**

**CO-FLUMACTONE *SEE*: ALDACTIDE.**

**CO-MAGALDROX *SEE*: MAALOX.**

## CO-PHENOTROPE *SEE*: LOMOTIL.

## CO-PRENOZIDE *SEE*: TRASIDREX.

## CO-SIMALCITE *SEE*: ALTACITE PLUS.

## CO-TRIMOXAZOLE *SEE*: SEPTRIN.

## CO-ZIDOCAPT *SEE*: CAPOZIDE.

## CODAFEN CONTINUS

*Description*: a combined opiate analgesic and NSAID produced as pink/white, two-layered, capsule-shaped tablets containing 20mg codeine phosphate and 300mg of sustained-release ibuprofen.

*Used for*: relief of pain including post-operative, rheumatic/arthritic conditions, dental and period pain.

*Dosage*: adults, 2 tablets every 12 hours at first increasing to 3 tablets every 12 hours if needed. Maintenance dose is 1 to 3 tablets each 12 hours.

*Special care*: Pregnancy, breastfeeding, allergy to anti-inflammatory drugs or aspirin. Those with liver, kidney or heart disease, heart failure, hypotension, hypothyroidism, head injury, elevated intracranial pressure, high blood pressure, history of bronchospasm. Monitor those having long-term treatment.

*Avoid use*: children, patients with peptic ulcer or history of peptic ulcer, respiratory depression, breathing disorders, chronic constipation.

*Possible interaction*: anticoagulants taken by mouth, thiazides, MAOIs, quinolones.

*Side effects*: dizziness, blurring of vision, headache, gastrointestinal upset and bleeding, peptic ulcer, drowsiness. Rarely, disturbance of liver and kidney function, thrombocytopenia, agranulocytosis (abnormal blood disorder in which there is a reduction in the number of certain white blood cells), respiratory depression.

*Manufacturer*: Napp.

## CODALAX

*Description*: a preparation which combines a stimulant laxative and faecal softener produced in the form of a solution of 2 different strengths. It contains 200mg Poloxamer '188' and 25mg dantron per 5ml. **CODALAX FORTE** contains 1g Poloxamer '188' and 75mg dantron per 5ml.

*Used for*: treatment and prevention of constipation in terminally ill persons (which has been caused by analgesic drugs).

*Dosage*: adults, Codalax, 5–10ml taken at night; Codalax Forte, 5ml taken at night.

*Special care*: incontinence.

*Avoid use*: babies in nappies, children, pregnancy, breastfeeding, patients suffering from severe painful conditions of the abdomen or intestinal blockage.

*Side effects*: red discoloration of urine and skin with which urine comes into contact.

*Manufacturer*: Napp.

## CODEINE PHOSPHATE *SEE*: CODAFEN CONTINUS.

## COGENTIN

*Description*: an anticholinergic preparation produced as tablets and in ampoules for injection. Quarter-scored, white tablets, contain 2mg benzatropine mesylate and are coded MSD 60. **COGENTIN INJECTION** contains 1mg per ml in 2ml ampoules.

*Used for*: treatment of Parkinsonism including drug-induced symptoms of tremor and involuntary muscle movements (dyskinesia).

*Dosage*: tablets 0.5mg each day at first, increasing gradually as required by 0.5mg every 5 or 6 days. Maximum dose is 6mg daily (according to prescribing notes). Children over 3 years, consult manufacturer. Adults, injection (for emergency treatment), 1–2mg given intramuscularly or intravenously.

*Special care*: pregnancy, breastfeeding, narrow angle glaucoma, tachycardia, enlarged prostate gland, gastro-intestinal blockage. Drug should be withdrawn slowly.

*Avoid use*: patients with movement disorder (tardive dyskinesia) or children under 3 years.

*Possible interaction*: antidepressants, phenothiazines, antidopaminergic drugs.

*Side effects*: agitation and confusion, anticholinergic effects; with higher doses, rash.

*Manufacturer*: M.S.D.

## COLESTID

*Description*: a form of a resin which is a bile acid sequestrant acting as a lipid-lowering agent. Colestid is available as 5g of granules in sachets containing colestipol hydrochloride. Also, **COLESTID ORANGE** granules consisting of 5g orange-flavoured powder containing colestipol hydrochloride with aspartame.

*Used for*: type II hyperlipoproteinaemias (high fat/proteinlevels in blood).

*Dosage*: adults, 5–30g each day in 1 or 2 divided doses taken with liquid. Children, consult manufacturer.

*Special care*: pregnancy, nursing mothers, additional vitamins A, D and K may be needed.

*Possible interaction*: diuretics, digitalis, antibiotics. Any drug should be taken 1 hour before or 4 hours after Colestid as there may be interference with absorption.

*Side effects*: constipation.

*Manufacturer*: Pharmacia.

## COLESTIPOL *SEE*: COLESTID.

## COLIFOAM

*Description*: a corticosteroid produced in the form of an aerosol foam containing 10% hydrocortisone acetate in mucoadherent foam.

*Used for*: ulcerative colitis and inflammation of the bowel – granular proctitis, proctosigmoiditis.

*Dosage*: adults, 1 applicatorful into rectum once or twice

each day for 2 or 3 weeks. Afterwards the same dosage every second day.

*Special care*: pregnant women, patients with severe ulcerative disease. Avoid use for prolonged periods.

*Avoid use*: children, patients with intestinal obstruction, abscess, perforation, peritonitis. Also, patients with recent anastomoses within the intestine, or extensive fistulas. Patients suffering from fungal or viral infections or tuberculosis.

*Side effects*: systemic corticosteroid effects including mood changes, thinning of bones, mood swings, elevated blood sugar levels.

*Manufacturer*: Stafford-Miller.

## COLISTIN *SEE*: COLOMYCIN.

## COLOMYCIN

*Description*: a polymyxin antibiotic preparation produced in the form of powder in vials for reconstitution with water and injection, syrup, tablets and as a powder for topical application. Colomycin powder for injection consists of 500,000 units colistimethate sodium or 1 million units colistimethate sodium in vials. **COLOMYCIN SYRUP** contains 250,000 units colistin sulphate per 5ml. **COLOMYCIN TABLETS** are quarter-scored and white containing 1.5 million units colistin sulphate and are marked with P inside a hexagon. **COLOMYCIN POWDER** for topical application contains 1g colistin sulphate in vial. **COLOMYCIN SYRUP** contains 250,000 units per 5ml.

*Used for*: Injection: burns and wounds, surgery, skin infections, ENT infections, gram negative infections, aerosol therapy. Tablets and syrup: gastrointestinal infections caused by gram negative bacteria, pre-operatively in bowel surgery. Powder, for topical application to wounds.

*Dosage*: adults, (over 60kg body weight), injection, 2 mega units every 8 hours; children 50,000 units/kg body weight each day 8-hourly. Adults, tablets, 1 to 2 8-hourly; children, syrup, up to 15kg body weight, 5–10ml; 15–30kg, 15–30ml; over 30kg same as adult. All taken 8-hourly. Powder, consult manufacturer.

*Manufacturer*: Forest.

## CONVULEX

*Description*: an anticonvulsant carboxylic acid preparation produced in the form of soft enteric-coated gelatin capsules of 3 different strengths containing 150mg, 300mg and 500mg of valproic acid.

*Used for*: epilepsy.

*Dosage*: adults and children, 15mg per kg of body weight at first in divided doses, gradually increasing by 5–10mg/kg body weight each day, as required, until control of fits is achieved. The maximum daily dose is 30mg per kg of body weight.

*Special care*: pregnancy, false positives for ketones in urine. Liver function tests and various blood tests (coagulation, aggregation of thrombocytes, fibrinogen levels) are performed prior to treatment, at dose increases and every 8 weeks during treatment. Patients should be advised to be aware of signs of pancreatitis (severe abdominal pain, anorexia, sickness).

*Avoid use*: patients with liver disease.

*Possible interaction*: alcohol, barbiturates, antidepressants, other antiepileptic drugs, anticoagulants, neuroleptic drugs.

*Side effects*: gastro-intestinal upset, central nervous system effects, toxic effects on liver coagulation, weight gain, increased appetite, cessation of periods or disturbances to menstrual cycle, hair loss or abnormal hair growth. Drug should be withdrawn if there are toxic liver effects, pancreatitis, coagulation disturbances or low fibrinogen levels in blood.

*Manufacturer*: Pharmacia.

## CORACTEN XL

*Description*: an antianginal and antihypertensive preparation which is a class II calcium antagonist available as sustained-release capsules of 2 different strengths. Caramel coloured capsules contain 30mg nifedipine and orange capsules contain 60mg nifedipine. Both are marked with the strength and COR. *Also,* **CORACTEN SR**, sustained-release capsules in two different strengths; pink/grey containing 10mg of nifedipine and brown/pink containing 20mg, both marked with strength and name.

*Used for*: Coracten XL: prevention of angina which is stable and chronic, hypertension. Coracten SR: prevention of stable, chronic angina, treatment of Prinzmetal's angina (diagnosis established by cardiologist).

*Dosage*: adults, angina and hypertension, Coracten XL: 30mg once each day, titrated and increased if necessary to a maximum daily dose of 90mg. Coracten SR: 10mg every 12 hours, titrated and increased, if necessary, according to response to maximum of 40mg every 12 hours.

*Special care*: elderly persons, patients with weak hearts, heart failure, diabetes, liver disease, serious low blood pressure, receiving dialysis treatment.

*Avoid use*: children, pregnant women, patients with cardiogenic (heart) shock, unstable or acute angina, within one month of heart attack, serious aortic stenosis, secondary prevention of heart attack. Coracten XL only, history of obstruction in gastrointestinal tract, liver disease, inflammatory bowel disorders, acute porphyria (inherited conditions in which there is an increased production of porphyrins by the bone marrow or liver).

*Possible interaction*: cimetidine, quinidine, I.V. magnesium sulphate, antihypertensive drugs, digoxin, diltiazem, rifampicin, grapefruit juice.

*Side effects*: flushing, headache, dizziness, oedema, lethargy, nausea, rash, pain in eyes, frequency of urination, gum hyperplasia (increase in number of cells), enlargement of breasts, muscle pain, tiredness. Rarely, allergic jaundice; discontinue in the event of heart pain or heart attack.

*Manufacturer*: Celltech.

## CORDARONE X

*Description*: a class III antiarrhythmic preparation produced in the form of tablets of 2 different strengths. White, scored tablets, marked with strength and action potential symbol contain 100mg or 200mg of amiodarone hydrochloride. Also, **CORDARONE X I.V** intravenous injection comprising 50mg of amiodarone per ml of solution in ampoules for injection.

*Used for*: various heart rhythm disorders especially those which do not respond to other drugs. Tachycardia associated with Wolfe-Parkinson-White syndrome.

*Dosage*: adults, 200mg 3 times each day for first week then 200mg twice each day for the following week. Maintenance dose is usually in the order of 200mg each day and the minimum necessary should be used. Children, manufacturer should be consulted. Cordarone I.V, by intravenous infusion according to manufacturers' instructions and as directed by specialist physician.

*Special care*: pregnancy, heart failure; liver, kidney and thyroid function should be tested throughout the course of treatment. Eyes should also be monitored and therapy started in hospital and under supervision of specialist physician.

*Avoid use*: breast-feeding, patients with heart block, shock, history of thyroid disease, serious bradycardia, sensitivity to iodine. Cordarone injection, serious respiratory failure, serious hypotension involving the arterial circulation, congestive heart failure, disease of heart muscle.

*Possible interaction*: pentamidine, other antiarrhythmic drugs, lithium, ß-blockers, diuretics, digoxin, phenytoin, calcium antagonists, anticoagulants taken by mouth, erythromycin, drugs which extend QT interval, anaesthetics, co-trimoxazole. Also, anti-psychotics, anti-malarial drugs, TCADs, corticosteroids, ciclosporin, antihistamines, amphotericin, tetracosactide.

*Side effects*: sensitivity to light, effects on eyes, heart, thyroid, liver and nervous system, pulmonary toxicity.

*Manufacturer*: Sanofi -Synthelabo.

## CORDILOX

*Description*: an antihypertensive and antiarrhythmic preparation which is a class I calcium antagonist produced as tablets of 3 different strengths; yellow, film-coated tablets, marked with the name and strength, contain 40mg, 80mg and 120mg of verapamil hydrochloride. *Also*, **CORDILOX 160**, yellow, film-coated tablets marked Cordilox 160, contain 160mg of verapamil hydrochloride. *Also*, **CORDILOX INTRAVENOUS** contains 2.5mg verapamil hydrochloride per ml in ampoules for injection.

*Used for*: Cordilox: supraventricular heart arrhythmias, angina. Cordilox 160: mild to moderate high blood pressure; Cordilox I.V: supraventricular heart arrhythmias.

*Dosage*: Cordilox and Cordilox I.V., heart arrhythmias, adults: 40–120mg 3 times each day; children: under 2 years, 20mg 2 or 3 times daily; over 2 years, 40–120mg 2 or 3 times each day. Cordilox I.V., adults and children, according to manufacturers' specifications and under specialist supervision. Cordilox 160, hypertension, adults, 1 tablet twice each day; children, up to 10mg per kg of body weight each day in divided doses. Cordilox, angina, adults only, 120mg 3 times each day.

*Special care*: patients with weak heart should take digitalis and diuretics; persons with first degree heart block, kidney or liver disease, heart attack, heart conduction disorders, bradycardia, hypotension.

*Avoid use*: severe bradycardia, second or third degree heart block, uncompensated heart failure, heart shock, sick-sinus syndrome.

*Possible interaction*: ß-blockers, grapefruit juice,digoxin, quinidine.

*Side effects*: flushes, dizziness, headache, tiredness, constipation.

*Manufacturer*: IVAX.

## CORGARD

*Description*: an antihypertensive, non-cardioselective ß-blocker produced in the form of pale blue tablets of 2 different strengths containing either 40 or 80mg (scored tablet) of nadolol and marked 207 or 241, respectively.

*Used for*: heart arrhythmias, angina, hypertension, additional treatment in thyrotoxicosis, prevention of migraine.

*Dosage*: heart arrhythmias, 40mg each day at first increasing as required to maximum of 160mg; angina, 40mg each day at first increasing as required with usual daily dose of 160mg; hypertension, 80mg each day at first increasing as needed with usual daily dose in the order of 80–240mg; thyrotoxicosis, 80–160mg once each day; prevention of migraine, 40mg each day at first increasing if necessary to a usual daily dose in the order of 80–160mg.

*Special care*: pregnancy, breast-feeding, patients with weak hearts should receive diuretics and digitalis, liver or kidney disease, diabetes, metabolic acidosis, weakness, insufficient cerebral circulation, thyrotoxic crisis, tendency to exhibit allergic symptoms. Persons undergoing general anaesthesia, may need to be withdrawn before planned surgery. Withdraw drug gradually.

*Avoid use*: children, patients with obstructive airways disease or history of bronchospasm (asthma), various heart disorders including heart block, heart shock, heart failure, sick sinus syndrome, serious peripheral arterial disease, sinus bradycardia, disease of heart muscle, Prinzmetal's angina, hypotension, right ventricular failure resulting from pulmonary hypertension, untreated phaeochromocytoma (tumour of the adrenal glands).

*Possible interaction*: cardiac depressant anaesthetics, theophylline, antihypertensives, ergot alkaloids, diltiazem, sympathomimetics, verapamil, clonidine withdrawal, CNS depressants, class I antiarrhythmic drugs, rifampicin, cimetidine, class II calcium antagonists, warfarin, reserpine, ibuprofen, indometacin, hypoglycaemics.

*Side effects*: bradycardia, fatigue on exercise, cold hands and feet, central nervous system effects, disturbance of sleep, gastro-intestinal upset, bronchospasm, heart failure, low blood pressure, baldness, thrombocytopenia (reduction in blood platelets). Withdraw drug gradually if dry eyes or skin rash occur.

*Manufacturer*: Sanofi-Synthelabo.

## CORGARETIC 40

*Description*: a combined antihypertensive, non-cardioselective ß-blocker and thiazide diuretic produced as scored, mottled, white tablets marked 283, containing 40mg of nadolol and 5mg of bendroflumethiazide. *Also,* **CORGARETIC 80**, scored, mottled, white tablets marked 284, containing 80mg of nadolol and 5mg of bendroflumethiazide.

*Used for*: high blood pressure.

*Dosage*: adults, 1or 2 tablets each day, using lowest possible effective doses, to a maximum daily dose of 160mg of nadolol and 10mg bendroflumethiazide (2x Corgaretic 80).

*Special care*: pregnancy, breast-feeding, patients with weak hearts should receive digitalis and diuretics, history of bronchospasm, liver or kidney disease, diabetes, metabolic acidosis, raised blood lipid levels, gout, weakness, insufficient cerebral blood supply, tendency to allergy. Persons undergoing general anaesthesia, may require drug to be withdrawn before planned surgery. Electrolyte levels should be monitored. Drug should be gradually withdrawn.

*Avoid use*: children, patients with obstructive airways disease or history of bronchospasm (asthma), various heart disorders including heart block, heart shock, heart failure, sick sinus syndrome, serious peripheral arterial disease, sinus bradycardia, Prinzmetal's angina, low blood pressure, severe heart muscle disease, uncompensated heart failure. Also, untreated tumour of adrenal gland (phaeochromocytoma), failure of right ventricle secondary to pulmonary hypertension, severe or progressive kidney failure, anuria.

*Possible interaction*: cardiac depressant anaesthetics, antihypertensives, ergot alkaloids, ibuprofen, sympathomimetics, verapamil, clonidine withdrawal, central nervous system depressants, class I antiarrhythmic drugs, diltiazem, cimetidine, reserpine. Also, indometacin, theophylline, class II calcium antagonists, hypoglycaemics, lithium, warfarin, digitalis, rifampicin. Also, amantadine, NSAIDs, potassium-sparing diuretics, potassium supplements, allopurinol.

*Side effects*: bradycardia, fatigue on exercise, cold hands and feet, disturbance of sleep, gastro-intestinal upset, low blood pressure, bronchospasm, heart failure, blood changes, baldness, thrombocytopenia (low levels of blood platelets), blood changes, sensitivity to light, gout. Withdraw drug gradually if skin rash or dry eyes occur.

*Manufacturer*: Sanofi-Synthelabo.

## COVERSYL

*Description*: an antihypertensive preparation and ACE inhibitor produced as tablets of 2 different strengths. White tablets contain 2mg perindopril tert-butylamine and white, scored oblong tablets contain 4mg.

*Used for*: additional therapy with digitalis and/or diuretics in congestive heart failure, renovascular and essential hypertension.

*Dosage*: adults, heart failure, treatment should start in hospital under close supervision with 2mg once daily taken in the morning increasing to 4mg once each day. Withdraw any diuretic 3 days before the start of treatment and resume later, if needed. Hypertension, 2mg once each day before food increasing to daily maintenance dose of 4mg (8mg once each day is maximum dose). Elderly persons should take a reduced dose of 2mg each day under close medical supervision.

*Special care*: patients with kidney disorders or receiving dialysis. Kidney function should be monitored before and during treatment; patients undergoing anaesthesia and surgery.

*Avoid use*: children, pregnancy, breast-feeding.

*Possible interaction*: tricyclic antidepressants, lithium, potassium supplements, potassium-sparing diuretics, NSAIDs, neuroleptic agents, antidiabetic drugs, antihypertensives.

*Side effects*: hypotension, skin rashes and itching, flushing, loss of sense of taste, angioneurotic oedema, headache, malaise, fatigue, nausea, pain in abdomen, weakness, slight cough, blood changes, protein in urine.

*Manufacturer*: Servier.

## CROMOGEN EASI-BREATHE

*Description*: an anti-inflammatory, non-steroidal, bronchodilator produced as an aerosol for inhalation containing 5mg of sodium cromoglicate per breath-actuated inhaler. Also, **CROMOGEN INHALER**, available as an aerosol containing 5mg of sodium cromoglicate per metered dose. Also, **CROMOGEN STERI-NEB**, a preservative-free solution containing 10mg sodium cromoglicate per ml, available as a single dose for use with nebulizer.

*Used for*: asthma and prevention of asthma brought on by exercise.

*Dosage*: adults and children, Easi-Breathe and Inhaler, 2 puffs 4 times each day in first instance with a maintenance dose of 1 puff 4 times daily. Cromogen Steri-Neb, 20mg with power-operated nebulizer 4 times each day at 3 to 6 hourly intervals. If necessary frequency can be increased to 5 or 6 times each day and, to be effective, therapy must be continuous.

*Side effects*: irritation of throat and short-lived cough (due to inhalation of powder). Rarely, short-lived bronchospasm.

*Manufacturer*: IVAX.

## CRYSTAPEN

*Description*: a preparation of penicillin which is sensitive to penicillinase called penicillin G. It is an antibiotic which is inactivated by the penicillinase enzymes produced by certain bacteria. It is inactivated by stomach (gastric) juices and poorly absorbed from the gut and is produced as an unbuffered powder in vials for reconstitution and injection. Available in two strengths containing 600mg or 1200mg of penicillin G sodium.

*Used for*: gonorrhoea, septicaemia, endocarditis, osteomyelitis, meningitis, respiratory tract, ear, nose and throat, skin and soft tissue infections.

*Dosage*: adults, 600–1200mg by intravenous or intramuscular injection each day in 2, 3 or 4 divided doses. For meningitis, up to 14.4g daily in divided doses may be needed; for suspected meningitis, 1200mg by intravenous or intramuscular injection. Children, newborns under 1 week old, 50mg per kg of body weight in 2 divided doses; 1 week to 1 month, 75mg/kg of body weight each day in 3 divided doses; 1 month to 12 years, 100mg per kg each day in 4 divided doses. For meningitis, age less than 1 week 100mg per kg each day in 2 divided doses; 1 week to 1 month, 150mg per kg each day in 3 divided doses; 1 month to 12 years, 180–300mg per kg each day in 4, 5 or 6 divided doses (maximum dose is 12g each day). Suspected meningitis, aged less than 12 months, 300mg; aged 1 to 9 years, 600mg; more than 10 years, 1200mg. All doses are delivered by intravenous or intramuscular injection.

*Side effects*: allergic responses, gastrointestinal effects.

*Manufacturer*: Britannia.

## CD CYCLIMORPH

*Description*: a strong analgesic preparation which combines an opiate with an anti-emetic and is available as solutions of 2 different strengths in 1ml ampoules for injection. Cyclimorph 10 contains 10mg morphine tartrate and 50mg cyclizine tartrate per ml; **CYCLIMORPH 15** contains 15mg morphine tartrate and 50mg cyclizine tartrate per ml.

*Used for*: acute and chronic, severe, intractable pain where control of sickness/nausea is also required.

*Dosage*: adults, 10 to 20mg given by subcutaneous, intravenous or intramuscular injection with at least a 4 hour interval between doses. The maximum is 3 doses in 24 hours.

*Special care*: pregnancy, breastfeeding, women in labour, elderly, seriously ill patients, diabetes, hypothyroidism, serious heart failure, obstruction of gastrointestinal tract, shock, glaucoma, enlarged prostate gland, underactive pituitary gland, insufficient hormonal output from cortex of adrenal glands.

*Avoid use*: children, patients with blocked airways or respiratory depression, head injury, elevated pressure within skull, serious liver disease, moderate to serious kidney disorders, ulcerative colitis, heart failure associated with chronic lung disease, serious intoxication with alcohol.

*Possible interaction*: central nervous system sedatives, MAOIs, diuretics, anticholinergic drugs, phenothiazines, propanolol.

*Side effects*: drug dependence and tolerance may develop, constipation, dizziness, dry mouth, blurring of vision, low blood pressure on standing up, sleepiness.

*Manufacturer*: CeNeS.

## CYCLIZINE *SEE*: CYCLIMORPH, VALOID.

## CYCLO-PROGYNOVA 1MG

*Description*: a combined oestrogen/progestogen hormonal preparation available as tablets in 2 different strengths. Cyclo-Progynova 1mg consists of a course of sugar-coated tablets; 11 beige ones contain 1mg oestradiol valerate and 10 brown ones contain 1mg oestradiol valerate and 0.25mg levonorgestrel. **CYCYLO-PROGYNOVA 2mg** consists of a course of sugar-coated tablets; 11 white ones contain 2mg oestradiol valerate and 10 brown ones contain 2mg oestradiol valerate and 0.5mg norgestrel (= 0.25mg levonorgestrel).

*Used for*: menopausal symptoms (climacteric syndrome), osteoporosis arising after the menopause.

*Dosage*: 1 oestradiol tablet each day for 11 days (beginning on fifth day of period, if present), followed by 1 combined oestradiol/levonorgestrel tablet for 10 days. Then there are 7 tablet-free days before course is repeated. The lower strength preparation should be tried first.

*Special care*: women at any risk of thrombosis and those with liver disease. Liver function should be monitored every 2 to 3 months during treatment. Patients with diabetes, porphyria, migraine, epilepsy, hypertension, fibroids in the uterus, multiple sclerosis, otosclerosis, gallstones, tetany, kidney disorders, asthma, SLE. These persons should be closely monitored. Also, women with a family history of breast cancer or fibrocystic disease of the breast should be carefully monitored. Breasts and pelvic organs should be examined and blood pressure checked regularly before and during the period of treatment. There is a small increased risk of breast cancer with HRT treatment. Persistent breakthrough bleeding should be investigated.

*Avoid use*: pregnancy, breast-feeding, endometriosis, undiagnosed vaginal bleeding, hormone-dependent cancers, breast cancer, serious heart, liver or kidney disease, thromboembolism, deep-vein thrombosis, thrombophlebitis. Also, women with kidney, liver or heart disease and Rotor or Dubin–Johnson syndromes. Drug should be stopped 6 weeks before planned surgery and during any condition which makes thrombosis more likely.

*Possible interaction*: drugs which induce liver enzymes.

*Side effects*: breakthrough bleeding, weight gain, tenderness and enlargement of breasts, gastro-intestinal upset, dizziness, nausea, headache, lowering of glucose tolerance, itching, short-lived rashes, vomiting, raised blood pressure, liver effects, nosebleeds, cholestatic jaundice, Drug should be stopped immediately in the event of frequent severe headaches, migraine, disturbance of vision, itching of whole body, thromboembolism or thrombophlebitis, jaundice, hepatitis, or sudden blood pressure rise.

*Manufacturer*: Viatris.

## CYMEVENE

*Description*: an antiviral preparation which is a DNA polymerase inhibitor available as a powder in vials for reconstitution and injection containing 500mg ganciclovir. *Also*, **CYMEVENE CAPSULES,** available in two different strengths; green, containing 250mg of ganciclovir and yellow/green containing 500mg. All are marked with two lines, strength and CY.

*Used for*: Cymevene injection, CMV disease (serious infections caused by cytomegalovirus in AIDS patients and those with reduced immunity). Cymevene capsules, prevention of CMV disease in patients who have received a liver or kidney transplant, maintenance treatment of retinitis (eye disease) caused by CMV in AIDS patients.

*Dosage*: adults, injection, 5mg per kg of body weight given by intravenous infusion every 12 hours for a period of 14 to 21 days. Maintenance treatment is 6mg per kg of body weight each day by intravenous infusion for 5 days out of 7; alternatively, 5mg per kg of body weight for one week or longer. Children according to manufacturer's instructions and as directed by specialist physician. Capsules, adult AIDS patients, 1000mg 3 times each day or 500mg 6 times each day – capsules to be taken with food and following on from at least 3 weeks of treatment given intravenously. Adult transplant patients, 1000mg given 3 times each day. Children, according to manufacturer's instructions and as directed by specialist physician.

*Special care*: Regular blood counts required due to toxic effects on blood; potential carcinogen. Patients with kidney disease, those who have received a liver transplant. Reduced doses may be needed in event of anaemia/leucopenia.

*Avoid use*: pregnancy, breastfeeding; women should use effective contraception.

*Possible interaction*: other antiviral drugs, zidovudine, drugs suppressing muscle activity, probenecid, imipenem, didanosine.

*Side effects*: effects on blood including anaemia, leucopenia, thrombocytopenia (treatment may need to be halted until levels recover). Effects on liver function, anorexia, itching, headache, fever, rash, malaise.

*Manufacturer*: Roche.

## CYPROHEPTADINE *SEE*: PERIACTIN.

## CYPROSTAT

*Description*: an anti-androgen preparation used to treat prostate cancer, a type which is hormone-dependent and develops under the influence of the male sex hormone, androgen. The drug blocks androgens produced by the adrenal glands and testes. Cyprostat is available in the form of tablets of 2 strengths; white scored tablets, marked BV within a hexagon, contain 50mg cyproterone acetate. White scored tablets, marked LA within a hexagon, contain 100mg cyproterone acetate.

*Used for*: long-term palliative treatment of cancer of the prostate gland, short-term treatment for hormonal flare up (testosterone flare) associated with antagonists to LHRH in treatment of tumour, hot flushes occasioned by medical or surgical castration.

*Dosage*: adult men, long-term palliative treatment, 200 to 300mg each day in 2 or 3 divided doses taken immediately after meals; testosterone flare, 300mg each day in 2 to 3 divided doses immediately following meals; hot flushes, 50 to 150mg each day in 1 to 3 divided doses after meals.

*Special care*: diabetes, liver disease, history of thrombosis, severe persistent depression, Sickle cell anaemia. Tests on liver function and checks on haemoglobin levels are needed before and during course of treatment. Drug should be withdrawn if liver toxicity develops.

*Side effects*: weariness, infertility, depression, liver disorders and toxicity, breast enlargement, anaemia, weight changes, osteoporosis, allergic responses, shortness of breath, thromboembolic changes, alteration in pattern of hair growth.

*Manufacturer*: Schering HC.

## CYPROTERONE ACETATE *SEE*: CYPROSTAT.

## CYSTEINE *SEE*: CICATRIN.

## CYSTRIN

*Description*: an anticholinergic and antispasmodic preparation available as white tablets containing 3mg oxybutynin hydrochloride marked C3 and white scored tablets, marked C5, containing 5mg oxybutynin hydrochloride.

*Used for*: incontinence, urgency and frequency of urination due to neurogenic bladder disorders or other causes, night-time bedwetting in children.

*Dosage*: adults, 5mg 2 or 3 times each day (with a maximum daily dose of 20mg), in divided doses. Elderly persons, 3mg twice each day at first, adjusted according to response. Children, 5 years and over, 3mg twice each day in first instance, adjusted according to response to usual dose in the order of 5mg 2 or 3 times daily. For night-time bedwetting, last dose should be taken at bedtime.

*Special care*: pregnant women, disease of the autonomic nervous system, liver or kidney disease, heart arrhythmias, heart failure, coronary heart disease, enlarged prostate, tachycardia, hyperthyroidism, hiatus hernia.

*Avoid use*: children under 5 years, breast-feeding, blocked gastro-intestinal tract or bladder, other intestinal diseases, glaucoma, myasthenia gravis, severe ulcerative colitis, toxic megacolon.

*Possible interaction*: other anticholinergics, TCADs, digoxin, levodopa, amantadine, phenothiazines, butyrophenones.

*Side effects*: facial flushing, anticholinergic effects.

*Manufacturer*: Sanofi-Synthelabo.

## CYTOTEC

*Description*: a synthetic form of prostaglandin (a naturally occurring hormone-like substance present in many body tissues) which inhibits the secretion of gastric juice and promotes the healing of ulcers. It is produced in the form of white, hexagonal tablets, containing 200μg of misoprostol, and marked SEARLE 1461.

*Used for*: stomach and duodenal ulcers, ulceration caused by NSAIDs, prevention of NSAID ulceration.

*Dosage*: adults, 4 tablets each day with meals, in divided doses, with last taken at bedtime for 1 to 2 months. Prevention of ulcers, 1 tablet 2, 3 or 4 times each day during the period that NSAID is being taken.

*Special care*: women should use effective contraception, patients with circulatory diseases including peripheral or coronary vascular disease and cerebrovascular disease.

*Avoid use*: children, pregnancy, women planning pregnancy, breast-feeding.

*Side effects*: gastro-intestinal upset, diarrhoea, pain in abdomen, vaginal bleeding and disturbance of menstrual cycle, dizziness, rash.

*Manufacturer*: Pharmacia.

# D

## DALACIN C

*Description*: an antibacterial preparation which is a lincosamide, available as capsules in two different strengths. Purple capsules, marked P&U 331 contain 75mg of clindamycin as hydrochloride; purple/maroon capsules, marked P&U 225 contain 150mg of clindamycin as hydrochloride. *Also,* **DALACIN PHOSPHATE**, available as a solution in ampoules for injection containing 150mg per ml, of clindamycin phosphate.

*Used for*: serious infections sensitive to clindamycin.

*Dosage*: adults, 150–450mg every 6 hours. Children, 3 to 6mg per kg of body weight every 6 hours. Dalacin phosphate, adults, 600mg–2.7g in divided doses each day, by intramuscular injection or intravenous infusion. Children over 1 month, 15–40mg/kg daily in divided doses, in same way as for adults.

*Special care*: pregnancy, breastfeeding, kidney or liver disease; cease use should colitis or diarrhoea occur.

*Avoid use*: in cases of lincomycin sensitivity.

*Possible interaction*: neuromuscular blocking agents.

*Side effects*: jaundice and blood disorders, pseudomembranous colitis, gastro-intestinal upsets.

*Manufacturer*: Pharmacia.

## DALACIN T

*Description*: antibiotic preparation available as an aqueous lotion in a roll-on bottle containing 10mg of clindamycin phosphate per ml of liquid. *Also,* **DALACIN T LOTION** available as an alcohol-based solution containing 10mg of clindamycin phosphate per ml.

*Used for*: acne vulgaris.

*Dosage*: apply twice each day to affected areas.

*Special care*: pregnancy. When using solution avoid eyes and mucous membranes.

*Avoid use*: in cases of lincomycin sensitivity.

*Possible interaction*: topical preparations of benzoyl peroxide.

*Side effects*: dermatitis, dry skin, folliculitis (solution). Discontinue should colitis or diarrhoea occur.

*Manufacturer*: Pharmacia.

## DALMANE

*Description*: a long-acting benzodiazepine (a hypnotic) available as capsules in two different strengths containing flurazepam as hydrochloride. Yellow/grey capsules marked ICN 15 contain 15mg; black/grey capsules marked ICN 30 contain 30mg.

*Used for*: short-term treatment of severe or disabling insomnia.

*Dosage*: adults, 15–30mg at bedtime, elderly persons, 15mg.

*Special care*: chronic liver, kidney or lung disease, acute, narrow-angle glaucoma, elderly persons, bereavement. May impair dexterity and judgement. Should not be used as sole therapy for depression or anxiety. To be withdrawn gradually.

*Avoid use*: children, pregnancy, breastfeeding, labour, acute lung disease, depression of the respiration, obsessional and phobic states, chronic psychosis. Also, myasthenia gravis, severe liver disorders, sleep apnoea syndrome.

*Possible interaction*: anticonvulsants, CNS depressants, alcohol.

*Side effects*: confusion, vertigo, drowsiness, ataxia, light-headedness, gastro-intestinal upsets, skin rashes, weakness in muscles, hypotension, disturbance in vision. Urine retention, changes in libido, impaired ability to perform tasks and in exercise of judgement; rarely, jaundice and effects on blood. Dependence is possible especially at higher doses and with longer treatment periods.

*Manufacturer*: ICN.

## DANTRON *SEE*: CODALAX, NORMAX.

## DEMECLOCYCLINE *SEE*: DETECLO.

## DEPO-PROVERA

*Description*: a depot-injectable preparation of the progestogen, medroxyprogesterone aceta, available in vials as a suspension of 150mg per ml.

*Used for*: contraception for women who for a number of reasons cannot use other methods. Only to be prescribed following counselling.

*Dosage*: women, during first 5 days of monthly cycle, 150mg injection, repeated every 3 months. Following birth, 150mg during first 5 days, unless the woman is breastfeeding when treatment should be delayed until 6 weeks or later and barrier contraception used. Repeat every 3 months. All by deep intramuscular injection. Repeat injections should all be given during the 5 days following the 12 week interval – any delay requires pregnancy to be ruled out before a further injection is given and barrier contraception to then be additionally used for first 2 weeks.

*Special care*: diabetes, severe depression, disturbance of vision, migraine, circulatory or heart disorders, thromboembolic disorders. Injection should not be repeated if woman develops cerebral circulatory disease, thromboembolism or thrombosis on the retina of the eye. Treatment slightly increases the risk of developing breast cancer.

*Avoid use*: pregnancy, abnormal vaginal bleeding of unknown cause, hormone-dependent cancers.

*Side effects*: temporary infertility following continuous treatment after treatment is stopped, absent, irregular or heavy vaginal bleeding during early cycles, weight gain, pain in abdomen, fluid retention, headaches, weakness, dizziness.

*Manufacturer*: Pharmacia.

## DERMOVATE

*Description*: a highly potent topical steroid preparation available as ointment and cream containing 0.05% clobetasol proprionate. *Also,* **DERMOVATE SCALP APPLICATION**, available as an alcohol-based solution containing 0.05% clobetasol proprionate. *Also,* **DERMOVATE-NN,** combining a highly potent topical steroid with an antibacterial and an antifungal agent. Available as ointment and cream containing 0.05% clobetasol proprionate, 0.5% neomycin sulphate and 100,000 units per gram of nystatin.

*Used for*: Dermovate, inflamed dermatitis, severe, persistent eczema that is hard to control, psoriasis, discoid lupus erythematosus (an autoimmune disorder affecting the skin), lichen planus (a chronic skin disorder of unknown cause). Dermovate Scalp Application, skin disorders affecting the scalp. Dermovate-NN, as for Dermovate but when infection is also present or suspected to be present.

*Dosage*: Dermovate, adults, apply thinly once or twice each day for up to one month; children over 1 year, as for adult but use for no more than 5 days. Dermovate scalp application, adults and children over 1 year, apply sparingly each night and morning until symptoms improve. Dermovate-NN, adults and children over 1 year, apply thinly up to 2 times each day.

*Special care*: use on face or for children should be limited to 5 days maximum, infants when nappy area is being treated, psoriasis (monitor). Withdraw gradually after prolonged use.

*Avoid use*: children aged less than 1 year, on acne, leg ulcers, tuberculous, ringworm or viral skin disease, perioral dermatitis, untreated infections whether fungal or bacterial. Extensive or prolonged use during pregnancy.

*Side effects*: skin atrophy, striae (lines) and telangiectasia (permanent widening of superficial blood vessels), suppression of adrenal glands, Cushingoid changes (as in Cushing's syndrome).

*Manufacturer*: GlaxoSmithKline.

## DESOGESTREL *SEE*: MARVELON, MERCILON.

## DETECLO

*Description*: a compound antibiotic, (tetracycline) preparation available as blue film-coated tablets, marked LL, and 5422 on the reverse, containing 115.4mg of chlortetracycline hydrochloride, 115.4mg of tetracycline hydrochloride and 69.2mg of demeclocycline hydrochloride.

*Used for*: ear, nose and throat infections; infection of respiratory, gastro-intestinal and urinary tracts and soft tissues, severe cases of acne vulgaris.

*Dosage*: adults, 1 tablet every 12 hours, either 1 hour before a meal or 2 hours afterwards.

*Special care*: elderly patients, those with impaired liver function.

*Avoid use*: children, pregnancy, breastfeeding, kidney impairment, SLE.

*Possible interaction*: penicillins, anticoagulants, oral contraceptives, milk, antacids, mineral supplements.

*Side effects*: allergic reactions, gastro-intestinal effects, superinfection (i.e. one infection arising during the course of another); withdraw in the case of raised pressure within the skull.

*Manufacturer*: Goldshield.

## DEXAMETHASONE *SEE*: SOFRADEX.

## DEXAMFETAMINE *SEE*: DEXEDRINE.

## DEXEDRINE CD

*Description*: a controlled drug and a form of amfetamine which is a sympathomimetic (i.e. something that mimics the effect of organ stimulation by the sympathetic nervous system which is part of the autonomic nervous system). It is available as scored, white tablets containing 5mg of dexamfetamine sulphate, marked EVANS DB5.

*Used for*: narcolepsy (a condition in which a person suddenly, abnormally and uncontrollably falls asleep), hyperkinetic (impulsive/hyperactive) conditions in children receiving specialist treatment and supervision.

*Dosage*: elderly persons, 5mg each day at first, increasing by 5mg after 1 week, if required to optimal dose, as advised by physician. Adults, 10mg each day in divided doses at first, increasing after 1 week by 10mg per day, if required and then at further weekly intervals until optimal dose is achieved. The maximum daily dose is 60mg each day in divided doses. Children aged 3 to 5 years, 2.5mg each day at first, increasing, if required, at weekly intervals by 2.5mg; children aged 6 to 12 years, 5 to 10mg each day at first, increasing, if required, at weekly intervals by 5mg each day to a usual maximum of 20mg daily.

*Special care*: pregnancy, epilepsy, family history of impairment in muscle tone (dystonia).

*Avoid use*: porphyria (an inherited disorder involving

abnormal production of porphyrins), glaucoma, high blood pressure, heart and circulatory disease, over-active thyroid gland, Gilles de la Tourette syndrome (an abnormal condition characterized by tics and grimaces, involuntary limb movements and sometimes, grunting, shouting or snorting), dystonias, hyperexcitability, history of substance abuse.

*Possible interaction*: alpha methyltyrosine, guanethidine, adrenoreceptor blocking drugs, MAOIs, lithium, methyltyrosine, TCADs.

*Side effects*: central nervous system effects, dry mouth, gastrointestinal disturbances, sleeplessness, kidney damage, raised blood pressure, sweating, rapid heart beat, damage to heart muscle, restlessness, slowed growth in children, anorexia, euphoria, dependence, muscle effects.

*Manufacturer*: Celltech.

## DEXKETOPROFEN *SEE*: KERAL.

## DEXTRAN *SEE*: TEARS NATURALE.

## DIAMOX

*Description*: a diuretic preparation which is a carbonic anhydrase inhibitor available as scored, white tablets containing 250mg of acetazolamide marked LEDERLE 4395. *Also,* **DIAMOX SR,** available as sustained-release, orange capsules containing 250mg of acetazolamide.

*Used for*: Diamox: congestive heart failure and oedema, epilepsy, glaucoma. Diamox SR: glaucoma.

*Dosage*: adults, Diamox, for heart failure, oedema: 250–375mg to start, each morning or on alternate days. For premenstrual oedema, 125–375mg in 1 dose taken 5 to 10 days before menstruation. For epilepsy, adults, 250–1000mg each day in divided doses. Epilepsy, children, 8 to 30mg per kg of body weight each day in divided doses to a maximum of 750mg. For glaucoma, adults, 250–1000mg each day in divided doses. Children, 125–750mg daily; infants, 125mg daily. Diamox SR, adults, glaucoma, 1 to 2 tablets each day.

*Special care*: breastfeeding, emphysema, pulmonary obstruction. Monitoring of blood, electrolytes and fluid is required. Any unusual rashes to be reported to doctor.

*Avoid use*: children, except for epilepsy, pregnancy, certain kidney conditions, chronic closed angle glaucoma, adrenal insufficiency, hypersensitivity to sulfonamides, depletion of sodium or potassium. Also, for glaucoma treatment liver impairment.

*Possible interaction*: oral anticoagulants, hypoglycaemics, folic acid antagonists.

*Side effects*: headache, drowsiness, thirst, flushing, polyuria, blood changes, rash, metabolic acidosis, paraesthesia (tingling, "pins and needles").

*Manufacturer*: Goldshield.

## DIAZEMULS

*Description*: a long-acting anxiolytic, benzodiazepine, available as an emulsion of 10mg in 2ml.

*Used for*: severe acute anxiety, delirium tremens,

anticonvulsant for status epilepticus (continual seizures resulting in brain damage if not stopped), acute muscular spasms, and as a premedication.

*Dosage*: adults, anxiety, delirium tremens, muscle spasms, 10mg by infusion or intravenous injection at 4-hourly intervals, elderly patients receive 5mg. Children, anxiety, delirium tremens, acute muscle spasms, 0.2mg per kg of body weight every 4 hours by same means as adults. Status epilepticus, adults and children, 0.15–0.25mg per kg of body weight by intravenous injection, repeated after half to one hour and then up to 3mg per kg over 24 hours, by intravenous infusion. For premedication, adults and children, 0.1–0.2mg per kg of body weight by intravenous injection.

*Special care*: chronic lung insufficiency, chronic liver or kidney disease, depression, glaucoma (acute, narrow angle), bereavement. Drug can affect dexterity and judgement. Long-term use is to be avoided and drug should be withdrawn gradually.

*Avoid use*: pregnancy, breastfeeding, labour, elderly persons, acute lung insufficiency, depression of respiration (except in cases of acute muscle spasms), sleep apnoea, severe liver insufficiency, myasthenia gravis (a severe autoimmune disorder). Also when treating anxiety, obsessional states or chronic psychosis.

*Possible interaction*: alcohol and other CNS depressants, anticonvulsants.

*Side effects*: vertigo, gastro-intestinal upsets, confusion, ataxia, drowsiness, light-headedness, hypotension,

disturbance of vision, skin rashes. Also urine retention, changes in libido. Dependence a potential problem.
*Manufacturer*: Alpharma.

## DIAZEPAM *SEE*: DIAZEMULS, DIAZEPAM RECTUBES.

## DIAZEPAM RECTUBES

*Description*: an anxiolytic preparation which is a long-acting benzodiazepine, available as an emulsion in three different strengths, for use with a rectal applicator, containing 2.5mg, 5mg or 10mg of diazepam, respectively.
*Used for*: serious anxiety, agitation, feverish and epileptic fits, muscular spasms in tetanus patients, sedation and premedication.
*Dosage*: for all conditions, adults, 0.5mg per kg of body weight every 12 hours as required, by rectal route; elderly persons, up to 0.25mg per kg every 12 hours. Children aged over 12 months, dosage depends upon body weight; weighing 10 to 15kg, 0.5mg per kg delivered with the applicator tube inserted half way into the rectum. Weighing more than 15kg, 0.5mg per kg delivered as for adult; all doses can be repeated after 12 hours.
*Special care*: chronic lung insufficiency, chronic liver or kidney disease, depression, glaucoma (acute, narrow angle), bereavement. Drug can affect dexterity and judgement. Long-term use is to be avoided and drug should be withdrawn gradually.
*Avoid use*: pregnancy, breastfeeding, labour, elderly persons,

acute lung insufficiency, depression of respiration (except in cases of acute muscle spasms), sleep apnoea, severe liver insufficiency, myasthenia gravis (a severe autoimmune disorder). Also when treating anxiety, obsessional states or chronic psychosis.

*Possible interaction*: alcohol and other CNS depressants, anticonvulsants.

*Side effects*: vertigo, gastro-intestinal upsets, confusion, ataxia, drowsiness, light-headedness, hypotension, disturbance of vision, skin rashes. Also urine retention, changes in libido. Dependence a potential problem.

*Manufacturer*: CP Pharm.

## DICLOFENAC *SEE*: ARTHROTEC, DICLOFLEX, DICLOMAX, MOTIFENE, VOLTAROL, VOLTAROL EMULGEL.

## DICLOFLEX

*Description*: a Non-steroidal anti-inflammatory drug (NSAID), phenylacetic acid, available as enteric-coated, brown tablets in two different strengths containing 25mg or 50mg of diclofenac sodium. *Also,* **DICLOFLEX RETARD,** available as sustained-release, pink tablets containing 100mg of diclofenac sodium. *Also,* **DICLOFLEX SR,** available as sustained-release pink tablets containing 75mg of diclofenac sodium, all marked DICL 75.

*Used for*: osteo- and rheumatoid arthritis, gout attacks, muscle and skeletal disorders, strains, sprains, back and joint pain.

*Dosage*: adults, Dicloflex, 75 to 100mg each day in divided doses; Dicloflex Retard, 1 tablet each day taken with a meal; Dicloflex SR, 1 to 2 tablets each day taken with a meal. Children, Dicloflex only, 1 to 3mg per kg of body weight each day in divided doses – not to be given to infants.

*Special care*: pregnancy, breastfeeding, elderly persons, liver, kidney or heart disorders, blood disorders or abnormalities, history of gastrointestinal ulcers or lesions, liver porphyria (inherited disorder involving the abnormal production of porphyrins). Patients receiving long-term treatment require monitoring.

*Avoid use*: final 3 months of pregnancy, known allergy to aspirin or NSAIDs, active peptic ulcer.

*Possible interaction*: diuretics, NSAIDs, salicylates, ciclosporin, antidiabetic drugs, steroids, quinolones, lithium, anticoagulants, methotrexate.

*Side effects*: short-lived stomach pain, fluid retention, headache. Rarely, stomach ulcer, blood changes, skin effects, liver and kidney dysfunction.

*Manufacturer*: Dexcel.

## DICLOMAX RETARD

*Description*: a Non-steroidal anti-inflammatory drug (NSAID), phenylacetic acid, available as sustained-release white capsules containing 100mg of diclofenac sodium, marked with name.

*Used for*: osteoarthritis, rheumatoid arthritis, ankylosing spondylitis, musculoskeletal disorders such as sprains and strains, back pains. Acute gout. *Also,* **DICLOMAX SR,** available as sustained-release, yellow capsules containing 75mg of diclofenac sodium.

*Dosage*: adults, Diclomax Retard, 1 capsule each day with food; Diclomax SR, 1 or 2 capsules each day, either as a single or divided dose.

*Special care*: pregnancy, breastfeeding, elderly persons, kidney, liver or heart disorders, blood disorders, hepatic porphyria (production of excess porphyrins in the liver producing abdominal pain, neuropathy and photosensitivity), and those with a history of gastro-intestinal ulcers or lesions. Patients on long-term treatment should be monitored.

*Avoid use*: children, active peptic ulcer, asthma, aspirin or anti-inflammatory drug-induced allergy, during last 3 months of pregnancy.

*Possible interaction*: steroids, NSAIDs, anticoagulants, antidiabetic drugs, quinolones, diuretics, salicylates, lithium, digoxin, methotrexate, ciclosporin.

*Side effects*: headache, fluid retention, gastro-intestinal upsets, short-lived stomach pain. Rarely, stomach ulcer, liver malfunction, skin reactions.

*Manufacturer*: Parke-Davis.

**DICYCLOVERINE HYDROCHLORIDE *SEE*: KOLANTICON.**

**DIFFLUSINAL *SEE*: DOLOBID.**

## DILTIAZEM *SEE*: TILDIEM.

## DIMETICONE *SEE*: KOLANTICON.

## DIMETICONE ACTIVATED *SEE*: ALTACITE PLUS, MAALOX.

## DIMOTANE PLUS

*Description*: a combined sympathomimetic (i.e. mimics effects of stimulation of the sympathetic (autonomic) nervous system)/antihistamine preparation available as a liquid containing 30mg of pseudoephedrine hydrochloride per 5ml and 4mg of brompheniramine maleate per 5ml. *Also,* **DIMOTANE ELIXIR,** containing 2mg of brompheniramine maleate per 5ml. *Also,* **DIMOTANE PLUS PAEDIATRIC,** containing 15mg of pseudoephedrine per 5ml and 2mg of brompheniramine maleate per 5ml.

*Used for*: allergic rhinitis (hayfever).

*Dosage*: Dimotane Plus, adults and children over 12 years, 10ml three times each day; children aged 6 to 12 years, 5ml three times each day. Dimotane Elixir, adults and children over 12 years, 10 to 20ml 3 to 4 times each day; children aged less than 3 years, 0.4 to 1mg per kg of body weight in 4 divided doses each day; aged 3 to 6 years, 5ml 3 to 4 times each day; aged 6 to 12 years, 5 to 10ml 3 to 4 times each day. Dimotane Plus Paediatric, children aged 2 to 5 years, 5ml three times each day; aged 6 to 12 years, 10ml three times each day.

*Special care*: pregnancy, asthma.

*Avoid use*: children under 2 years. Dimotane Plus, heart and circulatory disease, high blood pressure, overactive thyroid gland, glaucoma, epilepsy, brain damaged patients, those in comatose or pre-comatose states.

*Possible interaction*: anticholinergics, other sympathomimetics, MAOIs, NSAIDs, digoxin, tricyclic antidepressants, drugs that depress the central nervous system, agents that block adrenergic nerve transmission.

*Side effects*: impaired reactions and dexterity, drowsiness; stimulant in children and more rarely in adults.

*Manufacturer*: Goldshield.

## DIOCTYL

*Description*: a laxative preparation which acts as a faecal softener, available as white/yellow capsules containing 100mg of docusate sodium.

*Used for*: treatment and prevention of chronic constipation.

*Dosage*: adults, take lowest effective dose up to a maximum of 500mg each day in divided doses.

*Avoid use*: children.

*Manufacturer*: Schwarz.

## DIODERM

*Description*: a topical steroid with mild potency available as a cream containing 0.1% hydrocortisone.

*Used for*: allergic, itchy and inflammatory skin conditions.

*Dosage*: to be applied sparingly. Rub in well twice daily.

*Special care*: use on face or for children should be limited to 5 days maximum, infants when nappy area is being treated, psoriasis (monitor). Withdraw gradually after prolonged use.

*Avoid use*: children aged less than 1 year, on acne, leg ulcers, tuberculous, ringworm or viral skin disease, perioral dermatitis, untreated infections whether fungal or bacterial. Extensive or prolonged use during pregnancy.

*Side effects*: skin atrophy, striae (lines) and telangiectasia (permanent widening of superficial blood vessels), suppression of adrenal glands, Cushingoid changes (as in Cushing's syndrome).

*Manufacturer*: Dermal.

## DIPHENOXYLATE *SEE*: LOMOTIL.

## DIPIVEFRINE *SEE*: PROPINE.

## DISTACLOR MR

*Description*: an antibiotic/antibacterial preparation of cephalosporin, available as blue sustained-release tablets containing 375mg of cefaclor as monohydrate, marked Lilly TA4220 or Distaclor MR 375. *Also*, **DISTACLOR CAPSULES,** grey/purple capsules containing 500mg of cefaclor and marked Lilly 3062. *Also,* **DISTACLOR SUSPENSION,** available as granules for reconstitution with water, in two strengths, containing 125mg or 250mg cefaclor per 5ml of liquid.

*Used for*: infections of the skin, soft tissue and respiratory tract, otitis media, infections of the urinary tract.

*Dosage*: adults, Distaclor MR, 1 tablet twice each day; 2 twice each day for the treatment of pneumonia. Capsules and Suspension, 250mg every 8 hours up to a maximum of 4g per day. Children, Suspension, aged from 1 month to 1 year, 62.5mg; aged 1 to 5 years, 125mg; aged over 5 years, 250mg. All 3 times each day to a maximum of 1g.
*Special care*: pregnancy, breastfeeding, hypersensitivity to penicillins.
*Possible interaction*: anticoagulants, antacids, probenecid.
*Side effects*: gastro-intestinal upsets, hypersensitivity reactions, pseudomembranous colitis (a severe form of colitis).
*Manufacturer*: Dista.

## DISULFRAM *SEE*: ANTABUSE.

## DOCETAXEL *SEE*: TAXOTERE.

## DOCUSATE SODIUM *SEE*: DIOCTYL, FLETCHERS' ENEMETTE, NORGALAX, NORMAX.

## DOLOBID

*Description*: a salicylate analgesic and anti-inflammatory drug available as tablets in two different strengths, all capsule-shaped and film-coated. Peach coloured tablets contain 250mg of diflunisal, marked MSD 675 and orange tablets contain 500mg of diflunisal, marked MSD 697.
*Used for*: acute and chronic pain, osteoarthritis and rheumatoid arthritis.

*Dosage*: adults, for pain, 1000mg as first dose then 500mg every 12 hours, to a maximum daily dose of 1500mg. For arthritis, 500–1000mg daily, in 1 or 2 doses and varying according to the response.

*Special care*: elderly persons, kidney or liver disease, heart failure, a history of gastro-intestinal ulcers or haemorrhage, history of bronchial asthma, tendency for fluid retention. Patients with coagulation (blood) defects should be monitored during treatment and cause of eye conditions established. Kidneys and liver to be monitored during long-term treatment.

*Avoid use*: children, pregnancy, breastfeeding, serious kidney disorders, active stomach ulcer or bleeding in gut, aspirin or anti-inflammatory-induced allergy or asthma.

*Possible interaction*: anticoagulants, indometacin, codeine, aspirin, NSAIDs, antihypertensives, digoxin, methotrexate, furosemide, corticosteroids, quinolones, paracetamol, hydrochlorothiazide, lithium, mifepristone, antacids.

*Side effects*: diarrhoea, dyspepsia, headache, rash, tinnitus (ringing in ears), dizziness, gastro-intestinal pain, tiredness, kidney effects, central nervous system effects, disturbance of vision.

*Manufacturer*: M.S.D.

**DOMIPHEN BROMIDE *SEE*: BRADOSOL PLUS.**

**DORALESE**

*Description*: a selective a1 blocker, available as pale yellow, triangular, film-coated tablets containing 20mg of indoramin.

*Used for*: obstruction of urine outflow due to benign prostatic hypertrophy (enlarged prostate gland).

*Dosage*: adult men, 1 tablet twice each day at first, increasing if required every 2 weeks by 20mg to a daily maximum of 5 tablets (100mg), in divided doses.

*Special care*: liver or kidney disease, epilepsy, depression, Parkinsonism. Patients with poor heart function should be stabilised before treatment.

*Avoid use*: heart failure.

*Possible interaction*: antihypertensives, MAOIs.

*Side effects*: drowsiness, dry mouth, blocked nose, ejaculation failure, weight gain.

*Manufacturer*: SmithKline Beecham.

**DORZOLAMIDE *SEE*: TRUSOPT.**

**DOXAZOSIN *SEE*: CARDURA.**

**DOXEPIN *SEE*: SINEQUAN, XEPIN.**

**DOXYCYCLINE *SEE*: PERIOSTAT, VIBRAMYCIN.**

**DUOVENT**

*Description*: a selective ß2 agonist and antimuscarinic containing of 100µg of fenoterol hydrobromide and 40µg of ipratropium bromide per dose, available as a metered dose aerosol. Also **DUOVENT AUTOHALER**, containing

100μg of fenoterol hydrobromide and 40μg of ipratropium bromide per dose, available as a breath-activated, metered dose aerosol.

*Used for*: obstruction to airways in asthma or COPD, for bronchodilation.

*Dosage*: adults, 1 or 2 puffs 3 to 4 times each day; children aged over 6 years, 1 puff 3 times each day.

*Avoid use*: children under 6 years.

*Also,* **DUOVENT UDV**, containing 1.25mg fenoterol hydrobromide and 500μg of ipratropium bromide per 4ml of solution, in vials for use with nebuliser.

*Used for*: acute severe asthma.

*Dosage*: adults and children over 14 years, 1 vial nebulized immediately. Repeat under supervision. Maximum of 4 vials in 24 hours.

*Avoid use*: children under 14 years.

*Special care*: pregnancy, breastfeeding, severe heart and circulatory disorders, recent heart attack, hyperthyroidism, hypertension, glaucoma, enlarged prostate gland.

*Possible interaction*: sympathomimetics, **ß**-blockers, anticholinergics, corticosteroids, anaesthetics, xanthines, antidepressants, diuretics, digoxin.

*Side effects*: headache, dry mouth, nausea, dizziness, heart arrhythmias, trembling, raised heart beat rate, low blood calcium levels, nervousness.

*Manufacturer*: Boehringer Ingelheim.

## DUPHALAC

*Description*: a laxative preparation available as a solution containing 3.35g of lactulose per 5ml of liquid.

*Used for*: Portal systemic encephalopathy (PSE), constipation.

*Dosage*: adults, PSE, starting dose, 30 to 50ml 3 times each day; dose is adjusted according to response. Constipation, 15ml twice each day. Children, constipation, aged less than 12 months, 2.5ml twice each day; aged 1 to 4 years, 5ml twice each day; aged 5 to 10 years, 10ml twice each day.

*Special care*: patients with intolerance to lactose.

*Avoid use*: obstruction of the intestine, galactosaemia.

*Side effects*: wind, meteorism (build up of abdominal or intestinal gas, causing distention).

*Manufacturer*: Solvay.

## DYHYDROGESTERONE *SEE*: FEMAPAK, FEMOSTON, FEMOSTON-CONTI.

## DYSPAMET

*Description*: an H2 blocker available as a suspension containing 200mg of cimetidine per 5ml.

*Used for*: persistent, acid-related dyspeptic conditions, stomach and duodenal ulcer, borderline ulceration, oesophageal reflux, conditions in which a lowering of stomach acid is desirable.

*Dosage*: adults, 10ml twice each day, with breakfast and at bedtime. Minimum recommended course, 4 weeks.

Children over 12 months, 25 to 30mg per kg of body weight as divided dose.

*Special care*: exclude malignancy, pregnancy, breastfeeding, impaired kidneys. Monitor if treatment is long-term.

*Possible interaction*: phenytoin, theophylline, oral anticoagulants, lidocaine given intravenously.

*Side effects*: tiredness, dizziness, rash, diarrhoea, abnormal enlargement of breasts in males, confusion. Liver damage, which is reversible, may sometimes occur. Fever, muscle and joint pain, acute pancreatitis, headache, kidney inflammation, blood effects, heart block, raised or lowered heart beat and anaphylaxis have been rarely recorded.

*Manufacturer*: Goldshield.

# E

## EFCORTELAN

*Description*: a topical corticosteroid preparation available as a cream and ointment in 3 different strengths containing 0.5%, 1% or 2.5% hydrocortisone. Mildly potent.

*Used for*: dermatitis, eczema and intertrigo (inflammation and irritation caused when two skin surfaces rub together).

*Dosage*: rub into affected areas 2 or 3 times each day.

*Special care*: limit use in children or on face to 5 days. Withdraw gradually after prolonged use. Monitor in psoriasis patients. Special care in infants, if used in nappy area.

*Avoid use*: leg ulcers, scabies, peri-oral dermatitis, untreated fungal or viral infections, tuberculous, ringworm or viral skin diseases, acne. Lengthy or extensive use in pregnancy.

*Side effects*: skin striae (lines) and atrophy (dead skin), telangiectasia (multiple telangiectases, which are collections of distended blood capillaries), Cushingoid changes (Cushing's syndrome), adrenal gland suppression.

*Manufacturer*: GlaxoSmithKline.

## ELLESTE DUET 1MG

*Description*: a hormonal, HRT preparation containing oestrogen and progestogen, comprising a pack of film-coated tablets. 16 white tablets each contain 1mg of oestradiol, marked 01; 12 green tablets contain 1mg of oestradiol and 1mg of norethisterone acetate, each marked P1. *Also,* **ELLESTE DUET 2mg**, comprising a course of film-coated tablets. 16 orange ones contain 2mg of oestradiol marked 02 and 12 grey ones contain 2mg of oestradiol and 1mg of norethisterone acetate, marked P2.

*Used for*: menopausal symptoms; Elleste Duet is additionally used to prevent osteoporosis following the menopause.

*Dosage*: adult women, start course with 1 white or 1 orange tablet (depending upon preparation being used), waiting for 1st day of cycle if applicable, then follow with either the green or the grey tablets. Continue to take the tablets without a break, as directed by doctor.

*Special care*: patients considered to be at risk of thrombosis, those with diabetes, epilepsy, hypertension, multiple sclerosis, migraine, fibroids in uterus, fibrocystic disease, breast nodules, otosclerosis, tetany, liver disease (monitor liver function), porphyria, kidney disorder, cholelithiasis. All this group should be monitored closely. Regular examination of breasts and pelvic organs should be carried out and blood pressure checked. Persistent breakthrough bleeding. Women should self-examine breasts, attend for mammography (if applicable) and have cervical smear tests.

*Avoid use*: pregnancy, breast-feeding, hormone-dependent cancers, breast or uterus cancer, endometriosis, undiagnosed vaginal bleeding. Serious heart, kidney or liver disease, thrombophlebitis and thromboembolic diseases. Patients suffering from Dublin–Johnson syndrome or Rotor syndrome.

*Possible interaction*: drugs which induce liver enzymes.

*Side effects*: weight gain, enlargement and tenderness of breasts, fluid retention, cramps, gastro-intestinal upset, nausea and vomiting, headaches, breakthrough bleeding, dizziness. Cholestatic jaundice, effects on liver function, migraine, nose bleeds, worsening of varicose veins, lowered glucose tolerance, itching and reddening of skin (usually short-lived). Withdraw if migraines or other severe headaches occur for first time, or serious vision disturbances, signs of thromboembolic disorders, seizures, jaundice, hepatitis, serious, whole body itching, pregnancy. Stop 6 weeks before planned surgery or prolonged immobilisation.

*Manufacturer*: Pharmacia.

## ELLESTE DUET CONTI

*Description*: a hormonal HRT preparation containing oestrogen and progestogen, available as grey, film-coated tablets containing 2mg of oestradiol and 1mg of norethisterone acetate.

*Used for*: menopausal symptoms arising at least 1 year after cessation of periods in women who have not had a hysterectomy; prevention of osteoporosis following the menopause.

*Dosage*: adult women, 1 tablet daily, taken continuously, as directed by doctor.

*Special care*: patients considered to be at risk of thrombosis, those with diabetes, epilepsy, hypertension, multiple sclerosis, migraine, fibroids in uterus, fibrocystic disease, breast nodules, otosclerosis, tetany, liver disease (monitor liver function), porphyria, kidney disorder, cholelithiasis. All this group should be monitored closely. Regular examination of breasts and pelvic organs should be carried out and blood pressure checked. Persistent breakthrough bleeding. Women should self-examine breasts, attend for mammography (if applicable) and have cervical smear tests.

*Avoid use*: pregnancy, breast-feeding, hormone-dependent cancers, breast or uterus cancer, endometriosis, undiagnosed vaginal bleeding. Serious heart, kidney or liver disease, thrombophlebitis and thromboembolic diseases. Patients suffering from Dublin–Johnson syndrome or Rotor syndrome.

*Possible interaction*: drugs which induce liver enzymes.

*Side effects*: weight gain, enlargement and tenderness of breasts, fluid retention, cramps, gastro-intestinal upset, nausea and vomiting, headaches, breakthrough bleeding, dizziness. Cholestatic jaundice, effects on liver function, migraine, nose bleeds, worsening of varicose veins, lowered glucose tolerance, itching and reddening of skin (usually short-lived). Withdraw if migraines or other severe headaches occur for first time, or serious vision disturbances, signs of thromboembolic disorders, seizures, jaundice, hepatitis, serious, whole body itching, pregnancy. Stop 6 weeks before planned surgery or prolonged immobilisation.

*Manufacturer*: Pharmacia.

## ELLESTE SOLO

*Description*: a hormonal, HRT preparation comprising oestrogen alone, available as film-coated tablets in two strengths. White tablets contain 1mg of oestradiol and are marked 01; orange tablets contain 2mg, marked 02.

*Used for*: menopausal symptoms, mainly in women who have undergone a hysterectomy; prevention of osteoporosis after the menopause.

Dosage: adult women, 1 to 2mg each day, adjusting according to the response. May be taken without a break but women who have a uterus must also take additional progestogen for 12 to 14 days.

*Special care*: patients considered to be at risk of thrombosis, those with diabetes, epilepsy, hypertension, multiple sclerosis, migraine, fibroids in uterus, fibrocystic disease, breast nodules, otosclerosis, tetany, liver disease (monitor liver function), porphyria, kidney disorder, cholelithiasis. All this group should be monitored closely. Regular examination of breasts and pelvic organs should be carried out and blood pressure checked. Persistent breakthrough bleeding. Women should self-examine breasts, attend for mammography (if applicable) and have cervical smear tests.

*Avoid use*: pregnancy, breast-feeding, hormone-dependent cancers, breast or uterus cancer, endometriosis, undiagnosed vaginal bleeding. Serious heart, kidney or liver disease, thrombophlebitis and thromboembolic diseases. Patients suffering from Dublin–Johnson syndrome or Rotor syndrome.

*Possible interaction*: drugs which induce liver enzymes.

*Side effects*: weight gain, enlargement and tenderness of breasts, fluid retention, cramps, gastro-intestinal upset, nausea and vomiting, headaches, breakthrough bleeding, dizziness. Cholestatic jaundice, effects on liver function, migraine, nose bleeds, worsening of varicose veins, lowered glucose tolerance, itching and reddening of skin (usually short-lived). Withdraw if migraines or other severe headaches occur for first time, or serious vision disturbances, signs of thromboembolic disorders, seizures, jaundice, hepatitis, serious, whole body itching, pregnancy. Stop 6 weeks before planned surgery or prolonged immobilisation.

*Manufacturer*: Pharmacia.

## ELLESTE SOLO MX 40

*Description*: a hormonal preparation of oestrogen available as patches to stick onto the skin, each delivering 40μg of oestradiol over 24 hours. *Also,* **ELLESTE SOLO MX 80**, patches delivering 80μg of oestradiol over 24 hours.

*Used for*: HRT for oestrogen deficiency at and after the menopause; also, prevention of osteoporosis after the menopause (Elleste Solo MX 80).

*Dosage*: patches should be adhered to a clean and hairless area of skin below the waist and changed every 3 to 4 days, using a fresh area. For menopausal symptoms, a 40μg patch should be used at first, increasing to 80μg, if required. The maintenance dose should be at the lowest level that is effective. For prevention of osteoporosis, the

80μg patch should be used. When additional progestogen is needed, this should be taken for 12 to 14 days each month.

*Special care*: patients considered to be at risk of thrombosis, those with diabetes, epilepsy, hypertension, multiple sclerosis, migraine, fibroids in uterus, fibrocystic disease, breast nodules, otosclerosis, tetany, liver disease (monitor liver function), porphyria, kidney disorder, cholelithiasis. All this group should be monitored closely. Regular examination of breasts and pelvic organs should be carried out and blood pressure checked. Persistent breakthrough bleeding. Women should self-examine breasts, attend for mammography (if applicable) and have cervical smear tests.

*Avoid use*: pregnancy, breast-feeding, hormone-dependent cancers, breast or uterus cancer, endometriosis, undiagnosed vaginal bleeding. Serious heart, kidney or liver disease, thrombophlebitis and thromboembolic diseases. Patients suffering from Dublin–Johnson syndrome or Rotor syndrome.

*Possible interaction*: drugs which induce liver enzymes.

*Side effects*: weight gain, enlargement and tenderness of breasts, fluid retention, cramps, gastro-intestinal upset, nausea and vomiting, headaches, breakthrough bleeding, dizziness. Cholestatic jaundice, effects on liver function, migraine, nose bleeds, worsening of varicose veins, lowered glucose tolerance, itching and reddening of skin (usually short-lived). Withdraw if migraines or other severe headaches occur for first time, or serious vision disturbances, signs of thromboembolic disorders, seizures, jaundice, hepatitis, serious, whole body itching, pregnancy. Stop 6 weeks before planned surgery or prolonged immobilisation.

*Manufacturer*: Pharmacia.

## EMADINE

*Description*: an anti-inflammatory/antihistamine preparation available as eye drops containing 0.5mg of emedastine per ml.

*Used for*: seasonal conjunctivitis arising as a result of hayfever allergy.

*Dosage*: adults and children aged over 3 years, 1 drop into each affected eye twice each day.

*Special care*: infiltration of cornea – discontinue immediately; do not insert contact lenses for at least 10 to 15 minutes after inserting drops.

*Avoid use*: pregnancy, breastfeeding, elderly, children under 3 years, liver or kidney disorders.

*Side effects*: headache, blurring of vision, short-lived irritation, runny nose, pain fluid retention. Any adverse side effects should be reported to the Committee on the Safety of Medicines (CSM).

*Manufacturer*: Alcon.

## EMCOR

*Description*: an antianginal and anti-hypertensive preparation, which is a cardioselective ß-blocker, produced in the form of heart-shaped, orange, film-coated tablets containing 10mg bisoprolol fumarate. *Also,* **EMCOR LS,** yellow, scored, film-coated tablets containing 5mg of bisoprolol fumarate.

*Used for*: angina, hypertension.

*Dosage*: adults, 10mg once each day with a maximum daily dose of 20mg.

*Special care*: pregnancy, breast-feeding, liver or kidney disease, diabetes, metabolic acidosis, poor cerebral blood supply, history of bronchospasm, those undergoing anaesthesia; patients with weak hearts should be treated with digitalis and diuretics. Drug should be stopped gradually.

*Avoid use*: children, patients with asthma, heart diseases including heart block, heart shock, slow heartbeat rate, heart failure.

*Possible interaction*: cardiac depressants,anaesthetics, reserpine, sedatives, class II calcium antagonists, antihypertensives, sympathomimetics, cimetidine, indometacin, ergotamine, class I antiarrhythmic drugs, verapamil, clonidine withdrawal, hypoglycaemics, rifampicin, warfarin, ibuprofen.

*Side effects*: sleep disturbance, cold feet and hands, slow heartbeat, fatigue on exercise, wheeziness, heart failure, gastro-intestinal disorders; dry eyes or skin rash (stop use gradually), hair loss, low blood pressure, thrombocytopenia (abnormal decline in blood platelets).

*Manufacturer*: Merck.

## EMEDASTINE *SEE*: EMADINE.

## EMFLEX

*Description*: an indole NSAID which is a form of indometacin and is produced as orange/yellow capsules containing 60mg acemetacin.

*Used for*: osteoarthritis, rheumatoid arthritis, pain and inflammation following surgery and lower back pain.

*Dosage*: adults, 2 tablets daily in divided doses taken with meals, a glass of milk, or with an antacid preparation. The maximum daily dose is 3 capsules.

*Special care*: elderly patients, liver or kidney disease, congestive heart failure, septic infections, epilepsy, Parkinsonism, psychiatric illness, imbalance in fluid or electrolyte levels. Patients on long-term treatment should receive checks on liver and kidney function, blood count and eyes.

*Avoid use*: children, pregnancy, breast-feeding, certain gastro-intestinal disorders, peptic ulcer, angioneurotic oedema. Also, allergy to NSAID or aspirin.

*Possible interaction*: thiazides, salicylates, lithium, anticoagulants, furosemide, probenecid, ACE inhibitors, methotrexate, ß-blockers, triamterene haloperidol, quinolones.

*Side effects*: blood changes, dizziness, blurring of vision, headache, tinnitus (ringing in ears), gastro-intestinal upset, itching, chest pains, fluid retention.

*Manufacturer*: Merck.

## ENALAPRIL *SEE*: INNOVACE, INNOZIDE.

## ENOXAPARIN *SEE*: CLEXANE.

## ERGOTAMINE TARTRATE *SEE*: CAFERGOT.

## ERYMAX

*Description*: a preparation of an antibiotic macrolide, available as white and orange, enteric-coated pellets containing 250mg of erythromycin, contained in clear orange/opaque orange capsules.

*Used for*: infections sensitive to erythromycin, acne.

*Dosage*: adults, 250mg at 6-hour intervals or 500mg every 12 hours taken before or with food. For acne, 1 tablet twice each day for 1 month, then 1 tablet daily as maintenance dose. Children, for infections, 30–50mg per kg of body weight each day in divided doses at 6-hour intervals or twice daily.

*Special care*: myasthenia gravis (a severe autoimmune disorder affecting muscles), liver disease.

*Possible interaction*: digoxin, astemizole, alfentanil, anticoagulants taken by mouth, terfenadine, ciclosporin, carbamazepine, valproate, theophylline, phenytoin, statins, ergot derivatives, hexobarbital, cisapride, bromocriptine, disopyramide, midazolam, triazolam.

*Side effects*: allergic reactions, gastro-intestinal upset.

*Manufacturer*: Elan.

## ERYTHROCIN

*Description*: a preparation of an antibiotic macrolide, available in the form of oblong, white, film-coated tablets, containing 250mg and 500mg of erythromycin (as stearate), all marked with company symbol.

*Used for*: infections sensitive to erythromycin, acne.

*Dosage*: adults and children aged over 8 years, 1–2g each day in divided doses.

*Special care*: myasthenia gravis (a severe autoimmune disorder affecting muscles), patients with liver disease.

*Avoid use*: children under 8 years.

*Possible interaction*: digoxin, disopyramide, triazolam, pimozide, ergot derivatives, midazolam, valproate, bromocriptine, cisapride, tacrolimus, anticoagulants taken by mouth, astemizole, statins, ciclosporin, phenytoin, theophylline, terfenadine, zopiclone, carbamazepine, hexobarbital, alfentanil, quinidine.

*Side effects*: gastro-intestinal upset, cholestatic jaundice.

*Manufacturer*: Abbott.

## ERYTHROMYCIN *SEE*: AKENEMYCIN PLUS, ERYMAX, ERYTHROCIN, ERYTHROPED, ISOTREXIN, STIEMYCIN, TILORYTH, ZINERYT.

## ERYTHOPED A

*Description*: a preparation of an antibiotic macrolide, available as oval, film-coated yellow tablets containing 500mg of erythromycin as ethyl succinate; ERYTHROPED A sachets contain 1g in the form of granules. *Also,*

**ERYTHROPED SF,** a sugar-free suspension containing 125mg of erythromycin, as ethyl succinate, per 5ml. *Also,* **ERYTHROPED FORTE SF,** available as a sugar-free suspension containing 500mg of erythromycin as ethyl succinate per 5ml. *Also,* **ERYTHROPED P.I. SF,** a sugar-free suspension containing 125mg of erythromycin as ethyl succinate per 5ml.

*Used for*: infections sensitive to erythromycin, acne.

*Dosage*: adults and children over 8 years, 1g twice each day. Children under 2 years, 250mg; aged 2 to 8 years, 500mg, all twice each day. Alternatively, children may be given 30mg per kg of body weight (or up to 50mg per kg in severe cases) each day in divided doses.

*Special care*: myasthenia gravis (a severe autoimmune disorder affecting muscles), liver disease.

*Possible interaction*: digoxin, midazolam, zopiclone, anticoagulants taken by mouth, pimozide, phenytoin, astemizole, disopyramide, alfentanil, theophylline, terfenadine, triazolam, carbamazepine, ciclosporin, ergot derivatives, quinidine, cisapride, bromocriptine, hexobarbital, tacrolimus, statins.valproate,

*Side effects*: allergic reactions, gastro-intestinal upset, cholestatic jaundice.

*Manufacturer*: Abbott.

**ESMOLOL *SEE*: BREVIBLOC.**

**ESOMEPRAZOLE *SEE*: NEXIUM.**

## ESTRACOMBI

*Description*: a combined oestrogen, progestogen preparation available in the form of patches delivering either 50μg oestradiol per 24 hours, or 50μg of oestradiol and 250μg of norethisterone acetate per 24 hours, marked CG EFE and CG FNF, respectively.

*Used for*: hormone replacement therapy for menopausal women. Prevention of osteoporosis after the menopause.

*Dosage*: patch is applied to hairless skin below waist twice and changed every 3 to 4 days, being placed on a different area of skin each time. Start with oestradiol-only patch and apply twice weekly for two weeks, then use combined patch, in same way, for 2 weeks.

*Special care*: patients considered to be at risk of thrombosis, those with diabetes, epilepsy, hypertension, multiple sclerosis, migraine, fibroids in uterus, fibrocystic disease, breast nodules, otosclerosis, tetany, liver disease (monitor liver function), porphyria, kidney disorder, cholelithiasis. All this group should be monitored closely. Regular examination of breasts and pelvic organs should be carried out and blood pressure checked. Persistent breakthrough bleeding. Women should self-examine breasts, attend for mammography (if applicable) and have cervical smear tests.

*Avoid use*: pregnancy, breast-feeding, hormone-dependent cancers, breast or uterus cancer, endometriosis, undiagnosed vaginal bleeding. Serious heart, kidney or liver disease, thrombophlebitis and thromboembolic diseases. Patients suffering from Dublin–Johnson syndrome or Rotor syndrome.

*Possible interaction*: drugs which induce liver enzymes.
*Side effects*: weight gain, enlargement and tenderness of breasts, fluid retention, cramps, gastro-intestinal upset, nausea and vomiting, headaches, breakthrough bleeding, dizziness. Cholestatic jaundice, effects on liver function, migraine, nose bleeds, worsening of varicose veins, lowered glucose tolerance, itching and reddening of skin (usually short-lived). Withdraw if migraines or other severe headaches occur for first time, or serious vision disturbances, signs of thromboembolic disorders, seizures, jaundice, hepatitis, serious, whole body itching, pregnancy. Stop 6 weeks before planned surgery or prolonged immobilisation.
*Manufacturer*: Novartis.

## ESTRADERM MX.

*Description*: an oestrogen patch containing either 25, 50, 75 or 100μg of oestradiol. *Also*: **Estraderm TTS,** an oestrogen patch containing either 25, 50 or 100μg oestradiol.
*Used for*: hormone replacement therapy in menopausal women. Prevention of yfollowing menopause.
*Dosage*: patches are applied to area of hairless skin below waist and changed every 3 to 4 days, with a fresh site being used. For HRT, begin with 50μg patch and adjust after 1 month, as required. Maximum daily dose is 100μg. If a progestogen is required, this should be taken for 12 days in each 4 week treatment period. For prevention of osteoporosis, the 50μg patch is used.

*Special care*: patients considered to be at risk of thrombosis, those with diabetes, epilepsy, hypertension, multiple sclerosis, migraine, fibroids in uterus, fibrocystic disease, breast nodules, otosclerosis, tetany, liver disease (monitor liver function), porphyria, kidney disorder, cholelithiasis. All this group should be monitored closely. Regular examination of breasts and pelvic organs should be carried out and blood pressure checked. Persistent breakthrough bleeding. Women should self-examine breasts, attend for mammography (if applicable) and have cervical smear tests.

*Avoid use*: pregnancy, breast-feeding, hormone-dependent cancers, breast or uterus cancer, endometriosis, undiagnosed vaginal bleeding. Serious heart, kidney or liver disease, thrombophlebitis and thromboembolic diseases. Patients suffering from Dublin–Johnson syndrome or Rotor syndrome.

*Possible interaction*: drugs which induce liver enzymes.

*Side effects*: weight gain, enlargement and tenderness of breasts, fluid retention, cramps, gastro-intestinal upset, nausea and vomiting, headaches, breakthrough bleeding, dizziness. Cholestatic jaundice, effects on liver function, migraine, nose bleeds, worsening of varicose veins, lowered glucose tolerance, itching and reddening of skin (usually short-lived). Withdraw if migraines or other severe headaches occur for first time, or serious vision disturbances, signs of thromboembolic disorders, seizures, jaundice, hepatitis, serious, whole body itching, pregnancy. Stop 6 weeks before planned surgery or prolonged immobilization.

*Manufacturer*: Novartis.

## ESTROPIPATE *SEE*: HARMOGEN.

## ETHINYLESTRADIOL *SEE*: BINOVUM, BREVINOR, CILEST, EUGYNON 30, FEMODENE ED, FEMODENE, FEMODETTE, LOESTRIN 20, LOESTRIN 30, LOGYNON ED, LOGYNON, MARVELON, MERCILON, MICROGYNON 30 ED, MICROGYNON 30, MINULET, NORIMIN, OVRANETTE, OVYSMEN, SYNPHASE, TRINORDIOL, TRINOVUM.

## ETYNODIOL DIACETATE *SEE*: FEMULEN.

## EUCARDIC

*Description*: an a/ß-blocker available as scored tablets in 4 different strengths. Pink tablets, marked BM K1, contain 3.125mg of carvedilol; yellow tablets, marked BM F1, contain 6.25mg of carvedilol; peach coloured tablets, marked BM H3, contain 12.5mg of carvedilol and off-white tablets, marked BM D5, contain 25mg of carvedilol.

*Used for*: additional therapy for chronic heart failure which is stable in patients with euvolaemia, who are being treated with diuretics, digoxin or ACE inhibitors; prevention of angina, high blood pressure.

*Dosage*: adults, heart failure, treatment must be commenced in hospital under supervision of specialist and dosages only increased if patient's condition has not worsened. Start with 3.125mg dose twice each day taken with food, for two weeks. Then gradually increase, if drug is tolerated, at a minimum of 2 week intervals to 6.25mg, then to 12.5mg, then to 25mg, all twice each day. The maximum is 50mg twice each day in patients weighing over 85kg, or 25mg twice each day in those weighing less than 85kg who have mild to moderate heart failure. All patients with severe heart failure should receive lower dose. For prevention of angina, 12.5mg twice each day for 2 days, then 25mg twice each day. For hypertension, 12.5mg once each day at first, for 2 days, then increasing to 25mg once a day. If required, dose can be increased gradually every two weeks to a maximum of 50mg, either once each day or as a divided dose.

*Special care*: heart failure patients, monitor kidney and heart function and signs of deterioration in condition when dosages are being increased; also, when adjusting dose in ischaemic heart disease, insufficient kidney function, diffuse vascular disease. Stop drug gradually in ischaemic heart disease. Special care in patients with diabetes, unstable angina, hyperthyroidism (over-active thyroid).

*Avoid use*: children, pregnancy, breastfeeding, liver disorder, phaeochromocytoma (adrenal gland tumour), liver disease, metabolic acidosis, 2nd or 3rd degree heart block, severe low blood pressure, very slow heart beat rate, heart shock, extremely severe heart failure, COPD, asthma, sick sinus syndrome.

*Possible interaction*: rifampicin, general anaesthetics, cimetidine, clonidine withdrawal, verapamil, digoxin, class1 antiarrhythmics, diltiazem, drugs that lower blood pressure.

*Side effects*: dizziness, fall in blood pressure when rising up after lying down, gastrointestinal disturbance, fluid retention, slow heartbeat, disturbance of vision, dry eyes, headaches, angina, heart block, fall in blood circulation to peripheries. Any adverse reaction should be reported to the Committee on the Safety of Medicines (CSM).

*Manufacturer*: Roche.

## EUGYNON 30

*Description*: a combined oestrogen/progestogen and contraceptive produced as white, sugar-coated tablets containing 30 g ethinylestradiol and 250 g levonorgestrel.

*Used for*: oral contraception.

*Dosage*: 1 tablet each day for 21 days starting on first day of period followed by 7 tablet-free days.

*Special care*: patients with asthma, diabetes, Raynaud's disease, ulcerative colitis, Crohn's disease, Sydenham's chorea, tetanus, varicose veins, hypertension, serious kidney disease, multiple sclerosis, haemolytic uraemic syndrome, serious depression. Also, uterine fibroids, endometriosis, contact lenses, history of heart failure, gallstones. The risk of thrombosis increases with age and if woman smokes or is obese. Slight increased chance of breast cancer. Pelvic organs, breasts and blood pressure should be checked regularly during the time oral contraceptives are being taken.

*Avoid use*: pregnancy, history of thrombosis, those with

heart disease, heart valve disease and angina, some other circulatory conditions. Patient with sickle cell anaemia, infectious hepatitis, certain liver and kidney disorders, hormone-dependent cancers, undiagnosed vaginal bleeding. History of SLE and some other disorders that have previously occurred during pregnancy.

*Possible interaction*: tetracyclines, barbiturates, carbamazepine, primidone, griseofulvin, phenytoin, rifampicin, ampicillin, phenylbutazone, chloral hydrate, glutethimide, ethosuximide, dichloralphenazone, St John's Wort.

*Side effects*: nausea, headaches, bloatedness due to fluid retention, enlargement of breasts, cramps and leg pains, reduction in libido, depression, weight gain, bleeding, vaginal discharge, erosion of cervix.

*Manufacturer*: Schering H.C.

## EUMOVATE

*Description*: a moderately potent topical steroid in the form of cream and ointment containing 0.05% clobetasone butyrate.

*Used for*: dermatitis, eczema and skin conditions responsive to steroids.

*Dosage*: apply thinly to affected area up to 4 times each day.

*Special care*: should not be used on face or on children for more than 5 days. Should be stopped gradually.

*Avoid use*: prolonged or extensive use especially pregnant women or continual use as a preventative. Should not be used to treat acne, leg ulcers, scabies, peri-oral dermatitis, tuberculous skin conditions, skin disorders caused by viruses, ringworm, any untreated bacterial or fungal skin infections.

*Side effects*: thinning of skin, adrenal gland suppression, hair growth, Cushingoid type symptoms (Cushing's syndrome).

*Manufacturer*: GlaxoSmithKline.

## EVOREL

*Description*: oestrogen patches available in a number of different strengths delivering 25, 50, 75 or 100μg of oestradiol in each 24 hour period.

*Used for*: hormone replacement therapy in menopausal women. Prevention and treatment of post-menopausal osteoporosis, especially when there is a fracture risk.

*Dosage*: apply patch to hairless area of skin below waist and change for a new patch in a different site after 3 or 4 days. Women who have not had a hysterectomy should also receive a progestogen preparation for 12 out of each 28 day period of treatment. For menopausal symptoms, start with the 50μg patch and adjust after one month, according to response. The lowest dose to be effective should be used for maintenance and the maximum is 100μg per 24 hour period. For osteoporosis, use 50, 75 or 100μg doses.

*Special care*: patients with history of or considered to be at risk of thrombosis, those with liver disease. Careful monitoring of women with any of the following is required: fibroids in uterus, otosclerosis, porphyria, tetany, epilepsy, gallstones, migraine, multiple sclerosis, hypertension, diabetes. Regular examination of pelvic organs and breasts required during course of therapy, especially in women with family history of breast cancer.

*Avoid use*: pregnancy, breast-feeding, women with breast cancer or other cancers which are hormone-dependent, e.g. of genital tract; serious heart, liver or kidney disease, endometriosis, thrombosis, Dublin–Johnson or Rotor syndrome, undiagnosed vaginal bleeding.

*Possible interaction*: drugs that induce liver enzymes.

*Side effects*: enlargement and tenderness of breasts, nausea and vomiting, weight gain, breakthrough bleeding, gastro-intestinal upset, headache, giddiness. Withdraw drug immediately if any sign of thrombosis, rise in blood pressure, severe and frequent headaches, migraines, disturbance of vision, jaundice, pregnancy. Stop before planned surgery.

*Manufacturer*: Janssen-Cilag.

## EVOREL SEQUI

*Description*: a combined oestrogen/progestogen preparation available in two forms of skin patch, delivering 50μg of oestradiol hemihydrate every 24 hours or 50μg of oestradiol hemihydrate and 170μg of norethisterone acetate every 24 hours.

*Used for*: hormone replacement therapy in menopausal women who have not undergone hysterectomy. Prevention and treatment of osteoporosis after the menopause, especially in women at risk of fractures.

*Dosage*: apply patch to hairless area of skin below waist and change for a new patch in a different site after 3 or 4 days.

Start with oestradiol only patch and use for first 2 weeks, then use combined patch for following 2-week period.

*Special care*: patients with history of or considered to be at risk of thrombosis, those with liver disease. Careful monitoring of women with any of the following is required: fibroids in uterus, otosclerosis, porphyria, tetany, epilepsy, gallstones, migraine, multiple sclerosis, hypertension, diabetes. Regular examination of pelvic organs and breasts required during course of therapy, especially in women with family history of breast cancer.

*Avoid use*: pregnancy, breast-feeding, women with breast cancer or other cancers which are hormone-dependent, e.g. of genital tract; serious heart, liver or kidney disease, endometriosis, thrombosis, Dublin–Johnson or Rotor syndrome, undiagnosed vaginal bleeding.

*Possible interaction*: drugs which induce liver enzymes.

*Side effects*: enlargement and tenderness of breasts, nausea and vomiting, weight gain, breakthrough bleeding, gastro-intestinal upset, headache, giddiness. Withdraw drug immediately if any sign of thrombosis, rise in blood pressure, severe and frequent headaches, migraines, disturbance of vision, jaundice, pregnancy. Stop before planned surgery.

*Manufacturer*: Janssen-Cilag.

## EVOREL - PAK

*Description*: a combined oestrogen/progestogen preparation available as a skin patch and tablets. Skin patches deliver 50μg of oestradiol every 24 hours and white tablets contain 1mg of norethisterone, each marked C over 1. A pack comprises 8 patches and 12 tablets.

*Used for*: hormone replacement therapy in menopausal women who have not undergone hysterectomy. Prevention and treatment of osteoporosis after the menopause, especially in women at risk of fractures.

*Dosage*: apply patch to hairless area of skin below waist and change for a new patch in a different site after 3 or 4 days. For menopausal symptoms, start with 50µg patch; adjust dose after 1 month if necessary. Use minimum effective dose with maximum of 100µg once each day. 1 tablet should be taken each day (by women who have not had a hysterectomy), on days 15 to 26 of cycle. For osteoporosis, use 50µg dose.

*Special care*: patients with history of or considered to be at risk of thrombosis, those with liver disease. Careful monitoring of women with any of the following is required: fibroids in uterus, otosclerosis, porphyria, tetany, epilepsy, gallstones, migraine, multiple sclerosis, hypertension, diabetes. Regular examination of pelvic organs and breasts required during course of therapy, especially in women with family history of breast cancer.

*Avoid use*: pregnancy, breast-feeding, women with breast cancer or other cancers which are hormone-dependent, e.g. of genital tract; serious heart, liver or kidney disease, endometriosis, thrombosis, Dublin–Johnson or Rotor syndrome, undiagnosed vaginal bleeding.

*Possible interaction*: drugs which induce liver enzymes.

*Side effects*: enlargement and tenderness of breasts, nausea and vomiting, weight gain, breakthrough bleeding, gastro-intestinal upset, headache, giddiness. Withdraw drug immediately if any sign of thrombosis, rise in blood pressure, severe and frequent headaches, migraines, disturbance of vision, jaundice, pregnancy. Stop before planned surgery.

*Manufacturer*: Janssen-Cilag.

## EXOCIN

*Description*: a 4-quinolone antibiotic preparation produced as eyedrops containing 0.3% ofloxacin.

*Used for*: bacterial eye infections.

*Dosage*: 1 or 2 drops every 2 to 4 hours into eye during first 2 days. Then 1 or 2 drops 4 times daily. Use for a maximum period of 10 days.

*Special care*: pregnancy, breast-feeding.

*Avoid use*: patients with soft contact lenses.

*Side effects*: short-lived eye irritation.

*Manufacturer*: Allergan.

# F

## FAMOTIDINE *SEE*: PEPCID.

## FAVERIN

*Description*: an antidepressant drug of a type known as 5HT reuptake inhibitors, available as film-coated, scored, white tablets. Round tablets contain 50mg of fluvoxamine maleate, marked 291 and S; oval ones contain 100mg of fluvoxamine maleate, marked 313 and S.

*Used for*: depression, obsessive compulsive disorder.

*Dosage*: adults, 100mg taken at night in first instance with a normal maintenance dose in the order of 100–200mg each day in divided doses. The maximum dose is 300mg each day. Review treatment of obsessive compulsive disorder after 10 weeks if no improvement has occurred.

*Special care*: pregnancy, breast-feeding, diabetes, kidney or liver disease, history of epilepsy, bleeding disorders, mania, hypomania. Drug should be gradually withdrawn.

*Avoid use*: children, patients who have stopped taking MAOIs in last two weeks or those who finished moclobemide on the previous day.

*Possible interaction*: alcohol, benzodiazepines, tryptophan, MAOIs, lithium, carbamazepine, drugs affecting blood platelets, serotonergic (affecting secretion of serotonin) drugs, propanolol, phenytoin, tryptophan, theophylline, tricyclic antidepressants, aminophylline, St John's Wort, warfarin, clozapine.

*Side effects*: gastro-intestinal upset, malaise, nausea, diarrhoea, vomiting, weakness, dry mouth, nervousness, sleepiness, anorexia, headaches, anxiety, convulsions, tremor, rapid heartbeat, palpitations.
*Manufacturer*: Solvay.

## FELDENE

*Description*: an NSAID and piroxicam, which is available in a number of different forms. **FELDENE CAPSULES** are available in two strengths, all containing piroxicam: blue/maroon capsules, marked FEL 10 and Pfizer, contain 10mg; maroon capsules, marked FEL 20 and Pfizer, contain 20mg. *Also,* **FELDENE DISPERSIBLE**: scored, white tablets for dissolving in water, containing either 10mg or 20mg of piroxicam, marked FEL 10 and Pfizer or FEL 20 and Pfizer, respectively, with the 20mg tablets being oblong in shape. *Also,* **FELDENE MELT**: fast dissolving, white tablets containing 20mg of piroxicam. *Also,* **FELDENE SUPPOSITORIES** containing 20mg of piroxicam. *Also,* **FELDENE INTRAMUSCULAR INJECTION**: available as a solution in ampoules containing 20mg piroxicam per ml. *Also,* **FELDENE GEL**: a topical gel containing 0.5% piroxicam.
*Used for*: all preparations except gel: arthritic diseases including juvenile arthritis, gout, rheumatoid arthritis, ankylosing spondylitis, osteoarthritis and other skeletal and muscle disorders. Gel: rheumatic pains and pains in muscles and joints e.g. from strains and sprains, back ache and neuralgia (nerve pain).

*Dosage*: adults, preparations taken by mouth or suppositories, depending upon condition being treated, but in the order of 20 to 40mg each day, depending upon medical advice. (Melt tablets are dissolved on tongue and dispersible tablets dissolved in water or swallowed whole.) Injection, used for acute attacks, 1 dose of 20 to 40mg by deep intramuscular injection into buttock. Then tablets should be taken for maintenance. Children over 6 years old, for juvenile arthritis only, using dispersible tablets; under 15kg of body weight, 5mg; 16–25kg of body weight, 10mg; 26–45kg body weight, 15mg; over 45kg body weight, 20mg. All are daily doses. Injection is not for use in children. Feldene Gel is for use by adults and children over 14 years. 3cm gel is applied to affected area, 3 or 4 times each day.

*Special care*: elderly patients, pregnancy, breastfeeding, heart failure, liver or kidney disease. Also, phenylketonuria (if melt tablets are being used).

*Avoid use*: patients with allergy to NSAID or aspirin, active stomach ulcer, history of ulcers, anal inflammation (do not use suppositories).

*Possible interaction*: aspirin, other NSAIDs, lithium, anticoagulants, hypoglycaemics.

*Side effects*: oral preparations and injection, gastro-intestinal upset, oedema, central nervous system disturbance, malaise, tinnitus, inflammation at injection site. Gel may cause skin irritation and reddening, rash and itching.

*Manufacturer*: Pfizer.

## FELODIPINE *SEE*: PLENDIL, TRIAPIN.

## FEMAPAK 40

*Description*: a hormonal preparation combining oestrogen and progestogen available in the form of a pack containing skin patches and tablets. Skin patches release 40µg of oestradiol every 24 hours; white tablets contain 10mg of dydrogesterone and are marked S and 155. *Also,* **FEMAPAK 80**, containing skin patches delivering 80µg of oestradiol per 24 hours and 10mg of dydrogesterone, marked S and 155.

*Used for*: hormone replacement therapy in menopausal women who retain an intact womb; prevention of osteoporosis following the menopause (Femapak 80).

*Dosage*: women, patches should be adhered to non-hairy area of skin below waist and changed every 3 or 4 days, using a new site. HRT, if period is still occurring, start treatment within 5 days of its onset. Use Femapak 40 to begin with and only increase to 80 strength if needed and advised; maintain on lowest effective dose. Prevention of osteoporosis, use Femapak 80. For both conditions, tablets should be taken for last 2 weeks of each monthly cycle.

*Special care*: patients with history of or considered to be at risk of thrombosis, those with liver disease. Careful monitoring of women with any of the following is required: fibroids in uterus, otosclerosis, porphyria, tetany, epilepsy, gallstones, migraine, multiple sclerosis, hypertension, diabetes. Regular examination of pelvic organs and breasts required during course of therapy, especially in women with family history of breast cancer.

*Avoid use*: pregnancy, breast-feeding, women with breast cancer or other cancers which are hormone-dependent, e.g. of genital tract; serious heart, liver or kidney disease, endometriosis, thrombosis, Dublin–Johnson or Rotor syndrome, undiagnosed vaginal bleeding.

*Possible interaction*: drugs which induce liver enzymes.

*Side effects*: enlargement and tenderness of breasts, nausea and vomiting, weight gain, breakthrough bleeding, gastro-intestinal upset, headache, giddiness. Withdraw drug immediately if any sign of thrombosis, rise in blood pressure, severe and frequent headaches, migraines, disturbance of vision, jaundice, pregnancy. Stop before planned surgery.

*Manufacturer*: Solvay.

## FEMATRIX

*Description*: a hormonal, oestrogen preparation available in the form of skin patches delivering 40μg of oestradiol per 24 hours. *Also,* **FEMATRIX 80**, an oestrogen preparation available as skin patches delivering 80μg of oestradiol per 24 hours.

*Used for*: hormone replacement therapy in menopausal and post-menopausal women. Fematrix 80 is additionally used for the prevention of post-menopausal osteoporosis.

*Dosage*: women, patches should be adhered to non-hairy area of skin below waist and changed every 3 or 4 days, using a new site. Start with 40μg patch and increase to

80μg if necessary, according to medical advice. Use lowest effective dose for maintenance. Use 80μg patch for prevention of osteoporosis. Women who have not undergone hysterectomy require a progestogen for the last 12 to 14 days of each monthly cycle.

*Special care*: patients with history of or considered to be at risk of thrombosis, those with liver disease. Careful monitoring of women with any of the following is required: fibroids in uterus, otosclerosis, porphyria, tetany, epilepsy, gallstones, migraine, multiple sclerosis, hypertension, diabetes. Regular examination of pelvic organs and breasts required during course of therapy, especially in women with family history of breast cancer.

*Avoid use*: pregnancy, breast-feeding, women with breast cancer or other cancers which are hormone-dependent, e.g. of genital tract; serious heart, liver or kidney disease, endometriosis, thrombosis, Dublin–Johnson or Rotor syndrome, undiagnosed vaginal bleeding.

*Possible interaction*: drugs which induce liver enzymes.

*Side effects*: enlargement and tenderness of breasts, nausea and vomiting, weight gain, breakthrough bleeding, gastro-intestinal upset, headache, giddiness. Withdraw drug immediately if any sign of thrombosis, rise in blood pressure, severe and frequent headaches, migraines, disturbance of vision, jaundice, pregnancy. Stop before planned surgery.

*Manufacturer*: Solvay.

## FEMODENE

*Description*: a combined oestrogen/progestogen hormonal oral contraceptive in the form of white, sugar-coated tablets containing 30μg of ethinylestradiol and 75μg of gestodene.

*Used for*: oral contraception.

*Dosage*: 1 tablet daily, beginning on day 1 of period, for 21 days followed by 7 tablet-free days.

*Special care*: hypertension, severe kidney disease receiving dialysis, Raynaud's disease, diabetes, multiple sclerosis, asthma, varicose veins, elevated levels of prolactin (a hormone) in the blood (hyperprolactinemia). Risk of thrombosis increases with smoking, age and obesity. Blood pressure, breasts and pelvic organs should be checked during period of treatment.

*Avoid use*: pregnancy, heart and circulatory diseases, angina, sickle cell anaemia, pulmonary hypertension. Also hormone-dependent cancers, undiagnosed vaginal bleeding, chorea, liver disease, history of cholestatic jaundice of pregnancy, infectious hepatitis, Dublin–Johnson syndrome, Rotor syndrome, recent trophoblastic disease.

*Possible interaction*: phenytoin, carbamazepine, tetracyclines, primidone, chloral hydrate, glutethimide, phenylbutazone, rifampicin, griseofulvin, ampicillin, dichloralphenazone, ethosuximide, barbiturates, St John's Wort.

*Side effects*: feeling of bloatedness due to fluid retention, leg pains, breast enlargement, erosion of cervix, muscular cramps, weight gain, breakthrough bleeding, depression, headaches, vaginal discharge, loss of libido, nausea, brown patches on skin (chloasma). Stop drug immediately in event of pregnancy, if frequent, severe headaches occur or signs of thromboses, severe pain in upper abdominal region, enlarged liver, jaundice, rise in blood pressure, severe depression, increased number of fits. Drug should be discontinued 6 weeks before major planned surgery and re-started 2 weeks afterwards, as long as woman is fully mobile. Should be discontinued during long periods of immobility.

*Manufacturer*: Schering H.C.

## FEMODENE E.D.

*Description*: a combined oestrogen/progestogen hormonal oral contraceptive preparation consisting of 21 white, sugar-coated tablets containing 30µg ethinylestradiol and 75µg gestodene and 7 larger, white, sugar-coated placebo tablets containing lactose.

*Used for*: oral contraception.

*Dosage*: 1 tablet daily starting on first day of period with numbered tablet from red part of pack. Tablets are taken each day without a break, either hormonal or placebo depending upon the time in the cycle.

*Special care*: hypertension, severe kidney disease receiving dialysis, Raynaud's disease, diabetes, multiple sclerosis, asthma, varicose veins, elevated levels of prolactin (a hormone) in the blood (hyperprolactinemia). Risk of thrombosis increases with smoking, age and obesity. Blood pressure, breasts and pelvic organs should be checked during period of treatment.

*Avoid use*: pregnancy, heart and circulatory diseases, angina, sickle cell anaemia, pulmonary hypertension. Also hormone-dependent cancers, undiagnosed vaginal bleeding, chorea, liver disease, history of cholestatic jaundice of pregnancy, infectious hepatitis, Dublin–Johnson syndrome, Rotor syndrome, recent trophoblastic disease.

*Possible interaction*: phenytoin, carbamazepine, tetracyclines, primidone, chloral hydrate, glutethimide, phenylbutazone, rifampicin, griseofulvin, ampicillin, dichloralphenazone, ethosuximide, barbiturates, St John's Wort.

*Side effects*: feeling of bloatedness due to fluid retention, leg pains, breast enlargement, erosion of cervix, muscular cramps, weight gain, breakthrough bleeding, depression, headaches, vaginal discharge, loss of libido, nausea, brown patches on skin (chloasma). Stop drug immediately in event of pregnancy, if frequent, severe headaches occur or signs of thromboses, severe pain in upper abdominal region, enlarged liver, jaundice, rise in blood pressure, severe depression, increased number of fits. Drug should be discontinued 6 weeks before major planned surgery and re-started 2 weeks afterwards, as long as woman is fully mobile. Should be discontinued during long periods of immobility.

*Manufacturer*: Schering H.C.

## FEMODETTE

*Description*: a combined hormonal preparation containing oestrogen and progestogen available as sugar-coated, white tablets containing 20μg. of ethinylestradiol and 75μg of gestodene.

*Used for*: oral contraception.

*Dosage*: women, starting on first day of cycle, take 1 tablet each day for 21 days followed by 7 days with no tablet.

*Special care*: hypertension, severe kidney disease receiving dialysis, Raynaud's disease, diabetes, multiple sclerosis, asthma, varicose veins, elevated levels of prolactin (a hormone) in the blood (hyperprolactinemia). Risk of thrombosis increases with smoking, age and obesity. Blood pressure, breasts and pelvic organs should be checked during period of treatment.

*Avoid use*: pregnancy, heart and circulatory diseases, angina, sickle cell anaemia, pulmonary hypertension. Also hormone-dependent cancers, undiagnosed vaginal bleeding, chorea, liver disease, history of cholestatic jaundice of pregnancy, infectious hepatitis, Dublin–Johnson syndrome, Rotor syndrome, recent trophoblastic disease.

*Possible interaction*: phenytoin, carbamazepine, tetracyclines, primidone, chloral hydrate, glutethimide, phenylbutazone, rifampicin, griseofulvin, ampicillin, dichloralphenazone, ethosuximide, barbiturates, St John's Wort.

*Side effects*: feeling of bloatedness due to fluid retention, leg pains, breast enlargement, erosion of cervix, muscular cramps, weight gain, breakthrough bleeding, depression, headaches, vaginal discharge, loss of libido, nausea, brown patches on skin (chloasma). Stop drug immediately in event of pregnancy, if frequent, severe headaches

occur or signs of thromboses, severe pain in upper abdominal region, enlarged liver, jaundice, rise in blood pressure, severe depression, increased number of fits. Drug should be discontinued 6 weeks before major planned surgery and re-started 2 weeks afterwards, as long as woman is fully mobile. Should be discontinued during long periods of immobility.

*Manufacturer*: Schering H.C.

## FEMOSTON 1/10

*Description*: a combined hormonal preparation containing oestrogen and progestogen, available as 14 white tablets containing 1mg of oestradiol and 14 grey tablets containing 1mg of oestradiol and 10mg of dydrogesterone. All tablets are marked 379 and S. *Also,* **FEMOSTON 2/10,** comprising 14 red tablets containing 2mg of oestradiol and 14 yellow tablets containing 2mg of oestradiol and 10mg of dydrogesterone, all marked 379 and S. *Also,* **FEMOSTON 2/20,** comprising 14 red tablets containing 2mg of oestradiol and 14 blue tablets containing 2mg of oestradiol and 20mg of dydrogesterone, all marked 379 and S.

*Used for*: treatment of menopausal symptoms in women who have not undergone hysterectomy; prevention of osteoporosis in postmenopausal women at risk of bone fractures.

*Dosage*: menopausal symptoms, start with Femoston 1/10 white tablets and begin within first 5days of period, if present; if response is inadequate, change to Femoston

2/10 at start of next course. If there is breakthrough bleeding (rare) or if progestogen dose is inadequate, change to Femoston 2/20, as advised by doctor. Prevention of osteoporosis, use Femoston 2/10 and take 1 tablet each day; dose should only be reduced to Femoston 1/10 if there are severe side effects, according to medical advice.

*Special care*: hypertension, severe kidney disease receiving dialysis, Raynaud's disease, diabetes, multiple sclerosis, asthma, varicose veins, elevated levels of prolactin (a hormone) in the blood (hyperprolactinemia). Risk of thrombosis increases with smoking, age and obesity. Blood pressure, breasts and pelvic organs should be checked during period of treatment.

*Avoid use*: pregnancy, heart and circulatory diseases, angina, sickle cell anaemia, pulmonary hypertension. Also hormone-dependent cancers, undiagnosed vaginal bleeding, chorea, liver disease, history of cholestatic jaundice of pregnancy, infectious hepatitis, Dublin–Johnson syndrome, Rotor syndrome, recent trophoblastic disease.

*Possible interaction*: phenytoin, carbamazepine, tetracyclines, primidone, chloral hydrate, glutethimide, phenylbutazone, rifampicin, griseofulvin, ampicillin, dichloralphenazone, ethosuximide, barbiturates, St John's Wort.

*Side effects*: feeling of bloatedness due to fluid retention, leg pains, breast enlargement, erosion of cervix, muscular cramps, weight gain, breakthrough bleeding, depression, headaches, vaginal discharge, loss of libido, nausea, brown patches on skin (chloasma). Stop drug immediately in event of pregnancy, if frequent, severe headaches

occur or signs of thromboses, severe pain in upper abdominal region, enlarged liver, jaundice, rise in blood pressure, severe depression, increased number of fits. Drug should be discontinued 6 weeks before major planned surgery and re-started 2 weeks afterwards, as long as woman is fully mobile. Should be discontinued during long periods of immobility.

*Manufacturer*: Solvay.

## FEMOSTON-CONTI

*Description*: a combined hormonal preparation containing oestrogen and progestogen available as film-coated, pink tablets containing 1mg of oestradiol and 5mg of dydrogesterone, all marked 379 and S.

*Used for*: menopausal symptoms in women who have not undergone a hysterectomy and who are at least 1 year beyond the menopause. Prevention of osteoporosis after the menopause.

*Dosage*: women, take 1 tablet each day continuously.

*Special care*: hypertension, severe kidney disease receiving dialysis, Raynaud's disease, diabetes, multiple sclerosis, asthma, varicose veins, elevated levels of prolactin (a hormone) in the blood (hyperprolactinemia). Risk of thrombosis increases with smoking, age and obesity. Blood pressure, breasts and pelvic organs should be checked during period of treatment.

*Avoid use*: pregnancy, heart and circulatory diseases, angina, sickle cell anaemia, pulmonary hypertension. Also hormone-dependent cancers, undiagnosed vaginal bleeding, chorea, liver disease, history of cholestatic jaundice of pregnancy, infectious hepatitis, Dublin–Johnson syndrome, Rotor syndrome, recent trophoblastic disease.

*Possible interaction*: phenytoin, carbamazepine, tetracyclines, primidone, chloral hydrate, glutethimide, phenylbutazone, rifampicin, griseofulvin, ampicillin, dichloralphenazone, ethosuximide, barbiturates, St John's Wort.

*Side effects*: feeling of bloatedness due to fluid retention, leg pains, breast enlargement, erosion of cervix, muscular cramps, weight gain, breakthrough bleeding, depression, headaches, vaginal discharge, loss of libido, nausea, brown patches on skin (chloasma). Stop drug immediately in event of pregnancy, if frequent, severe headaches occur or signs of thromboses, severe pain in upper abdominal region, enlarged liver, jaundice, rise in blood pressure, severe depression, increased number of fits. Drug should be discontinued 6 weeks before major planned surgery and re-started 2 weeks afterwards, as long as woman is fully mobile. Should be discontinued during long periods of immobility.

*Manufacturer*: Solvay.

## FEMSEVEN

*Description*: a hormonal, oestrogen preparation available as skin patches delivering either 50, 75 or 100µg of oestradiol per 24 hours.

*Used for*: treatment of menopausal symptoms, prevention of bone thinning following the menopause.

*Dosage*: women, patches should be adhered to non-hairy area of skin below waist and changed every 7 days, using a new site. The 50µg patch should be used at first, changing to higher doses gradually over a few months, only if necessary. Women who have not undergone hysterectomy need to take a progestogen for at least 10 days of each monthly cycle.

*Special care*: hypertension, severe kidney disease receiving dialysis, Raynaud's disease, diabetes, multiple sclerosis, asthma, varicose veins, elevated levels of prolactin (a hormone) in the blood (hyperprolactinemia). Risk of thrombosis increases with smoking, age and obesity. Blood pressure, breasts and pelvic organs should be checked during period of treatment.

*Avoid use*: pregnancy, heart and circulatory diseases, angina, sickle cell anaemia, pulmonary hypertension. Also hormone-dependent cancers, undiagnosed vaginal bleeding, chorea, liver disease, history of cholestatic jaundice of pregnancy, infectious hepatitis, Dublin–Johnson syndrome, Rotor syndrome, recent trophoblastic disease.

*Possible interaction*: phenytoin, carbamazepine, tetracyclines, primidone, chloral hydrate, glutethimide, phenylbutazone, rifampicin, griseofulvin, ampicillin, dichloralphenazone, ethosuximide, barbiturates, St John's Wort.

*Side effects*: feeling of bloatedness due to fluid retention, leg pains, breast enlargement, erosion of cervix, muscular cramps, weight gain, breakthrough bleeding, depression, headaches, vaginal discharge, loss of libido, nausea, brown patches on skin (chloasma). Stop drug immediately in event of pregnancy, if frequent, severe headaches occur or signs of thromboses, severe pain in upper abdominal region, enlarged liver, jaundice, rise in blood pressure, severe depression, increased number of fits. Drug should be discontinued 6 weeks before major planned surgery and re-started 2 weeks afterwards, as long as woman is fully mobile. Should be discontinued during long periods of immobility.

*Manufacturer*: Merck.

## FEMSEVEN SEQUI

*Description*: a combined, hormonal preparation available as skin patches containing either oestrogen alone or oestrogen and progestogen. Patches deliver either 50mg of oestradiol per 24 hours or 50mg of oestradiol and 10μg of levonorgestrel per 24 hours.

*Used for*: hormone replacement therapy at menopause in women who have not undergone hysterectomy.

*Dosage*: women, patches should be adhered to non-hairy area of skin below waist and changed every 7 days, using a new site. Start with oestradiol patch alone and use for 2 weeks and continue with combined patch for next 2 weeks.

*Special care*: hypertension, severe kidney disease receiving dialysis, Raynaud's disease, diabetes, multiple sclerosis, asthma, varicose veins, elevated levels of prolactin (a hormone) in the blood (hyperprolactinemia). Risk of thrombosis increases with smoking, age and obesity. Blood pressure, breasts and pelvic organs should be checked during period of treatment.

*Avoid use*: pregnancy, heart and circulatory diseases, angina, sickle cell anaemia, pulmonary hypertension. Also hormone-dependent cancers, undiagnosed vaginal bleeding, chorea, liver disease, history of cholestatic jaundice of pregnancy, infectious hepatitis, Dublin–Johnson syndrome, Rotor syndrome, recent trophoblastic disease.

*Possible interaction*: phenytoin, carbamazepine, tetracyclines, primidone, chloral hydrate, glutethimide, phenylbutazone, rifampicin, griseofulvin, ampicillin, dichloralphenazone, ethosuximide, barbiturates, St John's Wort.

*Side effects*: feeling of bloatedness due to fluid retention, leg pains, breast enlargement, erosion of cervix, muscular cramps, weight gain, breakthrough bleeding, depression, headaches, vaginal discharge, loss of libido, nausea, brown patches on skin (chloasma). Stop drug immediately in event of pregnancy, if frequent, severe headaches occur or signs of thromboses, severe pain in upper abdominal region, enlarged liver, jaundice, rise in blood pressure, severe depression, increased number of fits. Drug should be discontinued 6 weeks before major planned surgery and re-started 2 weeks afterwards, as long as woman is fully mobile. Should be discontinued during long periods of immobility.

*Manufacturer*: Merck.

## FEMULEN

*Description*: a hormonal preparation which is a progestogen only contraceptive in the form of white tablets containing

500µg etynodiol diacetate marked on both sides with Searle.

*Used for*: oral contraception.

*Dosage*: 1 tablet at same time each day starting on first day of period and continuing without a break.

*Special care*: patients with history of, or considered to be at risk of thrombosis, hypertension, focal migraine, cysts on ovaries, hormone dependent cancer, liver disease. Blood pressure, breasts and pelvic organs should be checked regularly during the course of treatment. Slight increased risk of breast cancer.

*Avoid use*: pregnancy, previous ectopic pregnancy, history of heart, arterial or thromboembolic disease or stroke, liver tumour, recent trophoblastic cancer, undiagnosed vaginal bleeding, cholestatic jaundice when previously taking oral contraceptives or which developed during pregnancy.

*Possible interaction*: meprobamate, chloral hydrate, rifabutin, ethosuximide, barbiturates, ritonavir, carbamazepine, chlorpromazine, griseofulvin, dichloralphenazone, primidone, rifampicin, phenytoin, glutethimide, St John's Wort.

*Side effects*: headache, breast tenderness, ovarian cysts, acne, disruption to normal pattern of menstrual bleeding, acne. Discontinue immediately in event of pregnancy or if frequent serious headaches arise or migraines which were not previously occurring, jaundice, signs of thrombosis or thrombophlebitis, disturbance of vision.

*Manufacturer*: Pharmacia.

## FENBID GEL

*Description*: an NSAID available in the form of a gel in two strengths containing either 5% or 10% ibuprofen.

*Used for*: strains, sprains, muscle and joint pains, neuralgia (nerve pain), rheumatic pains and backache.

*Dosage*: adults and children over 14 years, rub gel into skin over affected area 2 or 3 times each day.

*Avoid use*: children under 14 years, pregnancy, breastfeeding, people with known allergy to NSAIDs or aspirin.

*Manufacturer*: Goldshield.

## FENBID SPANSULE

*Description*: an NSAID which is a propionic acid produced in the form of sustained-release capsules. Maroon/pink capsules contain off-white pellets comprising 300mg ibuprofen.

*Used for*: pain and arthritic conditions including ankylosing spondylitis, rheumatoid arthritis, osteoarthritis and other disorders of the skeleton and joints.

*Dosage*: 2 capsules twice each day at first increasing to 3 capsules twice daily if required. The maintenance dose is in the order of 1 or 2 capsules twice each day.

*Special care*: pregnancy, breast-feeding, elderly, asthma, disease of the gastro-intestinal tract, heart, liver or kidney disorders. Patients taking the drug long-term require careful monitoring.

*Avoid use*: children, patients with known allergy to aspirin or other anti-inflammatory drugs, stomach ulcer.

*Possible interaction*: thiazide diuretics, quinolones, anti-coagulant drugs.
*Side effects*: rash, gastro-intestinal upset and bleeding, thrombocytopenia (abnormal decline in blood platelets). If a patient contracts aseptic meningitis, it must be reported to the Committee on the Safety of Medicines (CSM).
*Manufacturer*: Goldshield.

## FENBUFEN *SEE*: LEDERFEN.

## FENOPROFEN *SEE*: FENOPRON.

## FENOPRON

*Description*: an NSAID and propionic acid, available in the form of tablets of 2 different strengths. Oval-shaped, orange tablets, coded DISTA 4019, contain 300mg of fenoprofen, as calcium salt; orange tablets coded DISTA 4021, contain 600mg of fenoprofen as calcium salt.
*Used for*: pain and arthritic conditions including ankylosing spondylitis, rheumatoid arthritis and osteoarthritis.
*Dosage*: 300–600mg 3 to 4 times daily with a maximum daily dose of 3g.
*Special care*: pregnancy, breast-feeding, elderly, liver or kidney disease, heart failure, asthma, a history of disorders involving gastro-intestinal bleeding. Patients taking the drug long-term should receive careful monitoring.
*Avoid use*: children, patients with ulcers, known allergy to aspirin or anti-inflammatory drugs, serious kidney disorders.

*Possible interaction*: aspirin, quinolones, hypoglycaemics, loop diuretics, anticoagulants, hydantoins, phenobarbital, sulphonylureas.
*Side effects*: allergic responses, intolerance of gastro-intestinal tract, blood changes, kidney and liver disorders.
*Manufacturers*: Typharm.

## FENOTEROL *SEE*: DUOVENT.

## FENTICONAZOLE *SEE*: LOMEXIN.

## FEXOFENADINE *SEE*: TELFAST.

## FINASTERIDE *SEE*: PROPECIA, PROSCAR.

## FLAGYL

*Description*: an antibacterial preparation and metronidazole, which is effective against anaerobic bacteria and certain other infective organisms. It is produced in a variety of forms: Flagyl tablets, film-coated, off-white tablets contain 200mg and 400mg metronidazole, the higher strength being capsule-shaped. Both are marked with strength and tablet name. **FLAGYL-S SUSPENSION** contains 200mg metronidazole (as benzoate) per 5ml liquid. **FLAGYL SUPPOSITORIES,** in two strengths, contain 500mg and 1g metronidazole.
*Used for*: infections caused by anaerobic bacteria, amoebic dysentery and other amoebic diseases, elimination of the organism *E. histolytica* (which causes amoebic dysentery)

from patients who are known to be infected but are not showing symptoms, abscess of liver, trichomoniasis (of urogenital tract), vaginosis of bacterial origin, dental infections and severe ulcerative gingivitis.

*Dosage*: adults, infections caused by anaerobic bacteria, Flagyl tablets or Flagyl Suspension, begin with 800mg 3 times each day and then reduce dose to 400mg; Flagyl suppositories, 1g suppository every 8 hours for 3 days then treat with oral preparation. Amoebic dysentery and diseases, use tablets or suspension according to manufacturer's instructions. Vaginosis, tablets or suspension, 400mg twice each day for 1 week or 2g as a single dose; trichomonas, 400mg twice each day for 1 week or 200mg 3 times each day, or, 800mg as morning dose with 1200mg taken at night, for 2 days, or, a single dose of 2g. Acute, ulcerative gum infections, tablets or suspension, 200mg 3 times each day for 3 days; dental infections, same dose but continued for 1 week. Children, anaerobic bacterial infections, tablets or suspension, 7.5mg per kg of body weight 3 times each day; suppositories, same dose rectally every 8 hours for 3 days, then continue with tablets or suspension. Amoebic dysentery and infections, according to manufacturer's instructions. Trichomonas, tablets or suspension, age 12 months to 3 years, 50mg 3 times each day; age 3 to 7 years, 100mg twice each day; age 7 to 10 years, 100mg 3 times each day; all given for 1 week. Aged over 12 years, as adult; not suitable for infants under 1 year old. Vaginitis of combined origin, treat children aged over 12 years as adult; not suitable for those aged under 10 years; aged 10 to 12 years, with caution as directed by doctor. Acute gum infections, aged 12 months to 3 years, 50mg three times each day; aged 3 to 7 years, 100mg twice each day; aged 7 years and over, 100mg three times each day.

*Special care*: pregnancy, breast-feeding, liver disorders, hepatic encephalopathy (a liver disease in which toxic substances normally removed by the liver interfere with the function of the brain).

*Avoid use*: children under 12 months.

*Possible interaction*: phenobarbital, alcohol, lithium, anticoagulant drugs taken by mouth.

*Side effects*: central nervous system effects, dark coloured urine, unpleasant taste in mouth and furring of tongue, gastro-intestinal upset, rash, angioneurotic oedema (a form of short-lived swelling due to fluid retention in various parts of the body), leucopenia (disturbance of white blood cell count). Long-term therapy may cause neuropathy (nerve disorders) and epileptic-type fits. In extremely rare cases, there may be hallucinations and confusion.

*Manufacturer*: Hawgreen.

## FLETCHERS' ENEMETTE

*Description*: a preparation which is a faecal softener available as a single dose micro-enema containing 90mg of docusate sodium and 3.78g of glycerol in 5ml of solution.

*Used for*: constipation, clearance of bowel before and after obstetrics surgery and before such procedures as sigmoidoscopy, radiological examination and proctoscopy.

*Dosage*: adults, 1 enema as required; children over 3 years, proportion of 1 enema according to body weight.
*Manufacturer*: Forest.

## FLEXIN CONTINUS

*Description*: a NSAID available as continuous-release tablets of three strengths, all of which are capsule-shaped and marked with strength and 1C. Green, red and yellow tablets contain 25mg, 50mg and 75mg of indometacin respectively.
*Used for*: arthritic disorders of joints and skeleton including osteoarthritis, ankylosing spondylitis, rheumatoid arthritis, degenerative disease of the hip joint, other musculo-skeletal and back disorders which cause pain, dysmenorrhoea (period pain).
*Dosage*: adults, 25–200mg each day in 1 or 2 divided doses taken with food, milk or antacid preparation.
*Special care*: elderly persons, patients with heart failure, liver or kidney disease, coagulation defects, disorders of the central nervous system. Those taking the drug long-term require careful monitoring and eye tests.
*Avoid use*: pregnancy, breast-feeding, allergy to aspirin or anti-inflammatory drug, stomach ulcer or previous gastro-intestinal lesions.
*Possible interaction*: corticosteroids, mifepristone, ß-blockers, cardiac glycosides, quinolones, diuretics, ciclosporin, methotrexate, salicylates, lithium, probenecid, anticoagulants.
*Side effects*: rash, blood changes, effects on central nervous

system, giddiness, visual disturbance, gastrointestinal intolerance, acute respiratory distress, corneal deposits, blood in urine. Drug should be discontinued if recurring headaches or gastro-intestinal bleeding occur.
*Manufacturer*: Napp.

## FLIXONASE

*Description*: a corticosteroid nasal spray delivering 50μg fluticasone propionate per metered dose. *Also*, **FLIXONASE NASULES,** single dose nasal drops delivering 400μg of fluticasone proprionate.
*Used for*: Flixonase, prevention and treatment of allergic rhinitis (hay fever), nasal congestion. Flixonase nasules, nasal polyps with nasal obstruction.
*Dosage*: adults, Flixonase, 2 sprays into each nostril in the morning, with a maximum of 4 sprays into both nostrils daily. Maintenance should be lowest effective dose, usually 1 spray in each nostril once each day. Flixonase nasules, insert contents of 1 nasule into affected nostril once or twice each day; use minimum dose that is effective and if no improvement after 4 to 6 weeks, cease use. Children, Flixonase only, aged 4 to 11 years, 1 spray (maximum of 2) into each nostril daily. Aged 12 and over, as adult.
*Special care*: pregnancy, breast-feeding, nasal infections should be treated first, transferring from other (systemic) steroid drugs taken orally. Prolonged use with higher doses may lead to systemic steroid effects or adrenal gland suppression – monitor and use for as short a time as possible and take into account other steroid sources.

*Avoid use*: children under 4 years of age.

*Side effects*: nosebleeds (sometimes severe), irritation of nose, interference with sense of taste and smell, allergic reactions. Rarely, perforation of nasal septum, anaphylaxis.

*Manufacturer*: A & H.

## FLIXOTIDE DISKHALER

*Description*: a corticosteroid preparation containing fluticasone propionate for use with diskhaler. 50, 100, 250 and 500μg fluticasone propionate disks are for use with breath-operated diskhaler delivery system. *Also,* **FLIXOTIDE ACCUHALER** 50, 100, 250 and 500μg fluticasone propionate per dose are for use with a breath-actuated, delivery system. *Also,* **FLIXOTIDE INHALER,** delivering 25μg of fluticasone proprionate per metered dose, for use with inhaler. *Also,* **FLIXOTIDE EVOHALER,** delivering 50, 125 or 250μg of fluticasone proprionate per metered dose, for use with inhaler. *Also,* **FLIXOTIDE NEBULES,** single use ampoules for use with nebuliser containing 0.5mg or 2mg of fluticasone proprionate per 2ml.

*Used for*: all preparations except nebules, prevention of bronchial asthma. Flixotide Nebules are used for prevention of chronic severe asthma attacks in adults and for acute flare-up of asthma in children.

*Dosage*: adults, all preparations except Nebules, 100–1000μg twice each day; children over 4 years of age, 50–100μg twice each day. Flixotide Nebules, adults and children over 16 years, 2mg (2000µg) twice each day using nebuliser; children aged 4 to 16 years, 1mg (1000µg) twice each day using the 0.5mg Nebules

*Special care*: pregnancy, breastfeeding, transferring from other (systemic) steroid drugs taken orally, those with history of, or with active tuberculosis. Risk of systemic steroid effects and adrenal gland suppression on long-term treatment – monitoring required. Height of children on prolonged therapy should be monitored.

*Avoid use*: children under 4 years of age.

*Side effects*: candidiasis (a yeast-like fungal infection) of throat and mouth, hoarseness, occasional unexplained bronchospasm. Rarely, rash, fluid retention in peripheral tissues, local allergic responses. Any adverse side effects associated with Flixotide Evohaler should be reported to the Committee on the Safety of Medicines (CSM).

*Manufacturer*: A & H.

## FLOMAX MR

*Description*: a selective α 1A-blocker, available as orange/brown sustained-release capsules marked with strength, logo and 701, containing 400µg of tamsulosin hydrochloride.

*Used for*: benign enlargement of the prostate gland.

*Dosage*: men, 1 each day with water, taken at same time after a meal.

*Special care*: low blood pressure.

*Avoid use*: severe liver disorder, orthostatic hypotension (low blood pressure occurring when a person stands up).

*Possible interaction*: other α-blockers.

*Side effects*: headache, weakness, palpitations, abnormal ejaculation, dizziness, sneezing, postural hypotension.

*Manufacturer*: Yamanouchi.

## FLOXAPEN

*Description*: a penicillinase-resistant form of penicillin. (Penicillinase is an enzyme produced by some bacteria that renders penicillin inactive, hence the infection being treated will be resistant to the antibiotic.) Floxapen is produced in several forms: black/caramel-coloured capsules of 2 strengths containing 250mg and 500mg flucloxacillin sodium, each marked with strength and name. **FLOXAPEN SYRUP** contains 125mg or 250mg flucloxacillin (as magnesium salt) per 5ml, supplied as powder for reconstitution with water to make 100ml. **FLOXAPEN INJECTION** is supplied as powder in vials for reconstitution at strengths of 250mg, 500mg and 1g flucloxacillin (as sodium salt).

*Used for*: ear, nose, throat, soft tissue, skin infections caused by gram positive bacteria, other infections including those caused by staphylococci bacteria resistant to penicillin.

*Dosage*: adults, capsules and syrup, 250mg 4 times each day taken 1 hour to half an hour before meals. Osteomyelitis and endocarditis, up to 8g in divided doses each day, every 6 to 8 hours. Injection, 250mg – 1g given intravenously 4 times each day. Children, capsules, syrup and injection, age 2 years and under, quarter of adult dose; age 2 to 10 years, half adult dose; over 10 years, adult dose.

*Side effects*: gastro-intestinal upset, allergic responses; rarely, pseudomembranous colitis, cholestatic jaundice, hepatitis.
*Manufacturer*: GlaxoSmithKline.

**FLUNITTRAZEPAM *SEE*: ROHYPNOL.**

**FLUOROMETHALONE *SEE*: FML.**

**FLUOXETINE *SEE*: PROZAC.**

**FLUARAZEPAM *SEE*: DALMANE.**

**FLURBIPROFEN *SEE*: FROBEN, OCUFEN, STREFLAM.**

**FLUTICASONE *SEE*: FLIXONASE, FLIXOTIDE, SERETIDE.**

**FLUVASTATIN *SEE*: LESCOL.**

**FLUVOXAMINE *SEE*: FAVERIN.**

**FML**
*Description*: an anti-inflammatory corticosteroid in the form of eyedrops containing 0.1% fluorometholone.
*Used for*: eye inflammation in which no infection is present.
*Dosage*: adults and children over 2 years, 1 to 2 drops 2, 3 or 4 times daily directly into eye.

*Special care*: pregnancy, glaucoma, prolonged use.
*Avoid use*: infections of tuberculous, viral or fungal origin and those in which pus is present; soft contact lenses.
*Side effects*: rise in pressure within eye, thinning of cornea, secondary fungal infection, cataract.
*Manufacturer*: Allergan.

## FORADIL

*Description*: a bronchodilator and selective ß2 -agonist available as clear capsules containing 12µg of formoterol fumarate, for use with a breath-activated inhaler.
*Used for*: for long-term use in patients with reversible obstruction of the airways (ROAD) and chronic obstructive lung disease (COPD), who benefit from regular treatment with bronchodilators.
*Dosage*: adults, ROAD, 1 capsule inhaled in the morning and a second dose in the evening; in very severe cases, the dose may be doubles to 2 capsules night and morning. The maximum daily dose is 4 capsules. Adults and children over 5 years, COPD, 1 capsule inhaled in the morning with the dose repeated at night. In very severe cases, 2 capsules twice each day in the morning and at night.
*Special care*: pregnancy, breastfeeding, diabetes, serious heart and circulatory disease, thyrotoxicosis (toxicity of thyroid gland), severe asthma. Use for chronic conditions only and not to treat acute asthma attack; continue with steroid therapy.
*Avoid use*: children under 5 years.

*Possible interaction*: steroids, antidepressants, ß-blockers, antiarrhythmics, xanthines, sympathomimetics.

*Side effects*: headaches, trembling, palpitations; rarely, muscle and joint pains, anxiety, raised heartbeat rate, dizziness, insomnia, unexplained bronchospasm, low blood potassium levels.

*Manufacturer*: Novartis.

## FORMOTEROL *SEE*: FORADIL, OXIS TURBOHALER.

## FOSCARNET *SEE*: FOSCAVIR.

## FOSCAVIR

*Description*: an antiviral preparation which is a DNA polymerase inhibitor, acting in two stages to inhibit the replication of cytomegalovirus in AIDS. Available as a solution containing 24mg foscarnet sodium hexahydrate per ml, produced as bottles of isotonic infusion.

*Used for*: life-threatening infections of viral origin particularly those of the eyes in patients with AIDS (cytomegalovirus retinitis). Also, for infections of mucous membranes and skin caused by Herpes simplex virus (HSV) in immunocompromised or AIDS patients, which have not responded to treatment with aciclovir.

*Dosage*: according to manufacturer's specifications.

*Special care*: kidney disease – monitor kidney function and also blood levels of electrolytes, before and during treatment. Patients should be well-hydrated.

*Avoid use*: pregnancy, breast-feeding.

*Possible interaction*: pentamidine given intravenously, other kidney toxic drugs.

*Side effects*: disturbance of kidney function, decreased haemoglobin and electrolyte levels in blood, convulsions, inflammation and ulceration of genitals. See manufacturer's prescribing notes.

*Manufacturer*: AstraZeneca.

## FOSINOPRIL *SEE*: STARIL.

## FRAMYCETIN SULPHATE *SEE*: SOFRADEX, SOFRAMYCIN.

## FRANGULA *SEE*: NORMACOL PLUS.

## FROBEN

*Description*: an analgesic preparation which is a propionic acid produced in the form of tablets of 2 strengths. Yellow, sugar-coated tablets contain 50mg and 100mg flurbiprofen, marked F50 and F100 respectively. Also **FROBEN SR** which are yellow, sustained-release capsules marked FSR containing 200mg flurbiprofen. **FROBEN SUPPOSITORIES** contain 100mg flurbiprofen

*Used for*: musculoskeletal disorders, osteoarthritis and ankylosing spondylitis, rheumatoid and rheumatic diseases; suppositories are also used for pain and dysmenorrhoea (severe period pains).

*Dosage*: adults, 150 to 200mg in divided doses each day to a maximum daily dose of 300mg. Dysmenorrhoea, 100mg either orally or using suppositories at start then 50 to 100mg every 4 to 6 hours, to a daily maximum of 300mg.

*Special care*: pregnancy, breast-feeding, elderly, liver, heart or kidney disease, bleeding disorders, high blood pressure, heart failure, asthma. Those taking the drug long-term require monitoring of kidney function.

*Avoid use*: children, patients with allergy to aspirin or anti-inflammatory drugs, those with stomach ulcer, ulcerative colitis or gastro-intestinal bleeding. Do not use suppositories if rectal or peri-anal inflammation is present.

*Possible interaction*: anticoagulant drugs, furosemide, quinolones.

*Side effects*: rash, intolerance of gastro-intestinal system, rarely thrombocytopenia, jaundice.

*Manufacturer*: Abbott.

## FUROSEMIDE *SEE*: LASIX.

## FRUSENE

*Description*: a potassium-sparing and loop diuretic produced in the form of scored yellow tablets containing 40mg furosemide and 50mg triamterene.

*Used for*: oedema accompanying liver or heart disease, congestive heart failure.

*Dosage*: adults, half to 2 tablets each day with a daily maximum of 6 (in divided doses).

*Special care*: pregnancy, breastfeeding, gout, enlarged prostate gland, difficulty in urination, acidosis, liver or kidney disease, diabetes.

*Avoid use*: children, patients in precoma resulting from liver cirrhosis, hyperkalaemia (raised blood potassium levels), progressive kidney failure.

*Possible interaction*: other potassium-sparing diuretics and potassium supplements, aminoglycosides, cardiac glycosides, neuromuscular blocking drugs, lithium, theophylline, NSAIDs, cephalosporins.

*Side effects*: rash, gastro-intestinal upset, gout, malaise, blood changes.

*Manufacturer*: Orion.

## FUCITHALMIC

*Description*: an antibacterial preparation produced in the form of eye drops containing 1% fusidic acid.

*Used for*: conjunctivitis where bacteria are cause of infection.

*Dosage*: apply 1 drop into eye twice each day.

*Side effects*: allergic reaction, local irritation of short-lived nature.

*Manufacturer*: Leo.

## FYBOGEL MEBEVERINE

*Description*: a bulking agent and antispasmodic preparation, produced in the form of effervescent granules in sachets for dissolving in water, containing 135mg mebeverine hydrochloride and 3.5g ispaghula husk. *Also,* **FYBOGEL,** a bulking agent produced in the form of plain, lemon or orange-flavoured granules for dissolving in water, containing 3.5g of ispaghula husk.

*Used for*: Fybogel mebeverine, irritable bowel syndrome; Fybogel, diverticular disease, constipation due to insufficient dietary fibre, IBS, ulcerative colitis, ileostomy, haemorrhoids, colostomy.

*Dosage*: adults, Fybogel Mebeverine, 1 sachet every morning and evening half an hour before meals in water. Additional sachet before midday meal may also be taken. Fybogel, 1 sachet in water taken in the morning and at night. Children, Fybogel only, 2.5 to 5ml in water, taken in the morning and at night.

*Avoid use*: patients with intestinal obstruction, colon that is not functioning properly due to muscle weakness, serious heart, circulatory and kidney disorders.

*Manufacturer*: R&C.

# G

## GAMANIL

*Description*: a TCAD preparation available as scored, maroon-coloured, film-coated tablets containing 70mg lofepramine (as hydrochloride).

*Used for*: depression.

*Dosage*: adults, 1 tablet 2 or 3 times each day.

*Special care*: elderly (reduce dose), psychoses or suicidal tendencies. Persons with heart and circulatory disease, liver disorders, overactive thyroid gland (hyperthyroidism), epilepsy, diabetes, constipation, urine retention, glaucoma, tumour of the adrenal glands. Blood tests and monitoring of liver and heart function are advisable during therapy.

*Avoid use*: children, pregnancy, breastfeeding, patients with heart block, heart rhythm disorders, weak heart, mania, serious liver disease.

*Possible interaction*: MAOIs or within 14 days of their use, other antidepressant drugs, neuroleptics, anticholinergic drugs, alcohol, adrenaline, noradrenaline (or anaesthetics containing these), quinidine, carbamazepine, phenytoin, antihypertensive drugs, thyroid drugs, barbiturates, cimetidine, sympathomimetics, oestrogens.

*Side effects*: gastro-intestinal disturbances such as constipation, blurred vision, dry mouth, anxiety, ringing in ears (tinnitus), drowsiness, insomnia, urine retention, sweating, tremor, raised heartbeat rate, arrhythmias, conduction defects, palpitations, weight gain or loss. Also low blood pressure on rising upright, blood changes, allergic skin reactions, abnormal breast enlargement and milk production (gynaecomastia and galactorrhoea), alterations in blood sugar, jaundice, loss of libido and impotence may occur. Occasionally, symptoms of schizophrenia and mania may be activated, particularly in elderly persons.

*Manufacturer*: Merck.

## GANCICLOVIR *SEE*: CYMEVENE, VIRGAN.

## GARAMYCIN

*Description*: an antibiotic preparation available in the form of drops containing 0.3% gentamicin (as sulphate).

*Used for*: external ear, and eye infections.

*Dosage*: ear infections, 3 to 4 drops 3 to 4 times each day; eye infections, 1 to 2 drops into eye every 4 hours.

*Avoid use*: (ears), infections of viral, tuberculous or fungal origin or in which pus is present; perforated ear drum.

*Side effects*: superinfection, possible mild irritation of short-lived duration.

*Manufacturer*: Schering-Plough.

## GASTROCOTE

*Description*: a preparation which is an antacid and reflux suppressant available as white tablets containing 200mg of alginic acid, 80mg of dried aluminium hydroxide gel, 40mg of magnesium trisilicate and 70mg of sodium bicarbonate, all coded GASTROCOTE. *Also*, **GASTROCOTE**

**LIQUID,** a suspension containing 220mg of sodium alginate, 80mg of dried aluminium hydroxide, 40mg of magnesium trisilicate and 70mg of sodium bicarbonate per 5ml.

*Used for*: hiatus hernia, heartburn, acid indigestion, reflux oesophagitis.

*Dosage*: adults and children aged over 6 years, 1 or 2 tablets to be chewed rather than swallowed, or 5 to 15ml of suspension, taken 4 times each day, following each main meal and at bedtime.

*Manufacturer*: Thornton & Ross.

## GAVISCON ADVANCE

*Description*: a reflux suppressant preparation available as an aniseed or peppermint flavoured liquid containing 1000mg of sodium alginate and 200mg of sodium bicarbonate per 10ml. *Also,* **GAVISCON TABLETS,** sugar and gluten-free, lemon or mint flavoured, white tablets containing 500mg of alginic acid, 25mg of magnesium trisilicate, 100mg of dried aluminium hydroxide gel and 170mg of sodium bicarbonate, marked on both sides with sword symbol and name. *Also,* **GAVISCON LIQUID,** available as a mint or aniseed flavoured, sugar-free liquid containing 500mg of sodium alginate, 267mg of sodium bicarbonate and 160mg of calcium carbonate per 10ml. *Also,* **GAVISCON INFANT FORMULA,** available as a powder containing 225mg of sodium alginate and 87.5mg of magnesium alginate per dose, when reconstituted.

*Used for*: preparations other than infant formula, hiatus

hernia, acid indigestion due to reflux, reflux oesophagitis, heartburn. Infant formula, regurgitation and stomach reflux.

*Dosage*: adults, Gaviscon Advance, 5 to 10ml taken 4 times each day, after main meals and at bedtime; Gaviscon tablets, Gaviscon liquid, 1or 2 tablets or 10 to 20ml 4 times each day after main meals and at bedtime. Children, should take half adult doses in same way. Gaviscon Infant formula, breastfed babies, weighing under 4.5kg, 1 dose; weighing over 4.5kg, 2 doses. In both cases, mix powder with 5ml of cooled boiled water and then add another 15ml of cooled boiled water and give after feeding. Bottle-fed babies weighing less than 4.5kg, add 1 dose to 115ml of formula milk; weighing over 4.5kg, add 2 doses to 225ml of formula milk. Older infants/young children, mix 2 doses with 15ml of water and give after each main meal.

*Special care*: patients on sodium-restricted diet.

*Manufacturer*: Britannia.

## GEL TEARS

*Description*: eye drops comprising 0.2% carbomer 980 in gel form.

*Used for*: dry eyes.

*Dosage*: 1 drop into each affected eye 3 or 4 times each day.

*Avoid use*: persons wearing soft contact lenses.

*Manufacturer*: Chauvin.

## GENTAMYCIN SULPHATE *SEE*: CIDOMYCIN, GARAMYCIN, GENTICIN.

## GENTICIN

*Description*: an antibiotic and aminoglycoside preparation available in ampoules for injection containing 40mg of gentamicin, as sulphate. *Also,* in the form of eye/ear drops containing 0.3% gentamicin (as sulphate).

*Used for*: injection, urinary tract infections, serious, life-threatening systemic infections sensitive to gentamicin. Drops, ear and eye bacterial infections.

*Dosage*: adults, injection, 3 to 4mg per kg of body weight by bolus intravenous injection or intramuscular injection, each day in divided doses. For very severe, life-threatening infections, up to 5mg per kg of body weight in 24 hours may be given, with monitoring of blood levels of gentamicin. Children, aged under 2 weeks, 3mg per kg of body weight every 12 hours; over 2 weeks old, 2mg per kg of body weight every 8 hours. Drops, adults and children, ear, 2 to 3 drops 3 or 4 times each day; eye, 1 to 2 drops up to 6 times each day; if infection is severe, 1 to 2 drops every 15 to 20 minutes, increasing time interval as infection responds.

*Special care*: injection, pregnancy, breastfeeding, Parkinson's disease, kidney disorders. Serum levels must be monitored as risk of kidney toxicity and vestibular toxicity. Drops, ear infections, do not use for prolonged period.

*Avoid use*: injection, myasthenia gravis (serious, chronic

condition affecting skeletal muscles which may be an autoimmune disorder); drops, ear infections, ruptured ear drum.

*Possible interaction*: ototoxic and kidney toxic drugs; injection, anaesthetics, drugs that block neuromuscular activity, penicillins, cephalosporins, ethacrynic acid, piretanide, aminoglycosides, furosemide.

*Side effects*: injection, kidney toxicity, ototoxicity (toxic effects on the 8th cranial nerve and the organs of balance and hearing), pseudomembranous colitis (rare). Drops, superinfection (secondary infection) – discontinue use; ear/eye infections, slight irritation which is short-lived; eye, blurring of vision.

*Manufacturer*: Roche.

## GESTODENE *SEE*: FEMODENE ED, FEMODENE, FEMODETTE.

## GLUCAGEN

*Description*: a hyperglycemic preparation of glucagon (rys) produced as a powder in vials along with diluent for reconstitution and injection. Available as 1mg glucagon hydrochloride per ml in pre-prepared syringes.

*Used for*: patients in whom blood sugar level has fallen to seriously low levels (e.g. diabetics taking insulin) and who have become unconscious, i.e. acute hypoglycemia.

*Dosage*: adults and children, 0.5mg–1mg by intravenous, intramuscular or subcutaneous injection in patients who cannot be roused enough to take glucose or sucrose by mouth. If patient still does not wake up, an intravenous dose of glucose should be given. When patient is conscious, carbohydrate should be taken by mouth.

*Special care*: pregnancy, breast-feeding, glucagonoma, insulinoma (these are forms of pancreatic tumour).

*Avoid use*: phaeochromocytoma (adrenal gland tumour).

*Possible interaction*: warfarin.

*Side effects*: gastro-intestinal upset, allergic responses.

*Manufacturer*: Novo Nordisk.

## GLUCAGON *SEE*: GLUCAGEN.

## GLUCOPHAGE

*Description*: an antidiabetic drug belonging to the group known as biguanides, available as film-coated, white tablets in two different strengths containing 500mg and 850mg of metformin hydrochloride and marked with strength and GL.

*Used for*: Type II diabetes, as sole therapy or combined with other oral antidiabetic drugs or insulin, especially in patients who are overweight and whose diabetes has not responded to a diet/exercise regime alone.

*Dosage*: adults, 500mg three times each day at first, or 850mg twice daily taken with, or just following a meal. Dose may be gradually increased after 10 to 15 days, to a daily maximum of 3g according to response.

*Special care*: kidney failure, the elderly.

*Avoid use*: pregnancy, breastfeeding, juvenile, growth-onset or unstable brittle diabetes (all forms of insulin-dependent diabetes mellitus), severe liver or kidney disease, ketoacidosis, stress, infections, surgery, endocrine disorders.

*Possible interaction*: risk of hypoglycemia with: sulfonamides, fibrates, fluconazole, aspirin, alcohol, chloramphenicol, MAOIs, NSAIDs, miconazole, oral anticoagulants, ß-blockers, ACE inhibitors, probenecid, phenylbutazone, cimetidine. Risk of hyperglycemia with: diuretics, progestogens, oestrogens, contraceptive pills, phenothiazines, derivatives of nicotinic acid, thyroid hormones, phenytoin, danazol, sympathomimetics, calcium antagonists, corticosteroids, isoniazid.

*Side effects*: allergic reactions including skin rash, hypoglycemia, disturbance of vision, liver disorders, gastrointestinal effects, headache, abdominal pains, malaise, blood effects, trembling, dizziness, raised liver enzymes, confusion, drowsiness.

*Manufacturer*: Merck.

## GLURENORM

*Description*: an antidiabetic drug belonging to the group known as sulphonylureas, available as scored, white tablets containing 30mg gliquidone and marked G.

*Used for*: Type II diabetes.

*Dosage*: adults, in the order of 45–60mg each day in divided doses before meals. Maximum dose is 180mg each day.

*Special care*: kidney failure, the elderly.

*Avoid use*: pregnancy, breastfeeding, juvenile, growth-onset or unstable brittle diabetes (all forms of insulin-dependent diabetes mellitus), severe liver or kidney disease, ketoacidosis, stress, infections, surgery, endocrine disorders. Also, porphyria (an inherited metabolic disorder involving porphyrins).

*Possible interaction*: risk of hypoglycemia with: sulfonamides, fibrates, fluconazole, aspirin, alcohol, chloramphenicol, MAOIs, NSAIDs, miconazole, oral anticoagulants, ß-blockers, ACE inhibitors, probenecid, phenylbutazone, cimetidine. Risk of hyperglycemia with: diuretics, progestogens, oestrogens, contraceptive pills, phenothiazines, derivatives of nicotinic acid, thyroid hormones, phenytoin, danazol, sympathomimetics, calcium antagonists, corticosteroids, isoniazid.

*Side effects*: allergic reactions including skin rash, hypoglycemia, disturbance of vision, liver disorders, gastrointestinal effects, headache, abdominal pains, malaise, blood effects, trembling, dizziness, raised liver enzymes, confusion, drowsiness.

*Manufacturer*: Sanofi-Synthelabo.

## GLYCEROL *SEE*: RELAXIT.

## GLYCINE *SEE*: CICATRIN.

## GOPTEN

*Description*: an antihypertensive preparation and ACE inhibitor available as capsules of 3 strengths. Yellow/red, orange/red and red/red capsules contain 0.5mg, 1mg and 2mg trandolapril respectively.

*Used for*: dysfunction of left ventricle following a heart attack, mild to moderate high blood pressure.

*Dosage*: adults, left ventricular dysfunction, 0.5mg once each day in first instance, starting 3 days after heart attack then increase gradually to maintenance dose of 4mg once each day. Hypertension, 0.5mg once each day at first, gradually increasing to a maintenance dose of 1 to 2mg once each day. The maximum single daily dose is 4mg. In all cases, diuretic medication should be stopped 2 to 3 days before beginning Gopten but can be re-started once patient is established on drug, if required.

*Special care*: anaesthesia or surgery, congestive heart failure, liver or kidney disease, stenosis (narrowing) of renal arteries on both sides, kidney dialysis. Kidney function should be monitored before starting treatment and during its course.

*Avoid use*: children, pregnancy, breast-feeding, obstruction of heart outflow or aortic stenosis. Those with angioneurotic oedema (fluid retention) caused by previous treatment with ACE inhibitors, or which is hereditary or of unknown cause.

*Possible interaction*: NSAIDs, potassium-sparing diuretics, potassium supplements, TCADs, lithium, neuroleptics, antihypertensive drugs, antidiabetics.

*Side effects*: headache, cough, rash, giddiness, weakness, palpitations, hypotension. Rarely there may be depression of bone marrow, blood changes (agranulocytosis—

characterized by serious deficiency of certain white blood cells), angioneurotic oedema.

*Manufacturer*: Abbott.

## GRAMICIDIN *SEE*: NEOSPORIN, SOFRADEX, SOFRAMYCIN.

# H

## HALF SECURON SR *SEE*: SECURON SR.

## HALF-INDERAL LA *SEE*: INDERAL.

## HARMOGEN

*Description*: a hormonal oestrogen preparation produced in the form of long, peach-coloured, scored tablets containing 1.5mg estropipate (equivalent to 0.93mg of estrone), marked 3773 and U.

*Used for*: hormonal replacement therapy in menopausal women and prevention of osteoporosis following menopause.

*Dosage*: adults, 1 to 2 tablets each day, along with a progestogen preparation for the last 10 to 13 days of each 28 day cycle in women who have not had a hysterectomy.

*Special care*: hypertension, severe kidney disease receiving dialysis, Raynaud's disease, diabetes, multiple sclerosis, asthma, varicose veins, elevated levels of prolactin (a hormone) in the blood (hyperprolactinemia). Risk of thrombosis increases with smoking, age and obesity. Blood pressure, breasts and pelvic organs should be checked during period of treatment.

*Avoid use*: pregnancy, heart and circulatory diseases, angina, sickle cell anaemia, pulmonary hypertension. Also hormone-dependent cancers, undiagnosed vaginal bleeding, chorea, liver disease, history of cholestatic jaundice of pregnancy, infectious hepatitis, Dublin-Johnson syndrome, Rotor syndrome, recent trophoblastic disease.

*Possible interaction*: phenytoin, carbamazepine, tetracyclines, primidone, chloral hydrate, glutethimide, phenylbutazone, rifampicin, griseofulvin, ampicillin, dichloralphenazone, ethosuximide, barbiturates, St John's Wort.

*Side effects*: feeling of bloatedness due to fluid retention, leg pains, breast enlargement, erosion of cervix, muscular cramps, weight gain, breakthrough bleeding, depression, headaches, vaginal discharge, loss of libido, nausea, brown patches on skin (chloasma). Stop drug immediately in event of pregnancy, if frequent, severe headaches occur or signs of thromboses, severe pain in upper abdominal region, enlarged liver, jaundice, rise in blood pressure, severe depression, increased number of fits. Drug should be discontinued 6 weeks before major planned surgery and re-started 2 weeks afterwards, as long as woman is fully mobile. Should be discontinued during long periods of immobility.

*Manufacturer*: Pharmacia.

## HELICLEAR

*Description*: a composite pack for ulcer treatment comprising 14 Zoton tablets, each containing 30mg of lansoprazole, 14 Klaricid tablets, each containing 500mg of clarithromycin and 28 tablets each containing 500mg of amoxicillin.

*Used for*: elimination of H.pylori bacteria in patients with duodenal ulcer.

*Dosage*: adults, 1 Zoton tablet, 1 Klaricid tablet and 2 amoxicillin tablets, twice each day for 1 week.

*Special care*: breastfeeding, liver or kidney disease; rule out cancer as cause of symptoms before treatment starts.

*Avoid use*: children, pregnancy, serious kidney disease.

*Possible interaction*: digoxin, antacids, oral contraceptives, ergot derivatives, zidovudine, phenytoin, cisapride, theophylline, astemizole, drugs metabolised by P450, sucralfate, anticoagulants taken by mouth, statins, pimozide, carbamazepine, ritonavir, terfenadine.*Also, see* individual entries.

*Side effects*: see under individual entries; for amoxicillin, *See*: Amoxil.

*Manufacturer*: Wyeth.

## HELIMET

*Description*: a composite treatment pack comprising 14 Zoton tablets each containing 30mg of lansoprazole, 14 Klaricid tablets each containing 500mg of clarithromycin and 14 tablets containing 400mg of metronidazole.

*Used for*: elimination of *H. pylori* bacteria in patients with duodenal ulcer.

*Dosage*: adults, 1 Zoton tablet, 1 Klaricid tablet and 1metronidazole tablet, twice each day for 1 week.

*Special care*: breastfeeding, liver or kidney disease; rule out cancer as cause of symptoms before treatment starts.

*Avoid use*: children, pregnancy, serious kidney disease.

*Possible interaction*: digoxin, antacids, oral contraceptives, alcohol, ergot derivatives, zidovudine, phenytoin, cisapride, theophylline, lithium, astemizole, drugs metabolised by P450, sucralfate, cytotoxics, anticoagulants taken by mouth, statins, pimozide, cimetidine, carbamazepine, ritonavir, terfenadine. *Also, see* individual entries.

*Side effects*: see under individual entries; for metronidazole, *See*: Flagyl.

*Manufacturer*: Wyeth.

## HEPARIN *SEE*: CLEXANE.

## HEPARINOID *SEE*: LASONIL.

## HORMONIN

*Description*: a hormonal oestrogen preparation available in the form of scored, pink tablets containing 0.27mg estriol, 1.4mg estrone and 0.6mg oestradiol.

*Used for*: hormone replacement therapy in women with menopausal symptoms, prevention of osteoporosis after menopause.

*Dosage*: women, 1 to 2 tablets each day, taken either cyclically or continuously, with a progestogen for last 12 or 13 days of 28 day cycle unless patient has had a hysterectomy.

*Special care*: hypertension, severe kidney disease receiving dialysis, Raynaud's disease, diabetes, multiple sclerosis, asthma, varicose veins, elevated levels of prolactin (a hormone) in the blood (hyperprolactinemia). Risk of thrombosis increases with smoking, age and obesity. Blood pressure, breasts and pelvic organs should be checked during period of treatment.

*Avoid use*: pregnancy, heart and circulatory diseases, angina, sickle cell anaemia, pulmonary hypertension. Also hormone-dependent cancers, undiagnosed vaginal bleeding, chorea, liver disease, history of cholestatic jaundice of pregnancy, infectious hepatitis, Dublin–Johnson syndrome, Rotor syndrome, recent trophoblastic disease.

*Possible interaction*: phenytoin, carbamazepine, tetracyclines, primidone, chloral hydrate, glutethimide, phenylbutazone, rifampicin, griseofulvin, ampicillin, dichloralphenazone, ethosuximide, barbiturates, St John's Wort.

*Side effects*: feeling of bloatedness due to fluid retention, leg pains, breast enlargement, erosion of cervix, muscular cramps, weight gain, breakthrough bleeding, depression, headaches, vaginal discharge, loss of libido, nausea, brown patches on skin (chloasma). Stop drug immediately in event of pregnancy, if frequent, severe headaches occur or signs of thromboses, severe pain in upper abdominal region, enlarged liver, jaundice, rise in blood pressure, severe depression, increased number of fits. Drug should be discontinued 6 weeks before major planned surgery and re-started 2 weeks afterwards, as long as woman is fully mobile. Should be discontinued during long periods of immobility

*Manufacturer*: Shire.

## HUMALOG

*Description*: a preparation of insulin lispro which is a very rapid acting insulin, containing 100iu per ml, available in cartridges and preloaded pens.

*Used for*: diabetes.

*Dosage*: according to individual patient requirements, usually self-delivered by subcutaneous injection, or continuous subcutaneous infusion, or by intravenous infusion or intramuscular injection. Given shortly before or just after a meal. Begins to take effect within 15 minutes and activity continues for 2 to 5 hours.

*Special care*: kidney or liver disease, patients transferring from animal insulins (should be warned that early signs of hypoglycemia may not be so apparent). Infections, illnesses, stress, emotional upset, pregnancy, change in insulin source, type etc; in all these cases, dose adjustments may be needed.

*Possible interaction*: oral contraceptives, MAOIs, alcohol, ß-blockers, corticotrophin, diuretics, corticosteroids.

*Side effects*: lipodystrophy (changes involving fat deposition) at injection site.

*Manufacturer*: Lilly.

## HUMALOG MIX 25

*Description*: a combined preparation of very rapid-acting and slower-acting insulins, comprising 25% insulin lispro and 75% insulin lispro protamine suspension, 100iu per ml, available in preloaded pens and in cartridges for Humapen and Autopen devices. *Also*, **HUMALOG**

**MIX50**, comprising a biphasic mix of 50% insulin lispro and 50% insulin lispro protamine suspension, 100iu per ml, available in pre-loaded pen device.

*Used for*: diabetes

*Dosage*: according to individual patient requirements, usually self-delivered by subcutaneous injection either just before or just after meals. Starts to act within 15 minutes and effects continue for about 22 hours.

*Special care*: kidney or liver disease, patients transferring from animal insulins (should be warned that early signs of hypoglycemia may not be so apparent). Infections, illnesses, stress, emotional upset, pregnancy, change in insulin source, type etc; in all these cases, dose adjustments may be needed.

*Possible interaction*: oral contraceptives, MAOIs, alcohol, ß-blockers, corticotrophin, diuretics, corticosteroids.

*Side effects*: lipodystrophy (changes involving fat deposition) at injection site.

*Manufacturer*: Lilly.

## HUMAN ACTRAPID

*Description*: a preparation of short-acting, human neutral insulin (pyr) which is highly purified comprising 100iu per ml, available as preloaded pens and in Penfil cartridges for use in pen device.

*Used for*: diabetes.

*Dosage*: according to individual patient requirements, usually self-delivered by intravenous, intramuscular or subcutaneous injection.

*Special care*: kidney or liver disease, patients transferring from animal insulins (should be warned that early signs of hypoglycemia may not be so apparent). Infections, illnesses, stress, emotional upset, pregnancy, change in insulin source, type etc; in all these cases, dose adjustments may be needed.

*Possible interaction*: oral contraceptives, MAOIs, alcohol, ß-blockers, corticotrophin, diuretics, corticosteroids.

*Side effects*: lipodystrophy (changes involving fat deposition) at injection site.

*Manufacturer*: Novo Nordisk.

## HYDRALAZINE *SEE*: APRESOLINE.

## HYDROCHLORTHIAZIDE *SEE*: ACCURETIC, ACEZIDE, AMIL-CO, CAPOZIDE, CARACE PLUS, CO-BETALOC, INNOZIDE.

## HYDROCORTISONE *SEE*: ACTINAC, ALPHADERM, ANUSOL HC, CALMURID HC, CANESTEN-HC, COLIFOAM, DIODERM, EFCORTELAN, HYDROCORTONE.

## HYDROCORTISONE-17-BUTYRATE *SEE*: LOCOID.

## HYDROCORTONE

*Description*: a corticosteroid (glucocorticoid and mineralocorticoid) available as quarter-scored, white tablets containing 10mg or 20mg (oval shaped tablets) of hydrocortisone and coded MSD 619, MSD 625 respectively.

*Used for*: hormone replacement therapy due to reduced production of hormones from the adrenal cortex (adrenal glands).

*Dosage*: adults, 10 to 20mg each day – consult manufacturer's specifications. Children, 0.4 to 0.8mg per kg of body weight in 2 or 3 divided doses each day, adjusted according to individual response.

*Special care*: elderly, pregnancy, breastfeeding, only for short-term treatment in children. Infections, especially tuberculosis, fungal and viral. Liver failure, cirrhosis, kidney disorders, congestive heart failure, recent heart attack, diarrhoea of unknown cause, ulcerative colitis, stomach ulcer, diverticulitis, recent scar tissue affecting digestive tract, inflammatory conditions of the veins, glaucoma. Also, cancers that have spread, diabetes, certain skin diseases, high blood pressure, psychotic conditions, epilepsy, osteoporosis, herpes simplex infections affecting the eyes, cerebral malaria, under-active thyroid gland, stress, previous steroid myopathy, intercurrent illnesses, myasthenia gravis. Also, accidental injuries and planned surgery – patient must be monitored. Patients should avoid exposure to measles infection – if inadvertently exposed, preventative treatment with immunoglobulins may be needed. Likewise, exposure to chickenpox or herpes zoster should be avoided – treatment with varicella-zoster immunoglobulin may be required. Taking drug in morning or every second day helps to reduce risk of suppression of adrenal glands. Patients should carry a 'steroid treatment card'. Treatment should be short-term. Withdraw treatment gradually.

*Avoid use*: whole body fungal infections, unless particular counter measures are being employed.

*Possible interaction*: anticholinesterases, phenobarbital, cardiac glycosides, diuretics, carbamazepine, antihypertensives, anticoagulants taken by mouth, rifampicin, oestrogens, hypoglycaemics, phenytoin, aminoglutethimide, primidone, ephedrine, rifabutin. Also, salicylates, NSAIDs, ciclosporin, live vaccines, azole antifungals, carbenoxolone, erythromycin, methotrexate.

*Side effects*: depending upon dose and duration of treatment, steroid side effects including electrolyte disturbances and fluid imbalances, water retention, loss of potassium, gastrointestinal disturbance, central nervous system effects, salt retention, impaired wound healing, effects on bones, osteoporosis, cataracts, cushingoid effects, skin changes, depression, high blood pressure, glaucoma. Also, muscle weakness, stomach ulcer, hyperglycaemia, changes in sperm mobility, euphoria, mood swings. Also, retarded growth in children.

*Manufacturer*: M.S.D.

**HYDRFLUMETHIAZIDE *SEE*: ALDACTIDE.**

**HYDROTALCITE *SEE*: ALTACITE PLUS.**

## HYDROXYETHYLCELLULOSE *SEE*: MINIMS ARTIFICIAL TEARS.

## HYDROXYZINE *SEE*: ATARAX, UCERAX.

## HYPOTEARS

*Description*: eyedrops available as a solution containing 1% polyvinyl alcohol.
*Used for*: deficiencies in tear secretions.
*Dosage*: 1 or 2 drops as needed.
*Avoid use*: patients wearing soft contact lenses.
*Manufacturer*: Novartis.

## HYPOVASE

*Description*: an antihypertensive preparation which is a selective α1-blocker. It is produced as tablets of various strengths all containing prazosin hydrochloride. White 500μg tablets marked Pfizer; scored, orange 1mg tablets marked HYP/1; scored, white 2mg tablets marked HYP/2 and Pfizer.
*Used for*: congestive heart failure, high blood pressure, Raynaud's phenomenon, additional therapy in the treatment of urinary tract obstruction when the cause is benign enlargement of the prostate gland.
*Dosage*: adults, congestive heart failure, 500μg, 2, 3 or 4 times each day in first instance, increasing to 4mg in divided doses each day. Then a usual maintenance dose in the order of 4–20mg in divided doses. Hypertension, 500μg as evening dose at first, followed by 500μg 2 or 3

times each day for a period of 3 days to 1 week. Then, 1mg 2 or 3 times each day for 3 days to 1 week. The dose may be further increased gradually as required with a daily maximum of 20mg, as divided doses. Raynaud's phenomenon, 500µg as starting dose in evening, followed by 500µg twice each day for 3 days to 1 week, adjusted according to response. Then a maintenance dose of 1 or 2mg twice each day. Additional therapy in urine obstruction, 500µg taken as evening dose at first, then 500mg twice each day for 3 days to 1 week, adjusted according to response. Usual maintenance dose of 2mg twice each day.

*Special care*: pregnancy, breastfeeding, elderly persons, patients suffering from congestive heart failure caused by stenosis (narrowing of arteries), subject to fainting while passing urine.

*Avoid use*: children.

*Possible interaction*: other anti-hypertensive drugs.

*Side effects*: dry mouth, dizziness on rising from lying down (postural hypotension), fluid retention, headache, nausea, blocked, stuffy nose, palpitations, impotence, diarrhoea, weariness, skin rash, blurring of vision.

*Manufacturer*: Pfizer.

**HYPROMELLOSE *SEE*: ILUBE, ISOPTO ALKALINE, ISOPTO ATROPINE, ISOPTO CARBACHOL, ISOPTO FRIN, ISOPTO PLAIN, MAXITROL, TEARS NATURALE.**

## HYTRIN

*Description*: an antihypertensive preparation which is a selective α1-blocker produced as tablets of 4 different strengths, all containing terazosin (as hydrochloride). White 1mg, yellow 2mg, brown 5mg and blue 10mg tablets are all marked with triangle-shaped symbols and logo.

*Used for*: high blood pressure, additional therapy for urine obstruction caused by benign enlargement of the prostate gland.

*Dosage*: adults, high blood pressure, 1mg taken at bedtime at first then gradually doubling at weekly intervals. The usual maintenance dose is in the order of 2–10mg taken once each day. Additional therapy for urinary obstruction, 1mg taken at bedtime at first, increasing gradually once a week to 5 to 10mg each day, as needed.

*Special care*: in patients liable to fainting.

*Possible interaction*: other anti-hypertensive drugs, diuretics.

*Side effects*: initial dose may cause fainting, low blood pressure on rising from lying down (postural hypotension), dizziness, weariness, blocked, stuffy nose, blurring of vision, fluid retention and swelling of hands and feet, sleepiness, weakness, palpitations.

*Manufacturer*: Abbott.

# I

## IBUGEL

*Description*: an NSAID available as a gel containing 5% ibuprofen. *Also,* **IBUGEL FORTE,** a gel containing 10% ibuprofen.

*Used for*: sprains, strains and pains in back, muscles, joints; neuralgia (nerve pain), mild arthritis.

*Dosage*: adults, rub gel into skin over affected area up to 3 times each day.

*Avoid use*: children, pregnancy, breastfeeding, known allergy to aspirin or NSAIDs.

*Manufacturer*: Dermal.

## IBUMOUSSE

*Description*: an NSAID available as an aqueous mousse containing 5% ibuprofen.

*Used for*: sprains, strains and pains in back, muscles, joints; neuralgia (nerve pain), mild arthritis.

*Dosage*: adults, rub in 1 to 3g of mousse into skin over affected area, 3 or 4 times each day.

*Avoid use*: children, pregnancy, breastfeeding, allergy to aspirin or NSAIDs.

*Manufacturer*: Dermal.

**IBUPROFEN *SEE*: BRUFEN, CODAFEN CONTINUS, FENBID GEL, FENBID SPANSULE, IBUGEL, IBUMOUSSE, IBUSPRAY, MOTRIN, PROFLEX.**

## IBUSPRAY

*Description*: an NSAID available as a spray containing 5% ibuprofen.

*Used for*: sprains, strains and pains in back, muscles, joints; neuralgia (nerve pain), mild arthritis.

*Dosage*: adults, apply 5 to 10 sprays to skin over affected area and rub in well. Can be repeated 3 to 4 times each day.

*Avoid use*: children, pregnancy, breastfeeding, allergy to aspirin or NSAIDs.

*Manufacturer*: Dermal.

## ILUBE

*Description*: a lubricant eye preparation available in the form of drops containing 5% acetylcysteine and 0.35% hypromellose.

*Used for*: dry eyes caused by insufficient secretion of tears or abnormal mucus production.

*Dosage*: 1 or 2 drops into affected eye 3 or 4 times each day.

*Avoid use*: patients with soft contact lenses.

*Manufacturer*: Alcon.

## IMIDAPRIL *SEE*: TANATRIL.

## IMODIUM

*Description*: a colorectal and opiate preparation available as grey/dark green capsules containing 2mg of loperamide hydrochloride, marked Janssen and Imodium. *Also,* **IMODIUM SYRUP**, a sugar-free liquid containing 1mg of loperamide hydrochloride per 5ml.

*Used for*: diarrhoea.

*Dosage*: adults, acute attack, 4mg at first, then further 2mg with each episode; chronic diarrhoea, 4 to 8mg in 2 divided doses. Children, acute diarrhoea, aged 4 to 8 years, 5ml 3 to 4 times each day for up to 3 days; aged 9 to 12 years, 10ml or 1 capsule 4 times each day for up to 5 days.

*Special care*: pregnancy, breastfeeding, liver disorders, acute dysentery.

*Avoid use*: children under 4 years, abdominal bloating, pseudomembranous colitis, acute ulcerative colitis, ileus.

*Side effects*: paralytic ileus (absence of or decline in the normal passage of food along the gut), abdominal bloating and cramps, nausea, dry mouth, constipation, dizziness, rashes, tiredness.

*Manufacturer*: Janssen-Cilag.

## INDERAL

*Description*: a preparation which is a non-cardioselective ß-blocker produced as pink, film-coated tablets containing 10mg, 40mg and 80mg of propranolol hydrochloride all marked with name and strength. *Also*, **INDERAL INJECTION** containing 1mg of propranolol hydrochloride per ml in ampoules for injection.

*Used for*: heart arrhythmias, prevention of second heart attack, enlarged and weakened heart muscle, angina, Fallot's tetralogy (a congenital defect of the heart), high blood pressure, additional therapy in thyrotoxicosis (toxicity of thyroid gland), phaeochromocytoma (adrenal gland tumour), situational and generalized anxiety.

*Dosage*: tablets, adults, prevention of second heart attack, 40mg 4 times each day for 2 or 3 days starting from 5 to 21 days after first attack. Then a maintenance dose of 80mg twice each day. Arrhythmias and enlarged heart, 10 to 40mg 3 or 4 times each day. Angina, 40mg 2 or 3 times each day at first increasing at weekly intervals if required to a usual dose in the order of 120–240mg daily. Hypertension, 80mg twice each day at first increasing at weekly intervals if required to usual dose in the order of 160 to 320mg daily. Phaeochromocytoma, 60mg each day taken along with an alpha-blocker for 3 days before operation for removal. If tumour is inoperable, a 30mg daily dose should be taken. Situational anxiety, 40mg each day; generalized anxiety, the same dose twice daily increasing to 3 times each day if needed. Tablets, children, arrhythmias, 0.25 to 0.5mg per kg of body weight 3 to 4 times each day. Fallot's tetralogy, up to 1mg per kg of body weight 3 or 4 times each day. Phaeochromocytoma, 0.25 to 0.5mg per kg of body weight 3 or 4 times each day, dose varying according to needs of patient. Injection, adults and children, according to manufacturer's instructions.

*Special care*: pregnancy, breast-feeding, patients with weak hearts should receive diuretics and digitalis, liver or kidney disease, diabetes, metabolic acidosis, weakness, insufficient cerebral circulation, thyrotoxic crisis, tendency to exhibit allergic symptoms. Persons undergoing general anaesthesia may need to be withdrawn before planned surgery. Withdraw drug gradually.

*Avoid use*: children, patients with obstructive airways disease or history of bronchospasm (asthma), various heart disorders including heart block, heart shock, heart failure, sick sinus syndrome, serious peripheral arterial disease, sinus bradycardia, disease of heart muscle, Prinzmetal's angina, hypotension, right ventricular failure resulting from pulmonary hypertension, untreated phaeochromocytoma (tumour of the adrenal glands).

*Possible interaction*: cardiac depressant anaesthetics, theophylline, antihypertensives, ergot alkaloids, diltiazem, sympathomimetics, verapamil, clonidine withdrawal, CNS depressants, class I antiarrhythmic drugs, rifampicin, cimetidine, class II calcium antagonists, warfarin, reserpine, ibuprofen, indometacin, hypoglycaemics.

*Side effects*: bradycardia, fatigue on exercise, cold hands and feet, central nervous system effects, disturbance of sleep, gastro-intestinal upset, bronchospasm, heart failure, low blood pressure, baldness, thrombocytopenia (reduction in blood platelets). Withdraw drug gradually if dry eyes or skin rash occur.

*Manufacturer*: AstraZeneca.

## INDERAL LA

*Description*: an antianginal, antihypertensive and anxiolytic preparation which is a non-cardioselective ß-blocker. Available as pink/purple sustained-release capsules containing 160mg of propranolol hydrochloride marked INDERAL LA. *Also*, **HALF-INDERAL LA**, pink/purple sustained-release capsules containing 80mg propranolol hydrochloride marked HALF-INDERAL LA.

*Used for*: angina, high blood pressure, additional therapy in thyrotoxicosis, also treatment of symptoms of situational and generalised anxiety.

*Dosage*: angina, 80mg or 160mg each day with a maximum of 240mg; high blood pressure, 160mg each day at first increasing by 80mg, gradually if needed, until condition is controlled. Thyrotoxicosis, 80mg or 160mg each day with a maximum daily dose of 240mg. Situational anxiety, 80mg each day, generalized anxiety, 80–160mg each day.

*Special care*: pregnancy, breast-feeding, patients with weak hearts should receive diuretics and digitalis, liver or kidney disease, diabetes, metabolic acidosis, weakness, insufficient cerebral circulation, thyrotoxic crisis, tendency to exhibit allergic symptoms. Persons undergoing general anaesthesia may need to be withdrawn before planned surgery. Withdraw drug gradually.

*Avoid use*: children, patients with obstructive airways disease or history of bronchospasm (asthma), various heart disorders including heart block, heart shock, heart failure, sick sinus syndrome, serious peripheral arterial disease, sinus bradycardia, disease of heart muscle, Prinzmetal's angina, hypotension, right ventricular failure resulting from pulmonary hypertension, untreated phaeochromocytoma (tumour of the adrenal glands).

*Possible interaction*: cardiac depressant anaesthetics, theophylline, antihypertensives, ergot alkaloids, diltiazem, sympathomimetics, verapamil, clonidine withdrawal,

CNS depressants, class I antiarrhythmic drugs, rifampicin, cimetidine, class II calcium antagonists, warfarin, reserpine, ibuprofen, indometacin, hypoglycaemics.

*Side effects*: bradycardia, fatigue on exercise, cold hands and feet, central nervous system effects, disturbance of sleep, gastro-intestinal upset, bronchospasm, heart failure, low blood pressure, baldness, thrombocytopenia (reduction in blood platelets). Withdraw drug gradually if dry eyes or skin rash occur.

*Manufacturer*: AstraZeneca.

## INDIVINA

*Description*: a hormonal preparation of oestrogen and progestogen available as white tablets in 3 different strengths. White tablets marked 1+2.5 contain 1mg of oestradiol valerate and 2.5mg of medroxyprogesterone; white tablets marked 1+5 contain 1mg of oestradiol valerate and 5mg of medroxyprogesterone acetate; white tablets marked 2+5 contain 2mg of oestradiol valerate and 5mg of medroxyprogesterone acetate.

*Used for*: menopausal symptoms and prevention of osteoporosis after the menopause in women who have womb intact.

*Dosage*: women, start with lowest dose tablets and take one each day continuously; change to 1mg/5mg tablets if breakthrough bleeding occurs and is persistent. Change to 2mg/5mg tablets if symptoms caused by deficiency of oestrogen are not controlled with lower dose.

*Special care*: hypertension, severe kidney disease receiving

dialysis, Raynaud's disease, diabetes, multiple sclerosis, asthma, varicose veins, elevated levels of prolactin (a hormone) in the blood (hyperprolactinemia). Risk of thrombosis increases with smoking, age and obesity. Blood pressure, breasts and pelvic organs should be checked during period of treatment.

*Avoid use*: pregnancy, heart and circulatory diseases, angina, sickle cell anaemia, pulmonary hypertension. Also hormone-dependent cancers, undiagnosed vaginal bleeding, chorea, liver disease, history of cholestatic jaundice of pregnancy, infectious hepatitis, Dublin–Johnson syndrome, Rotor syndrome, recent trophoblastic disease.

*Possible interaction*: phenytoin, carbamazepine, tetracyclines, primidone, chloral hydrate, glutethimide, phenylbutazone, rifampicin, griseofulvin, ampicillin, dichloralphenazone, ethosuximide, barbiturates, St John's Wort.

*Side effects*: feeling of bloatedness due to fluid retention, leg pains, breast enlargement, erosion of cervix, muscular cramps, weight gain, breakthrough bleeding, depression, headaches, vaginal discharge, loss of libido, nausea, brown patches on skin (chloasma). Stop drug immediately in event of pregnancy, if frequent, severe headaches occur or signs of thromboses, severe pain in upper abdominal region, enlarged liver, jaundice, rise in blood pressure, severe depression, increased number of fits. Drug should be discontinued 6 weeks before major planned surgery and re-started 2 weeks afterwards, as long as woman is fully mobile. Should be discontinued

during long periods of immobility. Any adverse side effects should be reported to the Committee on the Safety of Medicines (CSM).
*Manufacturer*: Orion.

## INDOCID PDA

*Description*: a prostaglandin synthetase inhibitor produced as a powder in vials for reconstitution and injection containing 1mg indometacin (as sodium trihydrate).
*Used for*: patent ductus arteriosus (PDA) in premature babies (a condition in which there remains a connection between the aorta and pulmonary artery, the ductus arteriosus, which normally closes after birth).
*Dosage*: 3 intravenous infusions, each given over 20 minutes to half an hour, at intervals of 12 to 24 hours depending upon baby's age, condition and urinary output.
*Special care*: kidney function and plasma levels of electrolytes should be monitored; also monitor for bleeding. Coronary heart failure, liver dysfunction, sepsis; babies in whom extracellular volume is low are at increased risk of kidney failure. Signs of infection can be masked.
*Avoid use*: babies with serious kidney disorders, untreated infection, gastro-intestinal bleeding or bleeding within the brain, disorders of blood coagulation, thrombocytopenia (a blood disorder in which there are low levels of platelets), necrotising enterocolitis, conditions requiring preservation of patency.
*Possible interaction*: furosemide, aminoglycosides, digitalis.
*Side effects*: bleeding, kidney disorders, worsening

infections, retention of fluid, imbalance in electrolyte (salts) levels.
*Manufacturer*: M.S.D.

**INDOMETACIN *SEE*: FLEXIN CONTINUS, INDOCID, INDOCID PDA, INDOMOD.**

## INDOMOD

*Description*: an NSAID and indole, available in the form of capsules of 2 strengths containing enteric-coated, continuous-release pellets. Orange capsules, marked 27, contain 25mg of indometacin and brown capsules, marked 26, contain 75mg of indometacin.
*Used for*: joint and bone disorders, including ankylosing spondylitis, rheumatoid arthritis, osteoarthritis, tenosynovitis, tendinitis, bursitis, gout.
*Dosage*: adults, 50 to 75mg as single or as 2 doses each day, increasing once a week by 25 or 50mg to a maximum daily dose of 200mg.
*Special care*: elderly persons, heart failure, liver or kidney disease, disorders of central nervous system. Patients taking drug long-term require careful monitoring of liver and kidney function and occasional eye tests.
*Avoid use*: pregnancy, breast-feeding, history of ulcers or active stomach ulcer, bleeding disorders, allergy to NSAID or aspirin.
*Possible interaction*: salicylates, probenecid, ß-blockers, corticosteroids, lithium, diuretics, quinolones, anticoagulants.

*Side effects*: disturbance of vision, deposits in cornea, gastrointestinal upset, blood changes, dizziness, effects on central nervous system. If recurrent headaches or gastro-intestinal bleeding occur, drug should be withdrawn.

*Manufacturer*: Pharmacia.

## INFANT GAVISCON *SEE*: GAVISCON.

## INNOVACE

*Description*: an antihypertensive preparation which is an ACE inhibitor produced as tablets of different strengths. White, round tablets contain 2.5mg of enalapril maleate marked MSD 14; ; triangular, white, scored tablets contain 5mg of enalapril maleate marked MSD 712; scored, red, triangular tablets contain 10mg of enalapril maleate marked MSD 713; scored, peach, triangular tablets contain 20mg of enalapril maleate marked MSD 714.

*Used for*: congestive heart failure, with digitalis and potassium-sparing diuretics. Prevention of heart attack and progression of disease in left ventricle of heart. Essential and renovascular high blood pressure.

*Dosage*: adults, heart failure, prevention of heart attack and disease progression, 2.5mg once each day at first increasing to a usual maintenance dose in the order of 20mg, maximum is 40mg. Treatment should normally begin in hospital for high-risk patients or those with serious heart failure. Diuretics should be discontinued or reduced before therapy starts. High blood pressure, 5mg each day at start, increasing to usual maintenance dose in order of 10 to 20mg once each day. If diuretic is being taken, discontinue 2 to 3 days before starting Innovace and begin with 2.5mg dose, increasing gradually, as required. Elderly patients should receive starting dose of 2.5mg.

*Special care*: breast-feeding, patients undergoing anaesthesia, kidney disease, hypertension associated with kidney disorders, patients having kidney dialysis (drug should not be used in those dialysed with high-flux membranes), serious congestive heart failure. Patients undergoing desensitisation or apheresis (a procedure in which blood is temporarily drawn off so that components can be selectively removed before it is reinfused) should have ACE inhibitor stopped before the procedure is carried out. Kidney function should be monitored during course of therapy.

*Avoid use*: children, pregnancy, patients with obstruction to outflow of heart or aortic stenosis (narrowing of aorta).

*Possible interaction*: potassium supplements or potassium-sparing diuretics, other antihypertensives, lithium, antacids, immunosuppressants, procainamide, allopurinol, neuroleptics, ciclosporin, antidiabetic agents, sympathomimetics, corticosteroids, alcohol, narcotic agents, cytostatics.

*Side effects*: tiredness, headache, dizziness, cough, gastrointestinal upset, angioedema (a condition in which there is widespread swelling, usually short-lived), low blood pressure, kidney failure, cough. Very rarely, anaphylaxis during desensitisation and apheresis of low density lipoproteins in blood.

*Manufacturer*: M.S.D.

## INNOZIDE

*Description*: an antihypertensive preparation combining an ACE inhibitor and thiazide diuretic available as scored, yellow tablets containing 20mg enalapril maleate and 12.5mg hydrochlorothiazide marked MSD 718.

*Used for*: mild to moderate high blood pressure in patients who have become accustomed to the same components taken individually.

*Dosage*: adults, 1 tablet each day with a maximum of 2 if needed. Other diuretics should be discontinued 2 to 3 days before treatment starts.

*Special care*: electrolytes (salts) or fluid imbalance, kidney or liver disease, stenosis (narrowing) of renal artery, heart disease or disease of the blood vessels of the brain, kidney dialysis with high flux membranes, gout, diabetes, undergoing anaesthesia. Patients undergoing desensitisation or apheresis (a procedure in which blood is temporarily drawn off so that components can be selectively removed before it is reinfused) should have ACE inhibitor stopped before the procedure is carried out.

*Avoid use*: children, pregnancy, breastfeeding, angioneurotic oedema (a condition in which there is widespread swelling) resulting from previous treatment with ACE inhibitor, anuria (absence of urination).

*Possible interaction*: hypoglycaemics, ACTH, tubocurarine,

corticosteroids, potassium supplements, potassium-sparing diuretics, NSAIDs, central nervous system depressants, lithium, sympathomimetic amines, narcotic analgesics, barbiturates, allopurinol, alcohol, ciclosporin, phenothiazines, procainamide, antacids, cytostatics.

*Side effects*: cough, tiredness, headache, skin rash, cramps, low blood pressure, pain in chest, dizziness, weakness, kidney failure, impotence, pancreatitis, angioneurotic oedema (widespread swelling) – drug should be immediately stopped. In extremely rare cases, anaphylaxis during desensitisation with wasp or bee venom or during apheresis (a procedure in which blood is temporarily drawn off so that components can be removed before it is reinfused).

*Manufacturer*: M.S.D.

## IPRATROPIUM BROMIDE *SEE*: ATROVENT, DUOVENT.

## ISMELIN

*Description*: an antihypertensive and adrenergic neurone blocker, available as a solution in ampoules for injection containing 10mg of guanethidine sulphate per ml.

*Used for*: hypertensive crisis.

*Dosage*: adults, 10 to 20mg by intramuscular injection with a second injection after 3 hours, if necessary.

*Special care*: pregnancy, kidney disease, fever, asthma, stomach ulcer, arteriosclerosis, anaesthesia.

*Avoid use*: children, 1st 3 months of pregnancy and during

final 2 weeks, heart or kidney failure, phaeochromocytoma (a tumour of the adrenal glands).

*Possible interaction*: sympathomimetics, MAOIs, hypoglycaemics, digitalis, tricyclic antidepressants, oral contraceptives, TCADs, antiarrhythmics, antipsychotics, other antihypertensives, ß-blockers.

*Side effects*: depression, blocked nose, dry mouth, blood changes, headaches, sick-sinus syndrome (heart disorder involving the sinus node), fluid retention and bloating, vomiting, failure to achieve ejaculation, blurring of vision, dermatitis, uraemia (presence of excessive amounts of urea in blood), raised blood urea nitrogen (BUN) levels, tingling/numbness/'pins-and-needles' in fingers and toes, bradycardia (slow heart beat), diarrhoea, dizziness, low blood pressure when rising from lying down (postural hypotension), tiredness, peripheral claudication (weakness and cramps caused by poor blood circulation), heart failure.

*Manufacturer*: Sovereign.

## ISOGEL

*Description*: a laxative, bulking agent available as granules of ispaghula husk for adding to water.

*Used for*: irritable colon, constipation, diarrhoea, control of colostomy.

*Dosage*: adults, 2 x 5ml teaspoonfuls added to water taken once or twice each day with meals; children should take half the adult dose.

*Manufacturer*: Pfizer Consumer.

## ISONIAZID *SEE*: RIFATER, RIFINAH, RIMACTAZID.

## ISOPTO ALKALINE

*Description*: lubricant eye drops containing 1% hypromellose.

*Used for*: lubrication of the surface of the eyes.

*Dosage*: introduce 1 or 2 drops directly onto surface of eyes 3 times each day.

*Avoid use*: persons wearing soft contact lenses.

*Manufacturer*: Alcon.

## ISOPTO ATROPINE

*Description*: lubricant and anticholinergic eyedrops containing 1% atropine sulphate and 0.5% hypromellose.

*Used for*: to produce long-lasting mydriasis (the drug is mydriatic)—fixed dilation of the pupil of the eye, and cycloplegia (cycloplegic)—paralysis of the ciliary muscles of the eye. This is in order to allow detailed examination of the eye to be carried out.

*Dosage*: adults, for uveitis (inflammation of the uveal tract), 1 drop 3 times each day; for refraction, 1 to 2 drops, 1 hour before eye is examined. Children, uveitis, 1 drop 3 times each day; refraction, 1 drop twice each day for 1 to 2 days before eye is examined.

*Special care*: pressure should be applied over lachrymal (tear) sac for 1 minute.

*Avoid use*: patients with soft contact lenses, narrow angle glaucoma.

*Side effects*: dry mouth, sensitivity to light, stinging in eye,

blurring of vision, headache, rapid heartbeat. Also changes in behaviour and psychotic responses.
*Manufacturer*: Alcon.

## ISOPTO CARBACHOL

*Description*: lubricant and cholinergic eyedrops containing 3% carbachol and 1% hypromellose.
*Used for*: glaucoma.
*Dosage*: adults, 2 drops 3 times each day.
*Avoid use*: children, patients with severe iritis (inflammation of the iris), abrasion of the cornea, wearing soft contact lenses.
*Manufacturer*: Alcon.

## ISOPTO FRIN

*Description*: eyedrops containing 0.12% phenylephrine hydrochloride and 0.5% hypromellose.
*Used for*: minor irritation/redness in eye, temporary relief of soreness.
*Special care*: infants, narrow angle glaucoma.
*Manufacturer*: Alcon.

## ISOPTO PLAIN

*Description*: lubricant eyedrops containing 0.5% hypromellose.
*Used for*: deficiency in tears.
*Avoid use*: soft contact lenses.
*Manufacturer*: Alcon.

## ISOTRETINOIN *SEE*: ISOTREXIN.

## ISOTREXIN

*Description*: a retinoid and macrolide preparation available as an alcohol-based gel containing 2% erythromycin and 0.05% isotretinoin.

*Used for*: mild to moderate acne.

*Dosage*: adults, apply thinly to affected skin 1 to 2 times each day and use for at least 6 to 8 weeks.

*Special care*: pregnancy, breastfeeding, avoid mucous membranes, mouth, eyes, damaged or sunburnt areas, build up in skin creases.

*Avoid use*: children.

*Possible interaction*: keratolytics.

*Side effects*: local skin irritation.

*Manufacturer*: Stiefel.

## ISPAGHULA *SEE*: FYBOGEL, KONSYL, MANEVAC.

## ISTIN

*Description*: an antianginal and anti-hypertensive preparation which is a class II calcium antagonist. It is available as 5mg and 10mg white tablets containing amlodipine besylate, marked Pfizer and ITN 5 and ITN 10, respectively.

*Used for*: angina in myocardial ischaemia, high blood pressure.

*Dosage*: adults, 5mg once each day; maximum dose, 10mg daily.

*Special care*: hypertensive crisis, impaired liver function, within 4 weeks of heart attack.

*Avoid use*: children, pregnancy, breastfeeding, angina which is unstable, heart shock, aortic stenosis (narrowing of aortic valve).

*Side effects*: fluid retention, headache, dizziness, overgrowth of gum cells, tiredness, skin rash, nausea, flushing. In rare instances, muscle, joint, back and abdominal pains, acid indigestion, sleepiness, weakness, baldness, itching, dry mouth, sweating, fainting, disturbance of vision, peripheral neuropathy (nerve damage), angioedema (widespread swelling), changes in mood, pancreatitis, vasculitis, (inflammation of veins), thrombocytopenia (bleeding disorder caused by low levels of blood platelets), impotence, altered bowel habit, increased urination.

*Manufacturer*: Pfizer.

# K

**KEFLEX**

*Description*: a cephalosporin antibiotic preparation, cefalexin monohydrate, produced in a number of different forms. White/dark green capsules contain 250mg of cefalexin monohydrate and dark green/pale green capsules contain 500mg, coded LILLY H69 and LILLY H71 respectively. **KEFLEX TABLETS**, peach-coloured containing 250mg of cefalexin monohydrate, coded LILLY U57 and oval, peach tablets contain 500mg, coded LILLY U49. Also, **KEFLEX SUSPENSION** in 2 strengths containing 125mg or 250mg of cefalexin monohydrate per 5ml of solution.

*Used for*: urinary tract infections, inflammation of middle ear, infections of respiratory tract, skin, bone, soft tissue. Also, dental infections.

*Dosage*: adults, 1–4g each day in divided doses. Children, 25 to 50mg per kg of body weight each day in divided doses.

*Special care*: patients with kidney disorder and allergy to penicillins.

*Possible interaction*: loop diuretics.

*Side effects*: gastro-intestinal upset, allergic reactions.

*Manufacturer*: Lilly.

**KERAL**

*Description*: an NSAID available as film-coated, scored

white tablets containing 25mg of dexketoprofen, as trometamol.

*Used for*: pain in muscles and bones, toothache and dental pain, dysmenorrhoea (period pain).

*Dosage*: adults, 12.5mg every 4 to 6 hours or 25mg every 8 hours. Daily maximum is 75mg. If pain is severe, dose should be taken half an hour before eating a meal.

*Special care*: elderly, mild kidney or liver disease, heart disorders, allergies, history of asthma, connective tissue disorders, SLE (Systemic Lupus Erythematosus – an autoimmune disorder of connective tissues).

*Avoid use*: children, pregnancy, breastfeeding, serious heart failure, moderate to serious kidney or liver disease, history of acid indigestion or recurrent stomach ulcer, active stomach ulcer, known allergy to NSAIDs or aspirin, bleeding in gut or other bleeding disorders, ulcerative colitis, Crohn's disease.

*Possible interaction*: other NSAIDs, tacrolimus, sulfonamides, ACE inhibitors, ß-blockers, zidovudine, probenecid, anticoagulants, digoxin, diuretics, ciclosporin, antidiabetic agents taken by mouth, pentoxifylline, anticoagulants, methotrexate, hydantoins, lithium, quinolones.

*Side effects*: headache, haematological changes, gastrointestinal intolerance, dizziness.

*Manufacturer*: Menarini.

## KETOCID

*Description*: an NSAID and preparation of propionic acid

available as sustained-release, clear/pink capsules containing 200mg of ketoprofen, marked KET 200 CR.

*Used for*: inflammatory joint disease including rheumatoid and osteoarthritis, ankylosing spondylitis, acute articular and periarticular inflammatory disease, gout and also, dysmenorrhoea (menstrual pain).

*Dosage*: adults, 1 tablet each day taken with food.

*Special care*: pregnancy, elderly patients, liver or kidney disorders, heart failure, allergies, history of asthma. Patients taking drug long-term should receive monitoring.

*Avoid use*: children, breastfeeding, chronic acid indigestion, stomach ulcer or previous stomach ulcer, severe kidney disorders, known allergy to NSAID or aspirin, asthma.

*Possible interaction*: digoxin, quinolones, methotrexate, anticoagulants, hydantoins, diuretics, lithium, sulfonamides.

*Side effects*: effects on central nervous system, gastrointestinal intolerance.

*Manufacturer*: Trinity.

## KETOPROFEN *SEE*: KETOCID, ORUDIS, ORUVAIL GEL, POWERGEL.

## KLARICID

*Description*: a macrolide antibiotic preparation, available in a variety of forms: oval, yellow, film-coated tablets contain 250mg or 500mg of clarithromycin, all marked with logo; **KLARICID XL,** available as sustained-release, film-coated, yellow, oval tablets containing 500mg of clarithromycin, marked with logo; **KLARICID PAEDIATRIC SUSPENSION** containing 125mg or 250mg of clarithromycin per 5ml solution, when reconstituted (supplied as granules); **KLARICID INTRAVENOUS INJECTION** containing 500mg clarithromycin as powder in vials for reconstitution. **KLARICID SACHETS,** available as a powder in sachets containing 250mg of clarithromycin.

*Used for*: infections of respiratory tract, middle ear, soft tissue and skin. *Also,* Klaricid 500mg tablets are used in conjunction with omeprazole or lansoprazole to eliminate *H. pylori* in patients with duodenal ulcer.

*Dosage*: adults, tablets and sachets, 250mg twice each day for 1 week; serious infections, 500mg twice each day for up to 2 weeks. Klaricid XL, 1 tablet each day with food for 1 to 2 weeks; severe infections, 2 tablets with food, once each day. Injection, 1g by intravenous infusion in 2 divided doses each day for 2 to 5 days. Elimination of *H. pylori,* 500mg twice each day with 1g of amoxicillin twice daily, and either 40mg of omeprazole once each day for 1 week, or 20mg of omeprazole once each day for 10 days, or 30mg of lansoprazole twice each day for 1 to 2 weeks. Children, use Klaricid Paediatric Suspension, aged under 1 year, 7.5mg per kg of body weight; aged 1 to 2 years, 62.5mg; aged 3 to 6 years, 125mg; aged 7 to 9 years, 187.5mg; aged 10 to 12 years, 250mg. All twice each day in divided doses.

*Special care*: pregnancy, breast-feeding, liver or kidney disease.

*Possible interaction*: anticoagulants taken by mouth, statins, astemizole, carbamazepine, theophylline, ritonavir, terfenadine, digoxin, cisapride, drugs metabolised by P450, ergot derivatives.

*Side effects*: gastro-intestinal upset, allergic responses, short-lived central nervous system effects, headache, skin rash, muscle and joint pains, numbness/tingling/'pins-and-needles' in fingers and toes, mouth inflammation, oral thrush, discolouration of teeth or tongue, inflammation of tongue, liver disorders, reversible loss of hearing. In rare cases, kidney dysfunction, prolongation of QT interval, low blood sugar levels, blood changes (leucopenia – low levels of white blood cells, thrombocytopenia – low levels of blood platelets), pseudomembranous colitis.

*Manufacturer*: Abbott.

## KLIOFEM

*Description*: a hormonal preparation of oestrogen and progestogen available as yellow tablets marked NOVO 2862 containing 2mg of oestradiol and 1mg of norethisterone acetate.

*Used for*: symptoms of the menopause, prevention of osteoporosis after the menopause.

*Dosage*: women, 1 tablet each day continuously, beginning at least 12 months after cessation of periods.

*Special care*: hypertension, severe kidney disease receiving dialysis, Raynaud's disease, diabetes, multiple sclerosis, asthma, varicose veins, elevated levels of prolactin (a hormone) in the blood (hyperprolactinemia). Risk of thrombosis increases with smoking, age and obesity. Blood pressure, breasts and pelvic organs should be checked during period of treatment.

*Avoid use*: pregnancy, heart and circulatory diseases, angina, sickle cell anaemia, pulmonary hypertension. Also hormone-dependent cancers, undiagnosed vaginal bleeding, chorea, liver disease, history of cholestatic jaundice of pregnancy, infectious hepatitis, Dublin–Johnson syndrome, Rotor syndrome, recent trophoblastic disease.

*Possible interaction*: phenytoin, carbamazepine, tetracyclines, primidone, chloral hydrate, glutethimide, phenylbutazone, rifampicin, griseofulvin, ampicillin, dichloralphenazone, ethosuximide, barbiturates, St John's Wort.

*Side effects*: feeling of bloatedness due to fluid retention, leg pains, breast enlargement, erosion of cervix, muscular cramps, weight gain, breakthrough bleeding, depression, headaches, vaginal discharge, loss of libido, nausea, brown patches on skin (chloasma). Stop drug immediately in event of pregnancy, if frequent, severe headaches occur or signs of thromboses, severe pain in upper abdominal region, enlarged liver, jaundice, rise in blood pressure, severe depression, increased number of fits. Drug should be discontinued 6 weeks before major planned surgery and re-started 2 weeks afterwards, as long as woman is fully mobile. Should be discontinued during long periods of immobility.

*Manufacturer*: Novo Nordisk.

## KLIOVANCE

*Description*: a hormonal preparation of oestrogen and progestogen available as white, film-coated tablets containing 1mg of oestradiol and 0.5mg of norethisterone acetate.

*Used for*: symptoms of the menopause.

*Dosage*: women, 1 tablet each day with no break between packs, starting at least 12 months after last period.

*Special care*: hypertension, severe kidney disease receiving dialysis, Raynaud's disease, diabetes, multiple sclerosis, asthma, varicose veins, elevated levels of prolactin (a hormone) in the blood (hyperprolactinemia). Risk of thrombosis increases with smoking, age and obesity. Blood pressure, breasts and pelvic organs should be checked during period of treatment.

*Avoid use*: pregnancy, heart and circulatory diseases, angina, sickle cell anaemia, pulmonary hypertension. Also hormone-dependent cancers, undiagnosed vaginal bleeding, chorea, liver disease, history of cholestatic jaundice of pregnancy, infectious hepatitis, Dublin–Johnson syndrome, Rotor syndrome, recent trophoblastic disease.

*Possible interaction*: phenytoin, carbamazepine, tetracyclines, primidone, chloral hydrate, glutethimide, phenylbutazone, rifampicin, griseofulvin, ampicillin, dichloralphenazone, ethosuximide, barbiturates, St John's Wort.

*Side effects*: feeling of bloatedness due to fluid retention, leg pains, breast enlargement, erosion of cervix, muscular cramps, weight gain, breakthrough bleeding, depression, headaches, vaginal discharge, loss of libido, nausea, brown patches on skin (chloasma). Stop drug immediately in event of pregnancy, if frequent, severe headaches occur or signs of thromboses, severe pain in upper abdominal region, enlarged liver, jaundice, rise in blood pressure, severe depression, increased number of fits. Drug should be discontinued 6 weeks before major planned surgery and re-started 2 weeks afterwards, as long as woman is fully mobile. Should be discontinued during long periods of immobility.

*Manufacturer*: Novo Nordisk.

## KOLANTICON

*Description*: a deflatulent, antacid and anticholinergic preparation available as a gel containing 400mg of dried aluminium hydroxide gel, 200mg of magnesium oxide, 5mg of dicycloverine hydrochloride and 40mg of dimeticone per 10ml of gel.

*Used for*: wind, stomach ulcer, over-secretion of stomach acid, spasm of gastrointestinal tract.

*Dosage*: adults, 10 to 20ml every 4 hours.

*Special care*: enlarged prostate gland, glaucoma.

*Avoid use*: children, obstruction of gastrointestinal tract, obstructive uropathy, myasthenia gravis (a severe autoimmune disorder), serious ulcerative colitis.

*Possible interaction*: tetracyclines.

*Side effects*: anticholinergic effects.

*Manufacturer*: Peckforton.

## KONSYL

*Description*: a laxative, bulking agent available as a sugar-free powder containing 6g of ispaghula husk. *Also*, **KONSYL ORANGE,** orange-flavoured powder containing 3.5g of ispaghula husk. Both preparations available in sachets for adding to water.

*Used for*: irritable bowel syndrome, constipation.

*Dosage*: adults, 1 sachet added to water or liquid and taken 3 times each day; children over 6 years, half adult dose.

*Avoid use*: children under 6 years, obstruction of intestine.

*Side effects*: wind, swelling of abdomen.

*Manufacturer*: Eastern.

# L

**LABETALOL *SEE*: TRANDATE.**

**LACIDIPINE *SEE*: MOTENS.**

**LACRI-LUBE**

*Description*: a preservative-free ointment containing liquid paraffin, soft white paraffin and non-ionic hydrous wool fat.

*Used for*: lubrication of eyes and protection of cornea.

*Dosage*: introduce small quantity onto surface of eye, as needed.

*Manufacturer*: Allergan.

**LACTIC ACID *SEE*: CALMURID HC.**

**LACTUGAL**

*Description*: an osmotic, laxative preparation available as a solution containing 3.1 to 3.7g of lactulose per 5ml.

*Used for*: constipation, portal systemic encephalopathy (PSE).

*Avoid use*: obstruction of intestine, galactosaemia.

*Side effects*: wind.

*Manufacturer*: Intrapharm.

**LACTULOSE *SEE*: DUPHALAC, LACTUGAL**

## LANSOPRAZOLE *SEE*: HELICLEAR, HELIMET.

## LASIX

*Description*: a loop diuretic available as white, scored tablets marked DLF containing 20mg of furosemide and white, scored tablets marked DLI containing 40mg of furosemide, both also marked with manufacturer's symbol. *Also,* **LASIX 500**, available as quarter scored, yellow tablets marked with the manufacturer's symbol and DIX on the reverse, containing 500mg of furosemide. *Also,* **LASIX PAEDIATRIC LIQUID**, containing 1mg of furosemide per ml. *Also,* **LASIX INJECTION**, available in ampoules containing 10mg of furosemide per ml.

*Used for*: Lasix, fluid retention; other preparations, acute or chronic kidney disease.

*Dosage*: Lasix, adults, 20–80mg in 1 dose daily or every other day; Lasix 500, for hospital use only according to manufacturer's instructions. Lasix injection, 20 to 50mg as slow intravenous or intramuscular injection at first and according to manufacturer's instructions. Children, Lasix, 1 to 3mg per kg of body weight each day; Lasix paediatric liquid, 1 to 3mg per kg of body weight each day; Lasix injection, 0.5 to 1.5mg per kg of body weight each day, given in same manner as for adults.

*Special care*: pregnancy, breastfeeding, gout, diabetes, enlarged prostate gland, impaired urination, liver or kidney disease, Potassium supplements may be necessary. Children being treated with large doses of paediatric liquid may experience diarrhoea or abdominal wind.

*Avoid use*: Lasix 500 in children, pre-coma caused by liver cirrhosis.

*Possible interaction*: NSAIDs, antihypertensives, cephalosporins, aminoglycosides, lithium, digitalis.

*Side effects*: gout, rash, gastro-intestinal upset.

*Manufacturer*: Borg.

## LASONIL

*Description*: an anti-inflammatory preparation available as an ointment containing 50 units of heparinoid per gram.

*Used for*: soft tissue injuries, strains and sprains.

*Dosage*: apply generously to affected area 2 or 3 times each day.

*Special care*: early pregnancy (first 3 months).

*Avoid use*: mucous membranes, eyes, infected or open wounds, senile purpura.

*Possible interaction*: anticoagulants taken by mouth.

*Manufacturer*: Bayer.

## LATANOPROST *SEE*: XALACOM, XALATAN.

## LEDERFEN

*Description*: an NSAID and propionic acid available as light blue, film-coated, capsule-shaped tablets marked WY 050 containing 300mg of fenbufen and light blue film-coated tablets marked WY 051, containing 450mg of fenbufen. *Also*, **LEDERFEN CAPSULES**, available as dark blue capsules marked WY 052 containing 300mg of fenbufen.

*Used for*: osteoarthritis, rheumatoid arthritis, ankylosing spondylitis and acute muscle/bone disorders.

*Dosage*: adults, 300mg in the morning with 600mg at night, or 450mg twice each day.

*Special care*: pregnancy, elderly patients, heart failure, kidney or liver disease, asthma or previous occurrence of asthma. Monitor those on long-term treatment.

*Avoid use*: active peptic ulcers or history of gastro-intestinal lesions, allergy induced by aspirin or anti-inflammatory drug.

*Possible interaction*: anticoagulants, salicylates, quinolones, cardiac glycosides, methotrexate, ciclosporin, drugs bound to proteins, lithium, diuretics, antihypertensives, mifepristone, corticosteroids.

*Side effects*: gastro-intestinal intolerance, oedema affecting fac, dizziness, angioedema (condition in which there is widespread swelling), erythema multiforme (a skin condition in which there are inflamed patches), purpura (bleeding beneath skin), Stevens–Johnson syndrome, disturbance of vision, sensitivity to light, death of patches of epidermal skin cells, inflammation of veins. In rare cases, pulmonary alveolitis (inflammation of alveoli-air sacs – of lungs), pulmonary eosinophilia (increase in number of eosinophils-white blood cells-as a result of inflammation). If skin rash occurs, drug should be withdrawn.

*Manufacturer*: Goldshield.

## LERCANIDIPINE *SEE*: ZANDIP.

## LESCOL

*Description*: a suppressant of cholesterol production (a statin), available in two strengths: yellow/brown capsules containing 20mg of fluvastatin and orange/brown capsules containing 40mg of fluvastatin. All capsules are marked with XU, the strength and the company logo. *Also,* **LESCOL XL,** available as yellow tablets containing 80mg of fluvastatin as sodium salt, marked with strength and name.

*Used for*: primary hypercholesterolaemia (high blood cholesterol levels) and mixed dyslipidaemia in patients whose condition cannot be controlled by diet alone: reduction of overall cholesterol, LDL-cholesterol, triglycerides and apolipoprotein B. Also, in patients with primary hypercholesterolaemia and coronary heart disease, to hinder progression of atherosclerosis in coronary arteries.

*Dosage*: Lescol, adults aged over 18 years, a starting dose of 20 to 40mg once each day taken at bedtime, increasing if necessary at 4 week intervals to a maximum of 40mg twice each day. The usual dose is 20 to 40mg once each day. Lescol XL, 1 tablet each day in patients who have first been treated with Lescol.

*Special care*: history of liver disease, or alcoholism (test liver function and discontinue if certain enzyme levels are high), myalgias or muscle weakness particularly with fever or if generally unwell. Any condition predisposing to rhabdomyolysis.

*Avoid use*: children, pregnancy, breastfeeding, kidney or liver disease, persistent high blood levels of certain enzymes – transaminases.

*Possible interaction*: immunosuppressive drugs, rifampicin, erythromycin, nicotinic acid, gemfibrozil, other fibrates.

*Side effects*: headache, abdominal pain, insomnia, nausea, acid indigestion. In rare cases, muscle pain, tenderness or weakness, abnormal liver function tests.

*Manufacturer*: Novartis.

**LEVOBUNOLOL** ***SEE*****: BETAGAN.**

**LEVOCABASTINE** ***SEE*****: LIVOSTIN.**

**LEVONORGESTREL** ***SEE*****: CYCLO-PROGYNOVA, EUGYNON 30, FEMSEVEN SEQUI, LOGYNON ED, LOGYNON, MICROGYNON 30 ED, MICROGYNON 30, NORGESTON, NUVELLE, OVRANETTE, TRINORDIOL.**

## LIBRIUM

*Description*: an anxiolytic preparation which is a long-acting benzodiazepine, available as capsules in 2 strengths. Yellow/green capsules contain 5mg of chlordiazepoxide and black/green capsules contain 10mg of chlordiazepoxide, all marked with strength and LIB.

*Used for*: treatment of severe anxiety over the short-term, with or without insomnia, symptoms of acute alcohol withdrawal.

*Dosage*: adults, anxiety, up to 30mg per day at first in divided doses with a daily maximum of 100mg. For insomnia, 10 to 30mg at bedtime. For alcohol withdrawal, 25 to 100mg repeated in 2 to 4 hours if necessary. Elderly, 5mg per day to begin with.

*Special care*: chronic lung insufficiency, chronic liver or kidney disease, depression, glaucoma (acute, narrow angle), bereavement. Drug can affect dexterity and judgement. Long-term use is to be avoided and drug should be withdrawn gradually.

*Avoid use*: children, pregnancy, breastfeeding, labour, elderly persons, acute lung insufficiency, depression of respiration (except in cases of acute muscle spasms), sleep apnoea, severe liver insufficiency, myasthenia gravis (a severe autoimmune disorder). Also when treating anxiety, obsessional states or chronic psychosis.

*Possible interaction*: alcohol and other CNS depressants, anticonvulsants.

*Side effects*: vertigo, gastro-intestinal upsets, confusion, ataxia, drowsiness, light-headedness, hypotension, disturbance of vision, skin rashes. Also urine retention, changes in libido. Dependence a potential problem.

*Manufacturer*: ICN.

## LIDOCAINE *SEE*: BRADOSOL PLUS.

## LIPITOR

*Description*: a statin and cholesterol lowering preparation available as film-coated, white, elliptical tablets in 4 different strengths, all containing atorvastatin as calcium trihydrate. Tablets are available in 10mg, 20mg, 40mg and 80mg strengths marked PD 155, PD 156, PD 157 and PD 158, respectively.

*Used for*: additional therapy (with dietary measures) in various forms of hyperlipidaemia; to lower LDL:HDL ratios and raise HDL; to lower total cholesterol:HDL ratios.

*Dosage*: adults, start with 10mg once each day and increase as required at monthly intervals to a maximum dose of 80mg once each day. Little information is available for prescribing in children.

*Special care*: liver disease, alcohol abuse. Liver function tests should be carried out. Women of child-bearing age must use reliable contraception.

*Avoid use*: pregnancy, breastfeeding, persistent elevated liver enzymes, liver disease.

*Possible interaction*: digoxin, colestipol, warfarin, ciclosporin, drugs metabolised by P450 3A4, niacin, erythromycin, azole antifungals, antacids, fibrates, oral contraceptives.

*Side effects*: headache, weakness, muscle pain, elevated CPK and ALT (enzyme) levels, gastrointestinal upset, insomnia.

*Manufacturer*: Pfizer.

## LIPOSTAT

*Description*: a statin available as bi-convex, yellow tablets in 3 different strengths containing 10mg, 20mg or 40mg of pravastatin, as sodium salt, each marked with strength.

*Used for*: hypercholesterolaemia (high levels of blood cholesterol) which does not respond to dietary measures. In patients with hypercholesterolaemia but no apparent coronary disease, as additional treatment with dietary measures to reduce the risk of heart attack, future death related to heart or circulatory disease and to reduce future need for revascularisation procedures. In patients with elevated blood cholesterol levels who have previously had a heart attack or who have unstable angina, to reduce risk of further heart attack or stroke, need for future revascularisation procedures, to reduce risk of death from coronary heart disease or to shorten length of hospital stay. In patients with high blood cholesterol levels and coronary heart disease, as additional treatment with dietary measures to reduce the progression of atherosclerosis in coronary arteries and lessen the risk of heart/circulatory events.

*Dosage*: adults, 10 to 40mg taken as 1 dose at night.

*Special care*: history of liver disease. Liver function tests to be undertaken during treatment and drug to be withdrawn if certain enzyme levels (phosphokinase, creatine, AST, ALT) are notably high. Women of child-bearing age must use effective contraception.

*Avoid use*: pregnancy, breastfeeding, liver disease, homozygotic, familial hypercholesterolaemia (a genetically determined, inherited form of the disorder).

*Possible interaction*: fibrates, erythromycin, nicotinic acid, ciclosporin. Lipostat should be taken 1 hour before or 4 hours after colestipol or colestyramine.

*Side effects*: muscle pain, headache, rashes, gastrointestinal upset, tiredness, chest pains not related to the heart.
*Manufacturer*: BMS.

## LIQUID GAVISCON *SEE*: GAVISCON.

## LIQUIFILM TEARS

*Description*: a preparation of eye drops available as a preservative-free solution containing 1.4% polyvinyl alcohol, either in single dose or multi-dose format.
*Used for*: eye lubrication, as substitute for tears.
*Dosage*: add 1 or 2 drops to eyes as needed.
*Avoid use*: multi-dose preparation, soft contact lenses.
*Manufacturer*: Allergan.

## LISINOPRIL *SEE*: CARACE, CARACE PLUS, ZESTRIL.

## LITHIUM SALTS *SEE*: CAMCOLIT.

## LIVOSTIN

*Description*: an antihistamine preparation available as a nasal spray and eye drops, both containing 0.5mg of levocabastine per ml.
*Used for*: hayfever, allergic conjunctivitis.
*Dosage*: adults and children over 9 years, nasal spray, 2 sprays in each nostril twice each day, increasing if necessary to 3 to 4 sprays daily. Eye drops, 1 drop per eye twice each day, increasing to three or four times each day if required.

*Special care*: pregnancy, soft contact lenses (eye drops).
*Avoid use*: children under 9 years, kidney disorder.
*Side effects*: tiredness, headache, sleepiness, local irritation. Eye drops, fluid retention, itching, nettle rash, breathlessness.
*Manufacturer*: Novartis.

## LOCOID

*Description*: a strong steroid preparation, available as a cream and ointment containing 0.1% hydrocortisone 17-butyrate. *Also,* **LOCOID CRELO,** an emulsion containing 0.15 hydrocortisone 17-butyrate. *Also*, **LOCOID LIPOCREAM**, 0.1% hydrocortisone 17-butyrate in a base containing 70% oil. *Also,* **LOCOID SCALP LOTION**, 0.1% hydrocortisone 17-butyrate in an alcoholic solution. *Also,* **LOCOID C**, a strong steroid 0.1% hydrocortisone 17-butyrate with an antifungal and antibacterial, 3% chlorquinaldol, available as cream and ointment.
*Used for*: Locoid and Locoid Crelo, eczema, psoriasis, skin disorders. Locoid Lipocream, skin disorders responsive to steroids. Locoid scalp lotion, seborrhoea affecting the scalp. Locoid C, as for Locoid but when infection is also present
*Dosage*: Locoid and Locoid Crelo, Locoid Lipocream, apply to affected area 2 to 3 times each day; Locoid Scalp Lotion, apply to scalp twice each day; Locoid C, apply 2 to 4 times each day.
*Special care*: should not be used on face or on children for more than 5 days. Should be stopped gradually.

*Avoid use*: prolonged or extensive use especially pregnant women or continual use as a preventative. Should not be used to treat acne, leg ulcers, scabies, peri-oral dermatitis, tuberculous skin conditions, skin disorders caused by viruses, ringworm, any untreated bacterial or fungal skin infections.

*Side effects*: thinning of skin, adrenal gland suppression, hair growth, Cushingoid type symptoms (as in Cushing's syndrome).

*Manufacturer*: Yamanouchi.

## LODOXAMIDE *SEE*: ALOMIDE.

## LOESTRIN 20

*Description*: a hormonal, contraceptive preparation of oestrogen and progestogen available as film-coated, blue tablets containing 20μg of ethinylestradiol and 1mg of norethisterone acetate. *Also,* **LOESTRIN 30**, available as film-coated, green tablets containing 30mg of ethinylestradiol and 1.5mg of norethisterone acetate.

*Used for*: oral contraception.

*Dosage*: women, 1 tablet daily for 21 days, commencing on the first day of menstruation, then 7 days without tablets.

*Special care*: hypertension, severe kidney disease receiving dialysis, Raynaud's disease, diabetes, multiple sclerosis, asthma, varicose veins, elevated levels of prolactin (a hormone) in the blood (hyperprolactinemia). Risk of thrombosis increases with smoking, age and obesity. Blood pressure, breasts and pelvic organs should be checked during period of treatment.

*Avoid use*: pregnancy, heart and circulatory diseases, angina, sickle cell anaemia, pulmonary hypertension. Also hormone-dependent cancers, undiagnosed vaginal bleeding, chorea, liver disease, history of cholestatic jaundice of pregnancy, infectious hepatitis, Dublin–Johnson syndrome, Rotor syndrome, recent trophoblastic disease.

*Possible interaction*: phenytoin, carbamazepine, tetracyclines, primidone, chloral hydrate, glutethimide, phenylbutazone, rifampicin, griseofulvin, ampicillin, dichloralphenazone, ethosuximide, barbiturates, St John's Wort.

*Side effects*: feeling of bloatedness due to fluid retention, leg pains, breast enlargement, erosion of cervix, muscular cramps, weight gain, breakthrough bleeding, depression, headaches, vaginal discharge, loss of libido, nausea, brown patches on skin (chloasma). Stop drug immediately in event of pregnancy, if frequent, severe headaches occur or signs of thromboses, severe pain in upper abdominal region, enlarged liver, jaundice, rise in blood pressure, severe depression, increased number of fits. Drug should be discontinued 6 weeks before major planned surgery and re-started 2 weeks afterwards, as long as woman is fully mobile. Should be discontinued during long periods of immobility.

*Manufacturer*: Pfizer.

## LOFEPRAMINE *SEE*: GAMANIL, LOMONT.

## LOGYNON

*Description*: a hormonal, contraceptive preparation containing oestrogen and progestogen available as sugar-coated tablets. 6 brown tablets contain 30μg of ethinylestradiol and 50μg of levonorgestrel; 5 white tablets contain 40μg of ethinylestradiol and 75μg of levonorgestrel; 10 ochre coloured tablets contain 30μg of ethinylestradiol and 125μg of levonorgestrel.

*Used for*: oral contraception.

*Dosage*: 1 tablet daily for 21 days starting on the first day of menstruation, in order directed on packet, then 7 days without tablets.

*Special care*: hypertension, severe kidney disease receiving dialysis, Raynaud's disease, diabetes, multiple sclerosis, asthma, varicose veins, elevated levels of prolactin (a hormone) in the blood (hyperprolactinemia). Risk of thrombosis increases with smoking, age and obesity. Blood pressure, breasts and pelvic organs should be checked during period of treatment.

*Avoid use*: pregnancy, heart and circulatory diseases, angina, sickle cell anaemia, pulmonary hypertension. Also hormone-dependent cancers, undiagnosed vaginal bleeding, chorea, liver disease, history of cholestatic jaundice of pregnancy, infectious hepatitis, Dublin–Johnson syndrome, Rotor syndrome, recent trophoblastic disease.

*Possible interaction*: phenytoin, carbamazepine, tetracyclines, primidone, chloral hydrate, glutethimide, phenylbutazone, rifampicin, griseofulvin, ampicillin, dichloralphenazone, ethosuximide, barbiturates, St John's Wort.

*Side effects*: feeling of bloatedness due to fluid retention, leg pains, breast enlargement, erosion of cervix, muscular cramps, weight gain, breakthrough bleeding, depression, headaches, vaginal discharge, loss of libido, nausea, brown patches on skin (chloasma). Stop drug immediately in event of pregnancy, if frequent, severe headaches occur or signs of thromboses, severe pain in upper abdominal region, enlarged liver, jaundice, rise in blood pressure, severe depression, increased number of fits. Drug should be discontinued 6 weeks before major planned surgery and re-started 2 weeks afterwards, as long as woman is fully mobile. Should be discontinued during long periods of immobility.

*Manufacturer*: Schering H.C.

## LOGYNON ED

*Description*: a hormonal contraceptive preparation containing oestrogen and progestogen available as sugar-coated tablets. 6 brown tablets contain 30µg of ethinylestradiol and 50µg of levonorgestrel; 5 white tablets contain 40µg of ethinylestradiol and 75µg of levonorgestrel; 10 ochre coloured tablets contain 30µg of ethinylestradiol and 125µg of levonorgestrel; 7 white tablets contain inert lactose (a form of sugar).

*Used for*: oral contraception.

*Dosage*: women, 1 tablet daily in order directed on packet, for 28 days starting on the first day of the cycle. Start new pack straight away.

*Special care*: hypertension, severe kidney disease receiving dialysis, Raynaud's disease, diabetes, multiple sclerosis, asthma, varicose veins, elevated levels of prolactin (a hormone) in the blood (hyperprolactinemia). Risk of thrombosis increases with smoking, age and obesity. Blood pressure, breasts and pelvic organs should be checked during period of treatment.

*Avoid use*: pregnancy, heart and circulatory diseases, angina, sickle cell anaemia, pulmonary hypertension. Also hormone-dependent cancers, undiagnosed vaginal bleeding, chorea, liver disease, history of cholestatic jaundice of pregnancy, infectious hepatitis, Dublin–Johnson syndrome, Rotor syndrome, recent trophoblastic disease.

*Possible interaction*: phenytoin, carbamazepine, tetracyclines, primidone, chloral hydrate, glutethimide, phenylbutazone, rifampicin, griseofulvin, ampicillin, dichloralphenazone, ethosuximide, barbiturates, St John's Wort.

*Side effects*: feeling of bloatedness due to fluid retention, leg pains, breast enlargement, erosion of cervix, muscular cramps, weight gain, breakthrough bleeding, depression, headaches, vaginal discharge, loss of libido, nausea, brown patches on skin (chloasma). Stop drug immediately in event of pregnancy, if frequent, severe headaches occur or signs of thromboses, severe pain in upper abdominal region, enlarged liver, jaundice, rise in blood pressure, severe depression, increased number of fits.

Drug should be discontinued 6 weeks before major planned surgery and re-started 2 weeks afterwards, as long as woman is fully mobile. Should be discontinued during long periods of immobility.

*Manufacturer*: Schering H.C.

## LOMONT

*Description*: a tricyclic antidepressant (TCAD), available as a suspension containing 70mg of lofepramine, as hydrochloride, per 5ml.

*Used for*: depression.

*Dosage*: adults, 5ml 2 to 3 times each day.

*Special care*: patients with psychoses or suicidal tendencies, elderly persons, pregnant and nursing mothers, people with cardiac disorders, epilepsy, hyperthyroidism, urine retention, closed angle glaucoma, liver disease, tumours of adrenal gland, diabetes.

*Avoid use*: children, patients with recent heart attack, heart arrhythmias, heart block, porphyria (rare blood disorder).

*Possible interaction*: alcohol, barbiturate drugs, local anaesthetics (containing adrenaline or noradrenaline), antihypertensive and sympathomimetic drugs, anticholinergic drugs, cimetidine, oestrogens.

*Side effects*: anticholinergic effects including urine retention, dry mouth, constipation, blurred vision, rapid heartbeat, palpitations, nervousness, insomnia, sweating, dizziness, fatigue, weight changes, jaundice, blood changes, allergic skin rashes, changes in libido, breast enlargement and impotence.

*Manufacturer*: Rosemont.

## LOMOTIL

*Description*: an opiate and anticholinergic preparation available as white tables marked SEARLE, containing 2.5mg of diphenoxylate hydrochloride and 25μg of atropine sulphate.

*Used for*: diarrhoea.

*Dosage*: adults, 4 tablets to begin with then half this dose every 6 hours until control is achieved. Children, aged 13 to 16 years, 2 tablets 3 times each day; aged 9 to 12 years, 1 tablet 4 times each day; aged 4 to 8 years, 1 tablet 3 times each day.

*Special care*: pregnancy, breastfeeding, liver disorder; severe dehydration or imbalance of electrolytes must be treated before therapy begins.

*Avoid use*: children under 4 years, acute ulcerative colitis, obstruction in the intestines, jaundice, pseudomembranous colitis (a severe form of colitis).

*Possible interaction*: drugs depressing the central nervous system, MAOIs (monoamine oxidase inhibitors).

*Side effects*: allergic reactions, gastro-intestinal upset, disturbances of the central nervous system, anticholinergic effects.

*Manufacturer*: Goldshield.

## LOPERAMIDE *SEE*: IMODIUM.

## LOPRESOR

*Description*: a cardioselective ß-blocker available as film-coated, scored tablets in 2 strengths; pink tablets contain

50mg of metoprolol tartrate and light blue tablets contain 100mg, all marked GEIGY. *Also,* **LOPRESOR SR**, available as scored, yellow, sustained-release capsule-shaped tablet marked CG/CG and CDC/CDC on the reverse, containing 200mg of metoprolol tartrate.

*Used for*: prevention of mortality after myocardial infarction (MI), supraventricular arrhythmias (Lopressor only), angina, high blood pressure, additional treatment in thyrotoxicosis, prevention of migraine.

*Dosage*: adults, Lopressor, see literature for initial dosage after MI, 200mg each day for maintenance with treatment continuing for at least 3 months. Arrhythmias, 50mg twice or 3 times each day to a daily maximum of 300mg. Angina, Lopressor, 50–100mg 2 or 3 times each day; Lopressor SR, 1 tablet each day, increasing to 2, once per day if necessary. High blood pressure, Lopressor, 100mg daily to begin with, increasing if necessary to 200mg in 1 or more divided doses; Lopressor SR, 1 tablet each day taken in the morning. Thyrotoxicosis, Lopressor, 50mg, 4 times each day or 1 tablet of Lopresor SR in the morning. Migraine, Lopressor, 100–200mg each day in divided doses or 1x Lopressor SR taken in the morning.

*Special care*: pregnancy, breast-feeding, liver or kidney disease, diabetes, metabolic acidosis, poor cerebral blood supply, history of bronchospasm, those undergoing anaesthesia; patients with weak hearts should be treated with digitalis and diuretics. Drug should be stopped gradually.

*Avoid use*: children, patients with asthma, heart diseases

including heart block, heart shock, slow heartbeat rate, heart failure.

*Possible interaction*: cardiac depressants,anaesthetics, reserpine, sedatives, class II calcium antagonists, antihypertensives, sympathomimetics, cimetidine, indometacin, ergotamine, class I antiarrhythmic drugs, verapamil, clonidine withdrawal, hypoglycaemics, rifampicin, warfarin, ibuprofen.

*Side effects*: sleep disturbance, cold feet and hands, slow heartbeat, fatigue on exercise, wheeziness, heart failure, gastro-intestinal disorders; dry eyes or skin rash (stop use gradually), hair loss, low blood pressure, thrombocytopenia (abnormal decline in blood platelets).

*Manufacturer*: Novartis.

## LORATADINE *SEE*: CLARITYN

## LORAZEPAM *SEE*: ATIVAN.

## LOSEC

*Description*: a proton pump inhibitor (limits the enzyme responsible for the final stage of stomach acid secretion), available as film-coated, oblong tablets in 3 different strengths, all containing enteric-coated pellets and marked with strength. Light pink tablets contain 10mg of omeprazole, darker pink tablets contain 20mg of omeprazole and brown-red tablets contain 40mg of omeprazole. *Also,* **LOSEC CAPSULES,** available in 3 different strengths, all containing enteric-coated granules.

Pink capsules, marked A/OS and 10, contain 10mg of omeprazole; brown/pink capsules marked A/OM and 20, contain 20mg of omeprazole; brown capsules, marked A/OL and 40, contain 40mg of omeprazole. *Also,* **LOSEC INFUSION,** available as a powder in vials for reconstitution containing 40mg of omeprazole. *Also,* **LOSEC INJECTION,** available as a powder in vials with solvent containing 40mg of omeprazole.

*Used for*: tablets and capsules, GORD (oesophageal reflux disease), reflux oesophagitis, duodenal and benign gastric ulcers, prevention and treatment of ulcers caused by NSAIDs in susceptible patients, relief of symptoms of acid indigestion, additional treatment with antibiotics to eliminate *H. pylori* in duodenal and stomach ulcers, Zollinger–Ellison (ZE) syndrome, in patients undergoing general anaesthesia, to prevent acid aspiration. Infusion and injection, prevention of aspiration of acid in patients undergoing general anaesthesia, short-term treatment of duodenal or stomach ulcers and reflux oesophagitis in patients unable to take tablets or capsules.

*Dosage*: adults, tablets or capsules: *GORD*, 20mg once each day for 4 weeks in first instance, then for further 4 to 8 weeks, if necessary, until completely healed. In cases that do not respond, 40mg can be taken. *Acid-reflux*, 10mg once each day for long-term treatment, increasing to 20mg once each day if flare-up occurs. *Ulcers associated with NSAIDs*, 20mg once each day. *Acid indigestion*, 10 to 20mg once each day for 2 to 4 weeks at first and then evaluate/investigate if response is poor. *To heal a duodenal ulcer*, usually 20mg (40mg in severe cases) once each day for 4 weeks; *prevention of relapse*, 10mg once each day, increasing to 20mg if relapse occurs. As component of *triple therapy in duodenal ulcer to eliminate H. pylori*, 40mg once each day or 20mg twice each day with 500mg of amoxicillin and 400mg of metronidazole, both 3 times each day for 1 week. Or, with 250mg of clarithromycin and 400mg of metronidazole twice each day for 1 week. Or, 1g of amoxicillin and 500mg of clarithromycin 3 times each day for 2 weeks. As component of *dual therapy in duodenal ulcer for elimination of H. pylori*, 20mg twice each day or 40mg once each day with 750mg to 1g of amoxicillin twice each day for 2 weeks, or with 500mg of clarithromycin 3 times each day for 2 weeks. *Treatment of stomach ulcer*, usually 20mg (40mg in severe cases) once each day for 8 weeks. As component of *dual therapy in stomach ulcer to eliminate H. pylori*, 20mg twice each day or 40mg once each day with 750mg to 1g of amoxicillin twice each day for 2 weeks. *Z-E syndrome*, 60mg once each day at first then adjusted according to response. Usual maintenance is in order of 20 to 120mg each day with higher doses over 80mg given as 2 divided doses. *Prevention of acid aspiration in anaesthesia*, 40mg on the night before surgery then 40mg 6 to 2 hours before operation. Children over 2 years, for treatment of severe GORD with ulceration only, 0.7 to 1.4mg per kg of body weight each day for 1 to 3 months with a maximum daily dose of 40mg. Adults, infusion or injection, *prevention of acid aspiration in patients undergoing anaesthesia*, 40mg by slow intravenous injection or infusion 1 hour before operation. *Other conditions,* 40mg once each day in same way for a maximum of 5 days. Not for children.

*Special care*: liver disease, in suspected stomach ulcer, malignancy must be excluded prior to treatment.

*Avoid use*: children (except for GORD), pregnancy, breastfeeding.

*Possible interaction*: warfarin, ketoconazole, digoxin, phenytoin, itraconazole, diazepam.

*Side effects*: dizziness, headache, skin rashes, gastrointestinal upset, muscle and joint pains, sleepiness, numbness/tingling/pins-and-needles extremities, raised liver enzymes, risk of infections in gastrointestinal tract. Any adverse side effects with infusion must be reported to the Committee on the Safety of Medicines (CSM).

*Manufacturer*: Novartis.

## LUDIOMIL

*Description*: a tetracyclic antidepressant available as film-coated tablets in 4 different strengths, all containing maprotiline hydrochloride. Pale yellow tablets contain 10mg, marked Co; greyish-red tablets contain 25mg, marked DP; light orange tablets contain 50mg, marked ER and brown-orange tablets contain 75mg, marked FS. All are also marked CIBA.

*Used for*: depression.

*Dosage*: adults, 25–75mg each day to start with in 1 or 3 divided doses, modifying after 1 or 2 weeks as required to a maximum of 150mg daily. Elderly, 30mg once each day at first or 3 doses of 10mg each day. Can be gradually increased over 1 to 2 weeks to 75mg once each day or 25mg 3 times each day.

*Special care*: pregnancy, breastfeeding, elderly, cardiovascular disease, cyclic affective disorder, receiving electroconvulsive therapy, schizophrenia, low blood pressure on rising upright, over-active thyroid gland, previous urine retention, chronic constipation, raised pressure within eye, suicidal tendencies, chronic constipation, contact lens wearers. Blood counts, liver and kidney function and teeth should be monitored along with indications of low blood sodium levels.

*Avoid use*: children, severe liver or kidney disease, narrow-angle glaucoma, mania, history of epilepsy, urine retention, recent heart attack, poisoning with drugs, alcohol or depressants of central nervous system, conduction defects.

*Possible interaction*: sympathomimetics, SSRIs, altretamine, barbiturates, ß-blockers, MAOIs, antiviral drugs, levacetylmethadol, antipsychotics, quinidine, anticholinergic drugs, tramadol, alcohol, opioids, methylphenidate, antihypertensives, anticonvulsants, neuroleptics, anaesthetics, diuretics, antidiabetic agents, cimetidine, phenytoin, benzodiazepines adrenergic neurone blockers, muscle relaxants, drugs that induce liver enzymes, coumarins, nefopam, rifampicin.

*Side effects*: skin rash, light-headedness, tiredness, fatigue, convulsions, headaches, dry mouth, cardiovascular, neurological and anticholinergic effects.

*Manufacturer*: Novartis.

## LUSTRAL

*Description*: an antidepressant and 5HT reuptake inhibitor, available as scored, white, capsule-shaped tablets in two strengths containing 50 or 100mg of sertraline hydrochloride and marked PFIZER with LTL-50 or LTL-100 respectively.

*Used for*: depression and anxiety, prevention of relapse or further bouts of depression, obsessive compulsive disorder, post-traumatic stress disorders in women.

*Dosage*: adults, depression with anxiety, 50mg each day to begin, with the dose being continued for maintenance; obsessive compulsive disorder, 50mg once each day at first with the usual maintenance being in the order of 50 to 200mg each day. Post-traumatic stress disorder, 25mg once each day at first for 1 week then a maintenance dose of 50mg once each day. Any dose increases should be implemented carefully by 50mg increments over several weeks to a daily maximum of 200mg. Then the lowest effective dose should be used for maintenance. Children, for obsessive compulsive disorder only and to be supervised by specialist physician, aged 6 to 12 years, 25mg each day at first for 1 week, then increasing to 50mg daily. Aged 13 to 17 years, 50mg each day at first, increasing if necessary at weekly intervals by 50mg increments to a daily maximum of 200mg.

*Special care*: pregnancy, breastfeeding, diabetes, epilepsy, anyone undergoing electroconvulsive therapy, kidney disease, mild to moderate liver disease, previous mania or hypomania, suicidal tendencies. Drug should be stopped if patient develops manic phase. Risk of bleeding disorders affecting skin (e.g. purpura) in patients with history of bleeding or those taking antiplatelet drugs. Drug should be gradually withdrawn.

*Avoid use*: children under 6 years, severe liver disorders.

*Possible interaction*: lithium, tryptophan, MAOIs, moclobemide, selegiline, sumatriptan, tramadol, TCADs, fenfluramine, cimetidine, NSAIDs, other serotonergic agents, tolbutamide, warfarin, drugs acting on central nervous system, drugs affecting blood platelets, St John's Wort.

*Side effects*: nausea, diarrhoea, tremor, increased sweating, indigestion, dry mouth, delay in ejaculation, insomnia, sleepiness, dizziness, muscle and joint pains, headaches, malaise, skin rashes, vision disturbance, rapid heartbeat, feelings of panic, low blood pressure on rising upright, nervousness, angioedema (in which there is widespread swelling) anaphylactoid reactions, raised prolactin levels in blood, symptoms of depersonalisation. Symptoms of serotonin syndrome, retention of urine, aggression, psychotic reactions, disordered movements. Withdraw drug immediately in event of fits occurring. In rare cases, pancreatitis, severe liver effects, low blood sodium levels, abnormal platelet function and laboratory test results, appearance of mania or hypomania. Withdrawal of symptoms when drug is stopped.

*Manufacturer*: Pfizer.

# M

## MMR II

*Description*: a combined preparation of live attenuated virus available as a powder in single dose vials with diluent for in pre-prepared syringes. Contains at least 1000 TCID50 of measles virus, at least 20000 TCID50 of mumps virus and at least 1000 TCID50 of rubella virus and 0.025mg of neomycin in each dose.

*Used for*: immunisation of children (and some adults) against measles, mumps and German measles

*Dosage*: children aged over 12 months, 1 full dose of vaccine by subcutaneous or intramuscular injection.

*Special care*: infections and fevers, brain injury, known allergy to egg proteins.

*Avoid use*: pregnancy, women should avoid conception within 3 months of receiving vaccine, previous anaphylactoid-type allergic reactions to vaccine or to neomycin, lowered immunity. Should not be given within 4 weeks of receiving other live vaccine or within 12 weeks of receiving blood transfusion or immunoglobulin.

*Side effects*: fever, nausea, rash, malaise, reactions at injection site, short-lived joint pains.

*Manufacturer*: Aventis Pasteur MSD.

## MAALOX

*Description*: an antacid preparation available as a suspension containing 220mg of dried aluminium hydroxide gel and 195mg of magnesium hydroxide (co-magaldrox 195/220) per 5ml. *Also,* **MAALOX PLUS SUSPENSION,** antacid and deflatulent preparation containing 220mg of dried aluminium hydroxide gel, 195mg of magnesium hydroxide and 25mg of activated dimeticone per 5ml. *Also,* **MAALOX TC SUSPENSION,** containing 600mg of dried aluminium hydroxide gel and 300mg of magnesium hydroxide (co-magaldrox 300/600) per 5ml.

*Used for*: Maalox and Maalox Plus, acid indigestion, heartburn, gastritis, over-secretion of stomach acid, wind. Maalox TC, treatment of duodenal ulcer and prevention of recurrence, stomach ulcer, heartburn, over-secretion of stomach acid.

*Dosage*: adults, Maalox and Maalox Plus, 5 to 10ml taken 20 minutes to 1 hour after a meal with a further dose at bedtime. Maalox TC, treatment of duodenal ulcer, 15ml 4 times each day taken 1 hour after meals and at bedtime; prevention, 15ml taken in morning after breakfast and a further 15ml dose in the evening. Over-secretion of stomach acid, 5 to 10ml 4 times each day, taken 20 minutes to 1 hour after meals and at bedtime.

*Possible interaction*: tetracyclines.

*Manufacturer*: R.P.R.

**MAGNESIUM ALGINATE *SEE*: GAVISCON INFANT.**

**MAGNESIUM HYDROXIDE *SEE*: MAALOX.**

**MAGNESIUM OXIDE *SEE*: KOLANTICON.**

## MAGNESIUM TRISILICATE *SEE*: GASTROCOTE, GAVISCON.

## MANEVAC

*Description*: a laxative preparation which is a bulking and stimulant agent, available as sugar-coated granules for adding to water containing 2.08g of plantago ovata seeds, 0.088g of ispaghula husks and 0.4 to 0.526g of senna pods per 5ml, when made up in solution.
*Used for*: constipation.
*Dosage*: adults, 5 to 10ml taken at night with a further dose before breakfast, if necessary; in severe cases, 10ml every 6 hours for a maximum of 3 days. Children over 5 years, 5ml each day.
*Avoid use*: children under 5 years, obstruction of intestine.
*Side effects*: wind, bloating, diarrhoea.
*Manufacturer*: Galen.

## MAPROTILINE HYDROCHLORIDE *SEE*: LUDIOMIL.

## MARVELON

*Description*: a hormonal, combined oestrogen/progestogen oral contraceptive preparation available as white tablets containing 30mg of ethinylestradiol and 150µg of desogestrel, marked ORGANON, TR over 5 and with *.
*Used for*: oral contraception.
*Dosage*: 1 tablet each day for 21 days, starting on first or fifth day of monthly cycle, followed by 7 tablet-free days.
*Special care*: hypertension, severe kidney disease receiving

dialysis, Raynaud's disease, diabetes, multiple sclerosis, asthma, varicose veins, elevated levels of prolactin (a hormone) in the blood (hyperprolactinemia). Risk of thrombosis increases with smoking, age and obesity. Blood pressure, breasts and pelvic organs should be checked during period of treatment.

*Avoid use*: pregnancy, heart and circulatory diseases, angina, sickle cell anaemia, pulmonary hypertension. Also hormone-dependent cancers, undiagnosed vaginal bleeding, chorea, liver disease, history of cholestatic jaundice of pregnancy, infectious hepatitis, Dublin–Johnson syndrome, Rotor syndrome, recent trophoblastic disease.

*Possible interaction*: phenytoin, carbamazepine, tetracyclines, primidone, chloral hydrate, glutethimide, phenylbutazone, rifampicin, griseofulvin, ampicillin, dichloralphenazone, ethosuximide, barbiturates, St John's Wort.

*Side effects*: feeling of bloatedness due to fluid retention, leg pains, breast enlargement, erosion of cervix, muscular cramps, weight gain, breakthrough bleeding, depression, headaches, vaginal discharge, loss of libido, nausea, brown patches on skin (chloasma). Stop drug immediately in event of pregnancy, if frequent, severe headaches occur or signs of thromboses, severe pain in upper abdominal region, enlarged liver, jaundice, rise in blood pressure, severe depression, increased number of fits. Drug should be discontinued 6 weeks before major planned surgery and re-started 2 weeks afterwards, as

long as woman is fully mobile. Should be discontinued during long periods of immobility.
*Manufacturer*: Organon.

## MAXITROL

*Description*: a compound preparation in the form of eyedrops combining a corticosteroid, aminoglycoside, lubricant and peptide. It contains 0.1% dexamethasone, 0.35% neomycin sulphate, 0.5% hypromellose, 6000 units polymyxin B sulphate/ml. Also MAXITROL OINTMENT containing 0.1% dexa-methasone, 0.35% neomycin sulphate and 6000iu polymixin B sulphate per gram.
*Used for*: infected and inflamed conditions of the eye.
*Dosage*: drops, insert 1 to 2 drops 4, 5 or 6 times each day; ointment, apply 3 or 4 times each day.
*Special care*: long-term use by pregnant women or in babies.
*Avoid use*: patients with glaucoma, tuberculous, viral or fungal infections or those producing pus; patients with soft contact lenses.
*Side effects*: cataract, thinning of cornea, rise in pressure within eye, fungal infection.
*Manufacturer*: Alcon.

## MEDROXYPROGESTERONE *SEE*: DEPO-PROVERA, INDIVINA, PREMIQUE, TRIDESTRA.

## MELOXICAM *SEE*: MOBIC.

## MELPHALAN *SEE*: ALKERAN.

## MENGIVAC (A + C)

*Description*: a vaccine preparation containing inactivated surface antigen of meningitis A and C. It is produced as a powder in vials, with diluent, containing 50μg of both group A and group C polysaccharide antigens of *Neisseria meningitidis*.

*Used for*: immunisation against meningitis, types A and C.

*Dosage*: adults and children over eighteen months, 0.5ml by deep subcutaneous or intramuscular injection.

*Special care*: pregnancy, breastfeeding.

*Avoid use*: patients with severe infections and feverish illnesses.

*Possible interaction*: agents which suppress the immune system.

*Side effects*: local skin reactions, slight fever.

*Manufacturer*: Aventis Pasteur MSD

## MENINGITEC

*Description*: a preparation of conjugated vaccine available as a suspension in vials comprising 10μg of meningococcal group C oligosaccharide per 0.5ml of suspension conjugated to *Corynebacterium diphtheriae* protein.

*Used for*: immunisation against meningitis, Type C.

*Dosage*: adults, 0.5ml by intramuscular injection; children aged 2 months to 1 year, 0.5ml by intramuscular injection with 2 further doses at intervals of at least 1 month; aged over 1 year, single 0.5ml dose given intramuscularly.

*Avoid use*: severe infections.

*Possible interaction*: immunosuppressant drugs.

*Side effects*: soreness at injection site, headache, feverishness, irritability, muscle pains, gastrointestinal upset, sleepiness. All adverse side effects should be reported to the Committee on the Safety of Medicines (CSM).

*Manufacturer*: Wyeth.

## MENOREST

*Description*: a hormonal, oestrogen preparation available as skin patches delivering either 37.5µg, 50µg or 75µg of oestradiol per 24 hours.

*Used for*: HRT for naturally occurring menopausal symptoms or those caused by surgery, prevention of osteoporosis after the menopause.

*Dosage*: all patches should be applied to clean, hairless area of skin below the waist and renewed every 3 or 4 days to a new area. Start with 50µg patch then adjust at 4 week intervals according to response, to achieve lowest effective dose. Continue to use 50µg strength for prevention of osteoporosis. In women with intact womb, a progestogen must also be taken for at least 12 days each month.

*Special care*: hypertension, severe kidney disease receiving dialysis, Raynaud's disease, diabetes, multiple sclerosis, asthma, varicose veins, elevated levels of prolactin (a hormone) in the blood (hyperprolactinemia). Risk of thrombosis increases with smoking, age and obesity. Blood pressure, breasts and pelvic organs should be checked during period of treatment.

*Avoid use*: pregnancy, heart and circulatory diseases, angina, sickle cell anaemia, pulmonary hypertension. Also hormone-dependent cancers, undiagnosed vaginal bleeding, chorea, liver disease, history of cholestatic jaundice of pregnancy, infectious hepatitis, Dublin–Johnson syndrome, Rotor syndrome, recent trophoblastic disease.

*Possible interaction*: phenytoin, carbamazepine, tetracyclines, primidone, chloral hydrate, glutethimide, phenylbutazone, rifampicin, griseofulvin, ampicillin, dichloralphenazone, ethosuximide, barbiturates, St John's Wort.

*Side effects*: feeling of bloatedness due to fluid retention, leg pains, breast enlargement, erosion of cervix, muscular cramps, weight gain, breakthrough bleeding, depression, headaches, vaginal discharge, loss of libido, nausea, brown patches on skin (chloasma). Stop drug immediately in event of pregnancy, if frequent, severe headaches occur or signs of thromboses, severe pain in upper abdominal region, enlarged liver, jaundice, rise in blood pressure, severe depression, increased number of fits. Drug should be discontinued 6 weeks before major planned surgery and re-started 2 weeks afterwards, as long as woman is fully mobile. Should be discontinued during long periods of immobility.

*Manufacturer*: Novartis.

## MERCILON

*Description*: a combined, hormonal oestrogen/progestogen preparation available as white tablets containing 20μg of ethinylestradiol and 150μg of desogestrel, marked TR over 4.

*Used for*: oral contraception.

*Dosage*: 1 tablet each day for 21 days starting on first or fifth day of monthly cycle, followed by 7 tablet-free days.

*Special care*: hypertension, severe kidney disease receiving dialysis, Raynaud's disease, diabetes, multiple sclerosis, asthma, varicose veins, elevated levels of prolactin (a hormone) in the blood (hyperprolactinemia). Risk of thrombosis increases with smoking, age and obesity. Blood pressure, breasts and pelvic organs should be checked during period of treatment.

*Avoid use*: pregnancy, heart and circulatory diseases, angina, sickle cell anaemia, pulmonary hypertension. Also hormone-dependent cancers, undiagnosed vaginal bleeding, chorea, liver disease, history of cholestatic jaundice of pregnancy, infectious hepatitis, Dublin–Johnson syndrome, Rotor syndrome, recent trophoblastic disease.

*Possible interaction*: phenytoin, carbamazepine, tetracyclines, primidone, chloral hydrate, glutethimide, phenylbutazone, rifampicin, griseofulvin, ampicillin, dichloralphenazone, ethosuximide, barbiturates, St John's Wort.

*Side effects*: feeling of bloatedness due to fluid retention, leg pains, breast enlargement, erosion of cervix, muscular cramps, weight gain, breakthrough bleeding, depression, headaches, vaginal discharge, loss of libido, nausea, brown patches on skin (chloasma). Stop drug immediately in event of pregnancy, if frequent, severe headaches

occur or signs of thromboses, severe pain in upper abdominal region, enlarged liver, jaundice, rise in blood pressure, severe depression, increased number of fits. Drug should be discontinued 6 weeks before major planned surgery and re-started 2 weeks afterwards, as long as woman is fully mobile. Should be discontinued during long periods of immobility.

*Manufacturer*: Organon.

**MESALAZINE *SEE*: ASACOL.**

**MESTRANOL *SEE*: NORINYL-1.**

**METHYLCELLULOSE *SEE*: CELEVAC.**

**METHYLDOPA *SEE*: ALDOMET .**

**METHYLPHENIDATE *SEE*: RITALIN**

**METHYLPREDNISOLONE *SEE*: MEDRONE, SOLU-MEDRONE.**

**METIPRANOLOL *SEE*: MINIMS METIPRANOLOL.**

**METOPROLOL *SEE*: BETALOC, CO-BETALOC, LOPRESOR.**

**METRONIDAZOLE *SEE*: FLAGYL, HELIMET.**

## MICRALAX

*Description*: a laxative preparation which is a lubricant and faecal softener, available as a micro-enema containing 450mg of sodium citrate, 45mg of sodium alkylsulphoacetate and 5mg of sorbic acid per 5ml of solution.

*Used for*: constipation, bowel clearance in advance of proctoscopy, sigmoidoscopy, x-ray examination.

*Dosage*: adults and children over 3 years, 1 enema inserted to full extent of applicator nozzle.

*Avoid use*: children aged under 3 years, inflammatory conditions of the bowel.

*Manufacturer*: Celltech.

## MICROGYNON 30

*Description*: a hormonal oestrogen/progestogen combined preparation in the form of beige, sugar-coated tablets containing 30µg ethinylestradiol and 150µg levonorgestrel.

*Used for*: oral contraception.

*Dosage*: 1 tablet each day starting on first day of period, followed by 7 tablet-free days.

*Special care*: hypertension, severe kidney disease receiving dialysis, Raynaud's disease, diabetes, multiple sclerosis, asthma, varicose veins, elevated levels of prolactin (a hormone) in the blood (hyperprolactinemia). Risk of thrombosis increases with smoking, age and obesity. Blood pressure, breasts and pelvic organs should be checked during period of treatment.

*Avoid use*: pregnancy, heart and circulatory diseases, angina, sickle cell anaemia, pulmonary hypertension. Also hormone-dependent cancers, undiagnosed vaginal bleeding, chorea, liver disease, history of cholestatic jaundice of pregnancy, infectious hepatitis, Dublin–Johnson syndrome, Rotor syndrome, recent trophoblastic disease.

*Possible interaction*: phenytoin, carbamazepine, tetracyclines, primidone, chloral hydrate, glutethimide, phenylbutazone, rifampicin, griseofulvin, ampicillin, dichloralphenazone, ethosuximide, barbiturates, St John's Wort.

*Side effects*: feeling of bloatedness due to fluid retention, leg pains, breast enlargement, erosion of cervix, muscular cramps, weight gain, breakthrough bleeding, depression, headaches, vaginal discharge, loss of libido, nausea, brown patches on skin (chloasma). Stop drug immediately in event of pregnancy, if frequent, severe headaches occur or signs of thromboses, severe pain in upper abdominal region, enlarged liver, jaundice, rise in blood pressure, severe depression, increased number of fits. Drug should be discontinued 6 weeks before major planned surgery and re-started 2 weeks afterwards, as long as woman is fully mobile. Should be discontinued during long periods of immobility.

*Manufacturer*: Schering H.C.

## MICROGYNON 30 ED

*Description*: a hormonal preparation combining oestrogen and progestogen, available as a course comprising 21 sugar-coated, beige coloured tablets containing 30μg of ethinylestradiol and 150μg of levonorgestrel and 7 white, sugar-coated tablets containing lactose.

*Used for*: oral contraception.

*Dosage*: women, 1 tablet each day beginning with pill marked 'start' and continuing to take 1 tablet each day without a break.

*Special care*: hypertension, severe kidney disease receiving dialysis, Raynaud's disease, diabetes, multiple sclerosis, asthma, varicose veins, elevated levels of prolactin (a hormone) in the blood (hyperprolactinemia). Risk of thrombosis increases with smoking, age and obesity. Blood pressure, breasts and pelvic organs should be checked during period of treatment.

*Avoid use*: pregnancy, heart and circulatory diseases, angina, sickle cell anaemia, pulmonary hypertension. Also hormone-dependent cancers, undiagnosed vaginal bleeding, chorea, liver disease, history of cholestatic jaundice of pregnancy, infectious hepatitis, Dublin–Johnson syndrome, Rotor syndrome, recent trophoblastic disease.

*Possible interaction*: phenytoin, carbamazepine, tetracyclines, primidone, chloral hydrate, glutethimide, phenylbutazone, rifampicin, griseofulvin, ampicillin, dichloralphenazone, ethosuximide, barbiturates, St John's Wort.

*Side effects*: feeling of bloatedness due to fluid retention, leg pains, breast enlargement, erosion of cervix, muscular cramps, weight gain, breakthrough bleeding, depression, headaches, vaginal discharge, loss of libido, nausea, brown patches on skin (chloasma). Stop drug immediately in event of pregnancy, if frequent, severe headaches occur or signs of thromboses, severe pain in upper abdominal region, enlarged liver, jaundice, rise in blood pressure, severe depression, increased number of fits. Drug should be discontinued 6 weeks before major planned surgery and re-started 2 weeks afterwards, as long as woman is fully mobile. Should be discontinued during long periods of immobility.

*Manufacturer*: Schering H.C.

## MINIMS ARTIFICIAL TEARS

*Description*: preservative-free eye drops containing 0.44% hydroxyethylcellulose and 0.35% sodium chloride in single dose units.

*Used for*: deficiency of tears/dry eyes.

*Dosage*: insert drops as often as is needed.

*Manufacturer*: Chauvin.

## MINIMS METIPRANOLOL

*Description*: a ß-blocker produced in the form of preservative-free, single dose eyedrops in 2 strengths containing 0.1% and 0.3% metipranolol.

*Used for*: control of raised pressure within eye following surgery. Also, for chronic glaucoma in patients wearing soft contact lenses or who are allergic to preservatives.

*Dosage*: chronic glaucoma, 1 drop into eye twice each day. Control of pressure within eye after surgery, consult manufacturer's instructions.

*Special care*: pregnancy, sinus bradycardia (slow heartbeat rate), 2nd or 3rd degree heart block.

*Avoid use*: obstructive airways disease, heart failure,

bradyarrhythmias (heart arrhythmias in which the heartbeat rate is slow).
*Possible interaction*: other ß-blockers, verapamil.
*Side effects*: slight stinging and irritation, headache.
*Manufacturer*: Chauvin.

## MINIMS PILOCARPINE

*Description*: a miotic preparation (one which causes contraction of the pupil) which is a cholinergic agonist and acts to cause constriction of the ciliary eye muscle. This helps to open drainage channels hence reducing pressure within the eye. It is produced as preservative-free, single dose eyedrops in 3 strengths containing 1%, 2% and 4% pilocarpine nitrate.
*Used for*: emergency treatment of glaucoma. To reverse the effect of weak mydriatic drugs.
*Dosage*: 1 drop every 5 minutes until the pupil is contracted.
*Manufacturer*: Chauvin.

## MINOCYCLINE *SEE*: AKNEMIN.

## MINULET

*Description*: a hormonal combined oestrogen/progestogen preparation available as sugar-coated white tablets containing 30µg of ethinylestradiol and 75µg of gestodene.
*Used for*: oral contraception.
*Dosage*: 1 tablet each day for 21 days beginning on first day of period followed by 7 tablet-free days.
*Special care*: hypertension, severe kidney disease receiving

dialysis, Raynaud's disease, diabetes, multiple sclerosis, asthma, varicose veins, elevated levels of prolactin (a hormone) in the blood (hyperprolactinemia). Risk of thrombosis increases with smoking, age and obesity. Blood pressure, breasts and pelvic organs should be checked during period of treatment.

*Avoid use*: pregnancy, heart and circulatory diseases, angina, sickle cell anaemia, pulmonary hypertension. Also hormone-dependent cancers, undiagnosed vaginal bleeding, chorea, liver disease, history of cholestatic jaundice of pregnancy, infectious hepatitis, Dublin-Johnson syndrome, Rotor syndrome, recent trophoblastic disease.

*Possible interaction*: phenytoin, carbamazepine, tetracyclines, primidone, chloral hydrate, glutethimide, phenylbutazone, rifampicin, griseofulvin, ampicillin, dichloralphenazone, ethosuximide, barbiturates, St John's Wort.

*Side effects*: feeling of bloatedness due to fluid retention, leg pains, breast enlargement, erosion of cervix, muscular cramps, weight gain, breakthrough bleeding, depression, headaches, vaginal discharge, loss of libido, nausea, brown patches on skin (chloasma). Stop drug immediately in event of pregnancy, if frequent, severe headaches occur or signs of thromboses, severe pain in upper abdominal region, enlarged liver, jaundice, rise in blood pressure, severe depression, increased number of fits. Drug should be discontinued 6 weeks before major planned surgery and re-started 2 weeks afterwards, as

long as woman is fully mobile. Should be discontinued during long periods of immobility.
*Manufacturer*: Wyeth.

## MISOPROSTOL *SEE*: ARTHROTEC, CYTOTEC, NAPRATEC.

## MIZOLASTINE *SEE*: MIZOLLEN.

## MIZOLLEN

*Description*: an antihistamine preparation available as white, scored, oblong, film-coated, sustained-release tablets containing 10mg of mizolastine marked MZI 10.
*Used for*: seasonal or perennial allergic rhinoconjunctivitis, (hayfever producing symptoms affecting the eyes and nose), urticaria (allergic nettle rash).
*Dosage*: adults, 1 tablet each day.
*Special care*: elderly persons, diabetes.
*Avoid use*: children, pregnancy, breastfeeding, heart disease including arrhythmias, low blood potassium levels, slow heartbeat, severe liver disorder, prolonged QT interval.
*Possible interaction*: antiarrhythmics, cimetidine, macrolides, azole antifungals, imidazole antifungal drugs, ciclosporin, nifedipine, drugs that prolong QT interval.
*Side effects*: weakness, drowsiness, dry mouth, headache, gastrointestinal upset, increased appetite. *Manufacturer*: Schwarz.

## MOBIC

*Description*: an NSAID and oxicam available as scored, yellow tablets in 2 strengths, containing 7.5mg and 15mg of meloxicam all marked with logo and 59D or 77C, respectively. *Also*, **MOBIC SUPPOSITORIES**, available in 2 strengths containing 7.5mg and 15mg of meloxicam.

*Used for*: Mobic, rheumatoid arthritis, acute osteoarthritis, ankylosing spondylitis. Mobic suppositories, osteoarthritis, rheumatoid arthritis.

*Dosage*: adults, Mobic, rheumatoid arthritis and ankylosing spondylitis, 15mg once each day; osteoarthritis, 7.5mg once each day, taken with food at mealtime, increasing if needed to 15mg once daily. Elderly, 7.5mg once each day at first. Suppositories, osteoarthritis, 1x7.5mg each day increasing to 15mg daily, if needed; elderly, 7.5mg each day at first. Rheumatoid arthritis, 15mg each day; elderly, 7.5mg daily.

*Special care*: previous gastrointestinal problems, especially bleeding, kidney failure, nephrotic syndrome (kidney disorder), low circulating blood volume, cirrhosis of the liver, congestive heart failure.

*Avoid use*: children, pregnancy, breastfeeding, inflammation of rectum and anus (proctitis) (suppositories only), stomach ulcer or history of such, severe kidney or liver failure, allergy to aspirin or NSAIDs.

*Possible interaction*: IUDs, colestyramine, antihypertensives, other NSAIDs, methotrexate, anticoagulants, ciclosporin, lithium, thrombolytics, diuretics.

*Side effects*: gastrointestinal upset, bleeding, ulceration or perforation of gut – patient must be monitored and advised to report symptoms, effects on heart, circulation and central nervous system, sensitivity to light, skin reactions including rash, itching, allergic nettle rash, erythema multiforme, Stevens Johnson syndrome, angioedema (in which there is widespread swelling) short-lived changes in liver tests, blood changes.
*Manufacturer*: Boehringer Ing.

## MOBIFLEX

*Description*: an NSAID belonging to the oxicam group available as film-coated, pentagonal-shaped brown tablets containing 20mg tenoxicam marked MOBIFLEX. *Also*, **MOBIFLEX INJECTION** available as powder in vials for reconstitution containing 20mg of tenoxicam.
*Used for*: rheumatoid arthritis, osteoarthritis, treatment of soft tissue injuries, (short-term only).
*Dosage*: adults, 1 tablet each day; injection, 20mg by intravenous or intramuscular injection for first 1 or 2 days, then patient should be transferred to tablets. Elderly patients should be treated with lowest dose to be effective and monitored for bleeding in the gut during the first month of treatment.
*Special care*: elderly patients, those with liver, kidney or heart disease or heart failure, high blood pressure. Patients with heart disorders should be monitored if receiving long-term treatment.
*Avoid use*: children, pregnancy, inflammation of gastro-

intestinal tract or bleeding, history of or active stomach ulcer, allergy to NSAID or aspirin.

*Possible interaction*: hypoglycaemics taken by mouth, antihypertensive drugs, lithium, anticoagulants, other NSAIDs, methotrexate, cardiac glycosides, corticosteroids, quinolones, mifepristone, diuretics.

*Side effects*: headache, blood changes, skin rash, gastrointestinal upset, rise in level of liver enzymes, jaundice, haemolytic anaemia, aplastic anaemia, allergic responses, fluid retention, disturbance of vision, kidney toxicity. In rare cases, vasculitis (inflammation of veins), vesiculobullous reactions (eruption of fluid-filled blisters on skin or mucous membranes).

*Manufacturer*: Roche.

## MOEXIPRIL *SEE*: PERDIX.

## MOGADON

*Description*: a long-acting benzodiazepine preparation available as scored, white tablets containing 5mg of nitrazepam marked ICN.

*Used for*: insomnia which is very severe, short-term treatment only.

*Dosage*: adults, 5 to 10mg, elderly persons, 2.5 to 5mg, with doses taken at bedtime.

*Special care*: chronic liver, kidney or lung disease, acute, narrow-angle glaucoma, elderly persons, bereavement. May impair dexterity and judgement. Should not be used as sole therapy for depression or anxiety. To be withdrawn gradually.

*Avoid use*: children, pregnancy, breastfeeding, labour, acute lung disease, depression of the respiration, obsessional and phobic states, chronic psychosis. Also, myasthenia gravis, severe liver disorders, sleep apnoea syndrome

*Possible interaction*: anticonvulsants, CNS depressants, alcohol.

*Side effects*: confusion, vertigo, drowsiness, ataxia, lightheadedness, gastro-intestinal upsets, skin rashes, weakness in muscles, hypotension, disturbance in vision. Urine retention, changes in libido, impaired ability to perform tasks and in exercise of judgement; rarely, jaundice and effects on blood. Dependence is possible especially at higher doses and with longer treatment periods.

*Manufacturer*: ICN.

## MOLIPAXIN

*Description*: an antidepressant preparation available as pink, film-coated, scored tablets containing 150mg of trazodone hydrochloride, marked MOLIPAXIN 150. *Also,* **MOLIPAXIN CAPSULES,** in 2 strengths: green/purple capsules containing 50mg of trazodone hydrochloride marked with logo and R365B; fawn/purple capsules containing 100mg of trazodone hydrochloride marked with logo and R365C. *Also,* **MOLIPAXIN LIQUID** containing 50mg of trazodone hydrochloride per 5ml.

*Used for*: depression which may be accompanied by anxiety.

*Dosage*: adults, 150mg each day as divided doses taken after meals or as single night-time dose. Dose may be increased to 300mg each day with a daily maximum of 600mg. Elderly persons, 100mg each day in divided doses after meals or as a single night-time dose. Maximum of 300mg each day.

*Special care*: serious kidney, liver or heart disease, epilepsy.

*Avoid use*: children.

*Possible interaction*: digoxin, CNS depressants, alcohol, clonidine, phenytoin, muscle relaxants, MAOIs, volatile anaesthetics.

*Side effects*: dizziness, nausea, headache, low blood pressure on rising upright (postural hypotension), drowsiness, priapism (abnormal, persistent erection of penis, which is painful and not associated with sexual arousal) occurs, blood changes. Drug should be withdrawn if liver dysfunction occurs.

*Manufacturer*: Hoechst.

## MONOCOR

*Description*: an antianginal and antihypertensive preparation which is a cardioselective ß-blocker available as film-coated tablets in two strengths; pink, scored tablets contain 5mg of bisoprolol fumarate, marked 5 on one side and LL on the other. White tablets contain 10mg of bisoprolol fumarate marked 10 on one side and LL on the other.

*Used for*: angina and high blood pressure.

*Dosage*: usual dose is 10mg once each day with a maximum of 20mg.

Lopressor SR taken in the morning.

*Special care*: pregnancy, breast-feeding, liver or kidney disease, diabetes, metabolic acidosis, poor cerebral blood supply, history of bronchospasm, those undergoing anaesthesia; patients with weak hearts should be treated with digitalis and diuretics. Drug should be stopped gradually.

*Avoid use*: children, patients with asthma, heart diseases including heart block, heart shock, slow heartbeat rate, heart failure.

*Possible interaction*: cardiac depressants,anaesthetics, reserpine, sedatives, class II calcium antagonists, antihypertensives, sympathomimetics, cimetidine, indometacin, ergotamine, class I antiarrhythmic drugs, verapamil, clonidine withdrawal, hypoglycaemics, rifampicin, warfarin, ibuprofen.

*Side effects*: sleep disturbance, cold feet and hands, slow heartbeat, fatigue on exercise, wheeziness, heart failure, gastro-intestinal disorders; dry eyes or skin rash (stop use gradually), hair loss, low blood pressure, thrombocytopenia (abnormal decline in blood platelets).

*Manufacturer*: Wyeth.

## MORPHINE *SEE*: CYCLIMORPH.

## MOTENS

*Description*: an antihypertensive preparation and class II calcium antagonist available as white, film-coated tablets in 2 strengths containing 2mg and 4mg of lacidipine, marked 10L and 9L respectively, and with logo.

*Used for*: high blood pressure.

*Dosage*: adults, 2mg once each day as morning dose; may be increased after 3 or 4 weeks to 6mg once each day if needed.

*Special care*: weak heart, liver disease, disturbances of conduction (of electrical nerve impulses).

*Avoid use*: children, pregnancy, breast-feeding.

*Possible interaction*: cimetidine.

*Side effects*: palpitations, flushing, headache, dizziness, rash, fluid retention, polyuria (passing of large quantities of pale urine), increase in amount of gum tissue. Drug should be withdrawn if chest pain occurs.

*Manufacturer*: Boehringer Ing.

## MOTIFENE

*Description*: an NSAID and phenylacetic acid available as dual release, clear/blue capsules containing enteric coated and sustained-release pellets, comprising 75mg of diclofenac.

*Used for*: osteoarthritis, rheumatoid arthritis, ankylosing spondylitis, orthopaedic and back pain, disorders of muscles and joints, strains and sprains, toothache, minor surgical pain.

*Dosage*: adults, 1 tablet taken in the morning before breakfast, increasing if necessary to 1 tablet twice each day every 8 to 12 hours.

*Special care*: elderly, pregnancy, breastfeeding, heart, kidney or liver disorders, previous gastrointestinal lesions, blood abnormalities. Patients taking drug long-term should be monitored.

*Avoid use*: children, last 3 months of pregnancy, stomach ulcer or bleeding in gastrointestinal tract, known allergy to aspirin or NSAID, asthma.

*Possible interaction*: diuretics, methotrexate, quinolones, antidiabetic agents, ciclosporin, other NSAIDs, salicylates, digoxin, lithium, steroids, anticoagulants.

*Side effects*: short-lived stomach pain, gastrointestinal upset, fluid retention, headaches. In rare cases, stomach ulcer, blood changes, skin reactions, abnormal kidney and liver function.

*Manufacturer*: Sankyo.

## MOTRIN

*Description*: an NSAID and propionic acid, available in the form of capsule-shaped, film-coated, white tablets containing 800mg of ibuprofen.

*Used for*: pain, rheumatism and other bone and muscle disorders including osteoarthritis, rheumatoid arthritis, Still's disease, non-rheumatoid arthropathies and ankylosing spondylitis.

*Dosage*: adults, 1200–1800mg each day in 3 divided doses, the maximum being 2400mg daily. Children, 20mg per kg of body weight each day with a maximum dose of 500mg in 24 hours for children weighing less than 30kg. For juvenile rheumatoid arthritis, 40mg per kg of body weight may be given each day.

*Special care*: elderly, liver or kidney disorders, high blood pressure, heart disease, defects of blood coagulation, asthma, previous disorders of gastro-intestinal tract.

*Avoid use*: pregnancy, patients with known allergy to NSAID or aspirin, stomach ulcer.

*Possible interaction*: thiazide diuretics, anticoagulants, quinolones, cardiac glycosides, corticosteroids, antihypertensives, mifepristone, lithium, methotrexate.

*Side effects*: rash, gastro-intestinal disorder or bleeding, fluid retention, thrombocytopenia. Drug should be withdrawn if symptoms affecting eyes occur. All cases of a septic meningitis must be reported to the Committee on the Safety of Medicines (CSM).

*Manufacturer*: Pharmacia.

## MOVICOL

*Description*: an iso-osmotic laxative preparation available as a powder in single dose sachets for reconstitution with water, containing 13.125g of polyethylene glycol, 178.5mg of sodium bicarbonate, 350.7mg of sodium chloride and 46.6mg of potassium chloride.

*Used for*: impacted faeces and chronic constipation.

*Dosage*: contents of sachet should be reconstituted with 125ml of water; adults, constipation, 1 to 3 sachets each day in divided doses; if using long-term, 1 to 2 sachets each day. Faecal impaction, 8 sachets within 6 hours each day for up to 3 days, in accordance with manufacturer's literature.

*Avoid use*: children, inflammation of bowel, perforation or obstruction in gastrointestinal tract, toxic megacolon, ulcerative colitis, ileus (any form of intestinal obstruction including twisting of the gut).

*Side effects*: nausea, abdominal extension. In rare cases, allergic reactions.
*Manufacturer*: Norgine.

**MUPIROCIN *SEE*: BACTROBAN.**

# N

## NABUMETONE *SEE*: RELIFEX.

## NADOLOL *SEE*: CORGARD, CORGARETIC.

## NAPRATEC

*Description*: an NSAID and propionic acid/prostaglandin analogue, available as 56 scored, yellow oblong tablets containing 500mg of naproxen, marked Searle N500, and 56 scored, white hexagonal shaped tablets containing 200µg of misoprostol, marked Searle 1461, in a combined pack.

*Used for*: osteoarthritis, rheumatoid arthritis, ankylosing spondylitis where the stomach has to be protected against the medication.

*Dosage*: adults, 1 of each type of tablet taken twice each day with food.

*Special care*: asthma, liver or kidney damage, elderly, ulcerative colitis, Crohn's disease, disease of blood vessels. Effective contraception must be used by women of child-bearing age. Monitoring required for those taking drugs long-term.

*Avoid use*: children, pregnancy, breastfeeding, duodenal or gastric ulcer, allergy induced by aspirin or anti-inflammatory drugs.

*Possible interaction*: diuretics, anticoagulants, sulphonylureas, ciclosporin, quinolones, sulfonamides, hydantoins, lithium, ß-blockers, probenecid, corticosteroids, methotrexate.

*Side effects*: diarrhoea, abdominal pain, gastro-intestinal upset, vaginal bleeding, menorrhagia (long or heavy menstruation), rash, allergic skin reactions, headache, dizziness, tinnitus (ringing in ears), vertigo, blood changes.

*Manufacturer*: Pharmacia.

## NAPROSYN SR

*Description*: a propionic acid, available as white, scored, film-coated, capsule-shaped tablets containing 500mg of naproxen as sodium salt, marked 500. *Also*, **NAPROSYN EC**, available as enteric-coated, white tablets in 3 strengths containing 250mg, 375mg and 500mg of naproxen, marked NPR EC 250, Naprosyn EC and NPR EC 500, respectively. *Also,* **NAPROSYN TABLETS**, available as scored, buff-coloured tablets in 2 strengths containing 250mg of naproxen, marked NPR LE 250 and oval-shaped tablets containing 500mg of naproxen, marked NPR LE 500.

*Used for*: osteoarthritis, rheumatoid arthritis, ankylosing spondylitis, musculoskeletal disorders, acute gout, dysmenorrhea (painful periods).

*Dosage*: adults, Naprosyn SR, 1 or 2 tablets once each day swallowed whole; Naprosyn EC, Naprosyn tablets, 500 to 1000mg each day either as single dose taken at night or in the morning or as 2 divided doses at 12 hour intervals. For gout, 750mg at first then 250mg every 8 hours; for musculoskeletal disorders and dysmenorrhoea, 500mg to start with and then 250mg every 6 to 8 hours, as needed to a maximum of 1250mg daily after first day of treatment. Children, for juvenile rheumatoid arthritis (JRA) only, use Naprosyn tablets and Naprosyn EC only, aged 5 to 16 years, 10mg per kg of body weight each day in 2 divided doses at 12 hour intervals.

*Special care*: elderly, liver or kidney damage, heart failure, asthma, a history of gastro-intestinal lesions. Patients being treated long-term require monitoring.

*Avoid use*: pregnancy, breastfeeding, stomach ulcer, allergy caused by aspirin or anti-inflammatory drugs.

*Possible interaction*: ACE inhibitors, corticosteroids, ß-blockers, lithium, mifepristone, cardiac glycosides, anticoagulants, adrenal function tests, ciclosporin, quinolones, sulphonylureas, hydantoins, furosemide, methotrexate, diuretics, probenecid.

*Side effects*: headache, kidney and liver disorders, gastrointestinal intolerance, rash, vertigo, blood changes, tinnitus (ringing in ears).

*Manufacturer*: Roche.

## NAPROXEN *SEE*: NAPRATEC, NAPROSYN, NYCOPREN, SYNFLEX.

## NEBILET

*Description*: an antihypertensive and cardioselective ß-blocker available as scored, white tablets containing 5mg of nebivolol hydrochloride.

*Used for*: high blood pressure.

*Dosage*: adults, 5mg each day; elderly patients should receive 2.5mg at first, increasing to 5mg each day if needed.

*Special care*: pregnancy, breast-feeding, liver or kidney disease, diabetes, metabolic acidosis, poor cerebral blood supply, history of bronchospasm, those undergoing anaesthesia; patients with weak hearts should be treated with digitalis and diuretics. Drug should be stopped gradually.

*Avoid use*: children, patients with asthma, heart diseases including heart block, heart shock, slow heartbeat rate, heart failure.

*Possible interaction*: cardiac depressants, anaesthetics, reserpine, sedatives, class II calcium antagonists, antihypertensives, sympathomimetics, cimetidine, indometacin, ergotamine, class I antiarrhythmic drugs, verapamil, clonidine withdrawal, hypoglycaemics, rifampicin, warfarin, ibuprofen.

*Side effects*: sleep disturbance, cold feet and hands, slow heartbeat, fatigue on exercise, wheeziness, heart failure, gastro-intestinal disorders; dry eyes or skin rash (stop use gradually), hair loss, low blood pressure, thrombocytopenia (abnormal decline in blood platelets).

*Manufacturer*: Menarini.

**NEBIVOLOL *SEE*: NEBILET .**

**NEDOCROMIL *SEE*: RAPITIL.**

**NEFOPAM HYDROCHLORIDE *SEE*: ACUPAN.**

## NEOMYCIN *SEE*: AUDICORT, BETNESOL-N, CICATRIN, DERMOVATE-NN, MAXITROL, NEOSPORIN, NIVEMYCIN, PREDSOL, SYNALAR-N.

## NEOSPORIN

*Description*: a peptide and aminoglycoside, available as eye drops containing 5000 units of polymixin B sulphate, 1700 units of neomycin sulphate and 25 units of gramicidin per ml.

*Used for*: bacterial eye infections, prevention of infections in the eye before and after surgery, removal of foreign bodies from the eye.

*Dosage*: 1 or 2 drops, 2 to 4 times each day.

*Special care*: do not allow access to fluids within eye.

*Manufacturer*: Dominion.

## NEXIUM

*Description*: a proton pump inhibitor available as film-coated, oblong, pink tablets in two strengths containing 20mg and 40mg of esomeprazole as magnesium trihydrate.

*Used for*: reflux oesophagitis which is causing erosion of the lining of the oesophagus, prevention of recurrence of reflux oesophagitis, treatment of symptoms of GORD. Also, with antibiotics, to eliminate *H. pylori* and to heal duodenal ulcers caused by *H. pylori*, prevention of recurrence of stomach ulcers associated with *H. pylori*.

*Dosage*: adults, reflux oesophagitis and erosion, 40mg once each day for 1 to 2 months; prevention of recurrence, 20mg once each day. GORD with no oesophagitis, 20mg once each day for 1 month then 20mg once each day, as needed, for maintenance. *H. pylori*, 20mg along with 1g of amoxicillin and 500mg of clarithromycin, all twice daily for 1 week. Tablets should be swallowed whole or mixed with plain water and drunk, but should not be chewed.

*Special care*: pregnancy, breastfeeding, severe kidney or liver disorders, long-term use. Possibility of malignancy should be ruled out before commencing treatment.

*Avoid use*: children.

*Possible interaction*: other drugs metabolised by CYP2C19, diazepam, phenytoin, warfarin, imipramine, ketoconazole, citalopram, itraconazole, clomipramine.

*Side effects*: dry mouth, gastrointestinal upset, skin effects, headache. In rare cases, anaphylaxis, angioedema (widespread swelling due to fluid retention).

*Manufacturer*: AstraZeneca.

## NICARDIPINE *SEE*: CARDENE.

## NICORETTE

*Description*: an alkaloid preparation available as skin patches in 3 strengths, releasing 5mg, 10mg or 15mg of nicotine every 16 hours.

*Used for*: as an aid to giving up smoking to replace nicotine. *Also*, **NICORETTE GUM,** plain or flavoured chewing gum containing 2mg and 4mg of nicotine. *Also*, **NICORETTE MICROTAB,** available as a tablet for placing beneath the tongue containing 2mg of nicotine. *Also,* **NICORETTE NASAL SPRAY,** available as a metered dose, nasal delivering 0.5mg per puff. *Also,* **NICORETTE INHALATOR,** available in a cartridges with a mouth-piece delivering 10mg of nicotine.

*Dosage*: adults, patches; 1x15mg patch applied to skin once each day for 2 months; then 1x10mg patch applied once each day for 2 weeks. Finally, 1x5mg patch once each day for 2 weeks. Patches should be adhered to a clean, non-hairy part of skin in morning, either on body or upper arm and removed after 16 hours, usually before going to bed. Gum, chew one piece slowly, as described in instructions, for half an hour, whenever there is a desire to smoke, to a maximum of 15 pieces each day. Slowly withdraw after using gum for 3 months. Microtabs, 1 or 2 tablets should be placed beneath the tongue, when there is an urge to smoke and allowed to dissolve slowly; maximum is 40 tablets daily for a minimum period of 3 months. Then, gradually reduce daily dose to 1 to 2 tablets each day before stopping completely. Inhalator, inhale 6 to 12 cartridges each day for 2 months then reduce the dose by half over the following 2 weeks. Finally, in next 2 weeks, reduce the daily dose to zero. Nasal spray, 1 spray into each side of nose, as needed, for first 2 months to a maximum of 64 daily or 1 in each nostril every half hour. Then, over following 2 weeks, reduce the dose gradually by half and then over next 2 weeks, further reduce to zero.

*Special care*: pregnancy, breastfeeding, diabetes, high blood pressure, peripheral disease of blood vessels, severe kidney disorders, recent heart attack, previous angina, serious heart arrhythmias, cerebrovascular event (stroke, etc.), overactive thyroid gland, gastritis, previous stomach ulcer, phaeochromocytoma (adrenal gland tumour). Patients should be advised not to smoke at all while using the product and not to combine with other preparations containing nicotine.

*Avoid use*: children under 18 years except under medical supervision.

*Possible interaction*: insulin, caffeine, adrenergic blockers and agonists, xanthines, oxazepam, paracetamol, pentazocine.

*Side effects*: gastrointestinal upset, hiccups, local irritation, over-production of saliva, palpitations, headaches, atrial fibrillation (heart flutter), dizziness, allergic reactions, dependence.

*Manufacturer*: Pharmacia.

## NICOTINE *SEE*: NICORETTE, NICOTINELL.

## NICOTINELL

*Description*: skin patches impregnated with nicotine at a concentration of 0.7mg per cm squared, in 3 sizes – 10, 20 and 30cm$^2$. *Also,* **NICOTINELL GUM,** fruit or mint-flavoured chewing gum containing 2mg and 4mg of nicotine.

*Used for*: to replace nicotine as an aid to giving up smoking.

*Dosage*: adults, patches, smoking more than 20 cigarettes daily, use one 30 square centimetre patch every 24 hours for 3 to 4 weeks, then reduce size of patch over next 3 to 4 week periods. Smoking less than 20 cigarettes each day, use one 20 square centimetre patch every 24 hours for 6 to 8 weeks, then one 10 square centimetre patch daily for next 3 to 4 weeks. In all cases, maximum period of treatment is 3 months. Patches should be adhered to clean, non-hairy area of skin on body or upper arm. Gum, chew one piece of gum slowly when there is a n urge to smoke, for half an hour to a maximum of 25 of 2mg strength or 15 of 4mg strength. Maximum treatment period is 3 months and then use of gum should be gradually stopped.

*Special care*: liver or kidney disease, angina, heart failure, peripheral vascular disease, high blood pressure, diabetes, overactive thyroid gland, cerebrovascular disease, stomach ulcer. Patients should not smoke while using the products and should carefully dispose of used patches.

*Avoid use*: children, pregnancy, breastfeeding, skin disorders, unstable angina, recent stroke, serious heart arrhythmias, people who smoke occasionally.

*Possible interaction*: warfarin, insulin, theophylline.

*Side effects*: dizziness, gastrointestinal upset, headache, local skin reactions with patches.

*Manufacturer*: Novartis Consumer.

**NIFEDIPINE *SEE*: ADALAT, BETA-ADALAT, CORACTEN.**

**NIMODIPINE *SEE*: NIMOTOP.**

## NIMOTOP

*Description*: a class II calcium antagonist available as film-coated, yellow tablets marked Bayer and SK, containing 30mg of nimodipine. *Also,* **NIMOTOP INFUSION**, a solution containing 0.2mg of nimodipine per ml in vials and bottles.

*Used for*: tablets, prevention of ischaemic, neurological defects after aneurysmal (ballooning in blood vessel) subarachnoid (intracranial) haemorrhage. Infusion, treatment of neurological deficits after aneurysmal subarachnoid haemorrhage.

*Dosage*: adults, 2 tablets every 4 hours commencing within 4 days of the haemorrhage and continuing for 21 days. Infusion, 1mg each hour by intravenous infusion for initial 2 hours, then 2mg per hour for 5 to 14 days. For bodyweights under 70kg, or for unstable blood pressure, start at 0.5mg per hour. Must be given with co-infusion running at 40ml per hour and should not be combined with Nimotop tablets.

*Special care*: pregnancy, raised intracranial pressure, cerebral oedema (fluid on the brain), kidney disease, low blood pressure (with infusion), liver cirrhosis. Check blood pressure. PVC apparatus should not be used—use polyethylene or polypropylene.

*Avoid use*: children.

*Possible interaction*: cimetidine, ß-blockers, anticonvulsants, nortriptyline, protease inhibitors, zidovudine, other calcium antagonists, methyldopa, azole antifungal drugs, sodium valproate, rifampicin, macrolides, fluoxetine, grapefruit juice, feeling of warmth, inflammation at injection site, short-lived rise in liver enzymes.

*Manufacturer*: Bayer.

## NISOLDIPINE *SEE*: SYSCOR MR.

## NITRAZEPAM *SEE*: MOGADON.

## NIVEMYCIN

*Description*: an antibacterial and aminoglycoside, available as tablets containing 500mg of neomycin sulphate.

*Used for*: preparation of bowel prior to surgery; additional therapy in hepatic (liver) coma.

*Dosage*: adults, beginning 2 to 3 days before operation, 2 tablets every hour for 4 hours then 2 tablets every 4 hours. Children, beginning 2 to 3 days before operation, aged 6 to 12 tears, 1/2 to 1 tablet every 4 hours; aged 12 years and over, 2 tablets every 4 hours.

*Special care*: pregnancy, breastfeeding, Parkinson's disease, kidney disorder, impaired motility of gastrointestinal tract, myasthenia gravis.

*Avoid use*: obstructed intestine.

*Possible interaction*: nephrotoxic (kidney) and ototoxic (affecting 8th cranial nerve or organs of balance and hearing) drugs, digoxin, contraceptive pill, neuromuscular blockers, penicillin V.

*Side effects*: gastrointestinal upset, nephrotoxicity, ototoxicity, allergic reaction, raised liver enzymes.

*Manufacturer*: Sovereign.

## NIZATIDINE *SEE*: AXID.

## NORETHISTERONE *SEE*: BINOVUM, BREVINOR, CLIMAGEST, CLIMESSE, ELLESTE DUET CONTI, ELLESTE DUET, ESTRACOMBI, EVOREL, EVOREL SEQUI, EVOREL - PAK, KLIOFEM, KLIOVANCE, LOESTRIN 20, LOESTRIN 30, NORIMIN, NORINYL -1, OVYSMEN, SYNPHASE, TRINOVUM.

## NORGALAX

*Description*: a laxative and faecal softener available as a single dose enema containing 120mg of docusate sodium in 10g.

*Used for*: constipation, emptying of bowel prior to endoscopic examination.

*Dosage*: adults, 1 enema as needed.

*Avoid use*: children, inflammation of bowel, obstruction of intestine.

*Side effects*: localised irritation.

*Manufacturer*: Norgine.

## NORGESTREL *SEE*: CYCLO-PROGYNOVA.

## NORIMIN

*Description*: a combined oestrogen/progestogen contraceptive available as white tablets containing 35μg of ethinylestradiol and 1mg of norethisterone tablet marked BX and SEARLE.

*Used for*: oral contraception.

*Dosage*: 1 tablet each day for 21 days, starting on 1st day of menstruation, then 7 days without tablets.

*Special care*: hypertension, severe kidney disease receiving dialysis, Raynaud's disease, diabetes, multiple sclerosis, asthma, varicose veins, elevated levels of prolactin (a hormone) in the blood (hyperprolactinemia). Risk of thrombosis increases with smoking, age and obesity. Blood pressure, breasts and pelvic organs should be checked during period of treatment.

*Avoid use*: pregnancy, heart and circulatory diseases, angina, sickle cell anaemia, pulmonary hypertension. Also hormone-dependent cancers, undiagnosed vaginal bleeding, chorea, liver disease, history of cholestatic jaundice of pregnancy, infectious hepatitis, Dublin–Johnson syndrome, Rotor syndrome, recent trophoblastic disease.

*Possible interaction*: phenytoin, carbamazepine, tetracyclines, primidone, chloral hydrate, glutethimide, phenylbutazone, rifampicin, griseofulvin, ampicillin, dichloralphenazone, ethosuximide, barbiturates, St John's Wort.

*Side effects*: feeling of bloatedness due to fluid retention, leg pains, breast enlargement, erosion of cervix, muscular cramps, weight gain, breakthrough bleeding, depression, headaches, vaginal discharge, loss of libido, nausea, brown patches on skin (chloasma). Stop drug immediately in event of pregnancy, if frequent, severe headaches occur or signs of thromboses, severe pain in upper abdominal region, enlarged liver, jaundice, rise in blood pressure, severe depression, increased number of fits.

Drug should be discontinued 6 weeks before major planned surgery and re-started 2 weeks afterwards, as long as woman is fully mobile. Should be discontinued during long periods of immobility.

*Manufacturer*: Pharmacia.

## NORINYL-1

*Description*: a combined oestrogen/progestogen contraceptive available as white tablets containing 50µg of mestranol and 1mg of norethisterone marked SEARLE and 1.

*Used for*: oral contraception.

*Dosage*: 1 tablet each day starting on 1st day of period, then 7 days without tablets.

*Special care*: hypertension, severe kidney disease receiving dialysis, Raynaud's disease, diabetes, multiple sclerosis, asthma, varicose veins, elevated levels of prolactin (a hormone) in the blood (hyperprolactinemia). Risk of thrombosis increases with smoking, age and obesity. Blood pressure, breasts and pelvic organs should be checked during period of treatment.

*Avoid use*: pregnancy, heart and circulatory diseases, angina, sickle cell anaemia, pulmonary hypertension. Also hormone-dependent cancers, undiagnosed vaginal bleeding, chorea, liver disease, history of cholestatic jaundice of pregnancy, infectious hepatitis, Dublin–Johnson syndrome, Rotor syndrome, recent trophoblastic disease.

*Possible interaction*: phenytoin, carbamazepine, tetracyclines, primidone, chloral hydrate, glutethimide, phenylbutazone, rifampicin, griseofulvin, ampicillin, dichloralphenazone, ethosuximide, barbiturates, St John's Wort.

*Side effects*: feeling of bloatedness due to fluid retention, leg pains, breast enlargement, erosion of cervix, muscular cramps, weight gain, breakthrough bleeding, depression, headaches, vaginal discharge, loss of libido, nausea, brown patches on skin (chloasma). Stop drug immediately in event of pregnancy, if frequent, severe headaches occur or signs of thromboses, severe pain in upper abdominal region, enlarged liver, jaundice, rise in blood pressure, severe depression, increased number of fits. Drug should be discontinued 6 weeks before major planned surgery and re-started 2 weeks afterwards, as long as woman is fully mobile. Should be discontinued during long periods of immobility.

*Manufacturer*: Pharmacia.

## NORMACOL

*Description*: a laxative and bulking agent, available as coated, white granules containing 62% sterculia, in 7g sachets. *Also,* **NORMACOL PLUS,** available as coated, brown granules containing 62% sterculia and 8% frangula in 7g sachets.

*Used for*: Normacol, constipation during pregnancy and that caused by a lack of fibre in the diet. Normacol Plus, constipation that has not responded to an initial increase in bulk in the diet.

*Dosage*: granules to be taken with a drink after meals and not chewed. Adults, 1 to 2 sachets or 1 to 2 heaped 5ml

spoonfuls, 1 to 2 times each day. Children, half adult dose, using Normacol or as advised, if using Normacol Plus.
*Special care*: do not take at bedtime; use of Normacol Plus during pregnancy.
*Avoid use*: total atony of colon (loss of muscle tone/flacidity), impacted faeces, obstruction of intestine.
*Manufacturer*: Norgine.

## NORMAX

*Description*: a bowel stimulant and faecal softener available as brown capsules containing 50mg of dantron and 60mg of docusate sodium (co-danthrusate), all marked NORMAX. *Also,* **NORMAX SUSPENSION,** available as a liquid containing 50mg of dantron and 60mg of docusate sodium (co-danthrusate).
*Used for*: constipation in patients who are terminally ill.
*Dosage*: adults, 1 to 3 capsules or 5 to 15ml of suspension, taken at night. Children aged over 6 years, 1 capsule or 5ml of suspension, taken at night.
*Special care*: faecal or urinary incontinence.
*Avoid use*: children aged under 6 years, pregnancy, breastfeeding, pains in abdomen, obstruction of the bowel.
*Side effects*: discoloured urine; possible risk of tumours developing in liver and bowel.
*Manufacturer*: Celltech.

## NORTRIPTYLINE *SEE*: ALLEGRON.

## NUVELLE

*Description*: a combined oestrogen/progestogen preparation available as sugar-coated tablets. 16 white tablets contain 2mg of oestradiol valerate and 12 pink tablets contain 2mg of oestradiol valerate and 75μg of levonorgestrel.

*Used for*: post-menopausal osteoporosis, hormone replacement therapy for climacteric syndrome (symptoms associated with the menopause).

*Dosage*: 1 white tablet each day for 16 days then 12 days of taking 1 pink tablet. Start on fifth day of menses (bleeding) if present.

*Special care*: hypertension, severe kidney disease receiving dialysis, Raynaud's disease, diabetes, multiple sclerosis, asthma, varicose veins, elevated levels of prolactin (a hormone) in the blood (hyperprolactinemia). Risk of thrombosis increases with smoking, age and obesity. Blood pressure, breasts and pelvic organs should be checked during period of treatment.

*Avoid use*: pregnancy, heart and circulatory diseases, angina, sickle cell anaemia, pulmonary hypertension. Also hormone-dependent cancers, undiagnosed vaginal bleeding, chorea, liver disease, history of cholestatic jaundice of pregnancy, infectious hepatitis, Dublin–Johnson syndrome, Rotor syndrome, recent trophoblastic disease.

*Possible interaction*: phenytoin, carbamazepine, tetracyclines, primidone, chloral hydrate, glutethimide, phenylbutazone, rifampicin, griseofulvin, ampicillin, dichloralphenazone, ethosuximide, barbiturates, St John's Wort.

*Side effects*: feeling of bloatedness due to fluid retention, leg pains, breast enlargement, erosion of cervix, muscular cramps, weight gain, breakthrough bleeding, depression, headaches, vaginal discharge, loss of libido, nausea, brown patches on skin (chloasma). Stop drug immediately in event of pregnancy.
*Manufacturer*: Schering H.C.

## NYCOPREN

*Description*: a propionic acid and NSAID, available as enteric-coated, white, oblong tablets containing 250 and 500mg of naproxen.
*Used for*: osteoarthritis, rheumatoid arthritis, acute gout, ankylosing spondylitis, inflammatory musculoskeletal disorders, juvenile rheumatoid arthritis (JRA).
*Dosage*: adults, 250 to 500mg twice each day. Gout, start with 750mg followed by 250mg every 8 hours. Musculo-skeletal conditions, 500mg to start then 250mg every 8 hours. Children, for JRA, weighing over 50kg, 250 to 500mg twice each day; not recommended for children weighing under 50kg.
*Special care*: elderly, pregnancy, kidney or liver disease, heart failure, history of gastro-intestinal lesions, asthma. Kidney and liver function should be monitored in patients on long-term therapy.
*Avoid use*: breastfeeding, allergy to aspirin or anti-inflammatory drugs, active stomach ulcer.
*Possible interaction*: sulfonamides, sulphonylureas, anticoagulants, quinolones, ß-blockers, lithium, hydantoins, furosemide, methotrexate, probenecid.

*Side effects*: headache, vertigo, blood changes, tinnitus (ringing in ears), rash, gastrointestinal intolerance.
*Manufacturer*: Ardern

## NYSTATIN *SEE*: DERMOVATE-NN, FLAGYL COMPAK.

# O

## OCUFEN

*Description*: an NSAID which is a propionic acid available in the form of eyedrops containing 0.03% flurbiprofen sodium.

*Used for*: to inhibit inflammation and constriction of the pupil (miosis) during operations of the eye. Also, to treat post-operative inflammation in the anterior segment of the eye when topical corticosteroids cannot be used.

*Dosage*: as directed by physician.

*Manufacturer*: Allergan.

## ODRIK

*Description*: an ACE inhibitor available as capsules in 3 strengths all containing trandolapril. Yellow/red capsules contain 0.5mg; orange/red capsules contain 1mg; red/red contain 2mg.

*Used for*: dysfunction of the left ventricle following heart attack, mild to moderate high blood pressure.

*Dosage*: adults, 0.5mg once each day at first (starting 3 days after heart attack, if being used for ventricular dysfunction), increasing every 2 to 4 weeks to a maximum of 4mg as a single daily dose. Maintenance dose is in the order of 1 to 2mg once each day. Any diuretics being taken should be discontinued 2 or 3 days before treatment starts, but can be resumed later, if needed.

*Special care*: liver or kidney disease, kidney dialysis, bilateral renal artery stenosis (narrowing of both renal arteries), undergoing anaesthesia or surgery, congestive heart failure, patients with low fluid and salt levels. Kidney function should be monitored before and during treatment.

*Avoid use*: pregnancy, breastfeeding, obstruction of blood outflow from heart or aortic stenosis (narrowing of aorta), angioneurotic oedema (widespread swelling due to fluid retention) caused by previous ACE inhibitor treatment, hereditary or of other cause.

*Possible interaction*: NSAIDs, potassium-sparing diuretics or supplements, TCADs, lithium, neuroleptics, antihypertensive drugs, antidiabetic agents.

*Side effects*: rash, cough, weakness, headache, dizziness, palpitations, hypotension. In rare cases, agranulocytosis (a blood disorder characterized by abnormal reduction in number of white blood cells (granulocytes), angioneurotic oedema, depression of bone marrow.

*Manufacturer*: Hoechst.

**OESTRADIOL *SEE*: AERODIOL, CLIMAGEST, CLIMAVAL, CLIMESSE, CYCLO-PROGYNOVA, ELLESTE DUET CONTI, ELLESTE DUET, ELLESTE SOLO, ELLESTE SOLO MX, ESTRACOMBI, ESTRADERM, EVOREL, EVOREL SEQUI, EVOREL - PAK, FEMAPAK, FEMATRIX, FEMOSTON, FEMOSTON-CONTI, FEMSEVEN, FEMSEVEN SEQUI, HORMONIN, INDIVINA, KLIOFEM, KLIOVANCE, MENOREST, NUVELLE,**

**OESTROGEL, PROGYNOVA, SANDRENA, TRIDESTRA, ZUMENON.**

**ESTRIOL *SEE*: HORMONIN, OVESTIN.**

## OESTROGEL

*Description*: an oestrogen preparation available as a gel for delivery with measured dose, pump device, containing 0.06% oestradiol.

*Used for*: HRT to treat vasomotor symptoms, atrophic urethritis and vaginitis (inflammation of urethra and vagina). Prevention of osteoporosis after the menopause.

*Dosage*: women, for menopausal symptoms, urethritis, vaginitis, 2 doses applied to arms, shoulders or inside of thighs once each day at first, continuing for 4 weeks. If no significant improvement, dose can be increased to 4 measures daily. Prevention of osteoporosis, 2 doses applied as above once each day. Women who have a womb should also take a progestogen for 12 days each month, as advised by doctor.

*Special care*: hypertension, severe kidney disease receiving dialysis, Raynaud's disease, diabetes, multiple sclerosis, asthma, varicose veins, elevated levels of prolactin (a hormone) in the blood (hyperprolactinemia). Risk of thrombosis increases with smoking, age and obesity. Blood pressure, breasts and pelvic organs should be checked during period of treatment.

*Avoid use*: pregnancy, heart and circulatory diseases, angina, sickle cell anaemia, pulmonary hypertension. Also hormone-dependent cancers, undiagnosed vaginal bleeding, chorea, liver disease, history of cholestatic jaundice of pregnancy, infectious hepatitis, Dublin–Johnson syndrome, Rotor syndrome, recent trophoblastic disease.

*Possible interaction*: phenytoin, carbamazepine, tetracyclines, primidone, chloral hydrate, glutethimide, phenylbutazone, rifampicin, griseofulvin, ampicillin, dichloralphenazone, ethosuximide, barbiturates, St John's Wort.

*Side effects*: feeling of bloatedness due to fluid retention, leg pains, breast enlargement, erosion of cervix, muscular cramps, weight gain, breakthrough bleeding, depression, headaches, vaginal discharge, loss of libido, nausea, brown patches on skin (chloasma). Stop drug immediately in event of pregnancy.

*Manufacturer*: Hoechst.

**OESTROGEN *SEE*: PREMARIN, PREMIQUE, PREMPAK - C.**

**ESTRONE *SEE*: HORMONIN.**

**OFLOXACIN *SEE*: EXOCIN.**

**OMEPRAZOLE *SEE*: LOSEC.**

## OPTILAST

*Description*: antihistamine preparation available as eyedrops containing 0.05% of azelastine hydrochloride.

*Used for*: seasonal and perennial allergic conjunctivitis.

*Dosage*: adults, 1 drop in each eye twice each day, if necessary, increasing to 4 times daily. Use should be for 6 weeks only in perennial conjunctivitis. Children aged over 4 years, for seasonal conjunctivitis only, dose as for adults.

*Avoid use*: children aged under 4 years.

*Side effects*: bitter taste in mouth, local irritation of eye.

*Manufacturer*: Viatris.

## ORCIPRENALINE *SEE*: ALUPENT.

## ORUDIS

*Description*: an NSAID available as capsules in 2 strengths both containing ketoprofen. Purple/green capsules and pink capsules contain 50mg and 100mg respectively, both marked with strength and name. *Also*, **ORUDIS SUPPOSITORIES** containing 100mg.

*Used for*: musculo-skeletal disorders, including osteoarthritis, rheumatoid arthritis, joint disorders, ankylosing spondylitis, gout, pain following orthopaedic surgery, dysmenorrhoea (period pain) – capsules only.

*Dosage*: adults, capsules, 50 to 100mg twice each day with meals; suppositories, 1 at night with capsules taken during the day, if needed.

*Special care*: pregnancy, elderly, heart failure, heart, liver or kidney disorders. Elderly patients should be started on lowest effective dose and carefully monitored for first 4 weeks for bleeding in gastrointestinal tract. Patients taking the drug long-term should receive careful monitoring.

*Avoid use*: children, patients with known allergy to aspirin or NSAID, history of or active stomach ulcer, asthma, serious kidney disease, proctitis (inflammation of rectum and anus) – suppositories only.

*Possible interaction*: hydantoins, mifepristone, ciclosporin, anticoagulants, sulfonamides, diuretics, high doses of methotrexate, quinolones, cardiac glycosides, corticosteroids, lithium, antihypertensives.

*Side effects*: rash, gastrointestinal intolerance, kidney toxicity, malaise, haematological and neurological effects, central nervous system effects, sensation of numbness/tingling/'pins and needles', fatigue, abnormal liver function, mouth inflammation and ulceration, allergic reactions.

*Manufacturer*: Hawgreen.

## ORUVAIL GEL

*Description*: an NSAID which is a propionic acid available in the form of a gel containing 2.5% ketoprofen.

*Used for*: sports injuries, painful injuries to muscles, bones, strains, sprains, bruises, etc.

*Dosage*: adults, 15g each day in 2 to 4 divided doses for up to 1 week; massage affected area after applying gel.

*Special care*: pregnancy, avoid mucous membranes, eyes and broken skin.

*Avoid use*: breastfeeding, children, patients with known allergy to NSAID or aspirin, history of asthma.

*Side effects*: slight local irritation of skin.

*Manufacturer*: R.P.R.

## OTRIVINE

*Description*: a sympathomimetic available as nasal drops containing 0.1% xylometazoline hydrochloride. *Also,* **OTRIVINE SPRAY,** containing 0.1% xylometazoline hydrochloride. *Also,* **OTRIVINE CHILDREN'S NASAL DROPS,** containing 0.05% xylometazoline hydrochloride.

*Used for*: stuffy nose and congestion of nasal passages.

*Dosage*: adults, 2 to 3 drops or 1 spray into each side of nose, 2 to 3 times each day. Children, using paediatric drops, aged over 3 months, 1 to 2 drops in each side of nose once or twice each day.

*Special care*: pregnancy.

*Avoid use*: children aged under 3 months, continuous use for more than 1 week.

*Side effects*: headache, irritation of nose, rapid heartbeat.

*Manufacturer*: Novartis Consumer.

## OTRIVINE-ANTISTIN

*Description*: a sympathomimetic and antihistamine preparation available as drops containing 0.05% xylometazoline hydrochloride and 0.5% antazoline sulphate.

*Used for*: allergic conjunctivitis.

*Dosage*: adults, 1 to 2 drops 2 to 3 times each day into affected eye(s); elderly and children aged over 5 years, 1 drop 2 to 3 times each day.

*Special care*: dry eyes, coronary artery disease, high blood pressure, overactive thyroid gland, diabetes.

*Avoid use*: children under 5 years, wearers of contact lenses, narrow angle glaucoma.

*Possible interaction*: clonidine.

*Side effects*: drowsiness, short-lived stinging, headache, blurred vision.

*Manufacturer*: Novartis Consumer.

## OVESTIN

*Description*: a hormonal oestrogen preparation available as white tablets containing 1mg of estriol coded DG7, ORGANON and with *. Also, **OVESTIN CREAM,** with applicator containing 0.1% of estriol.

*Used for*: tablets, disorders of genital and urinary tract arising when oestrogen is deficient, e.g. atrophic vaginitis, vaginal atrophy; also, recurrent infections. Cream, atrophic vaginitis, itching, dryness and atrophy of vulva in elderly women. Treatment of this area before vaginal operations.

*Dosage*: women, tablets, 0.5 to 3mg each day for 4 weeks then 0.5–1mg daily. Cream, 1 applicator dose into vagina each day for 3 weeks with a maintenance dose of 1 applicatorful twice weekly. Use lowest effective dose for shortest possible time. Stop using for 4 weeks every 2 to 3 months and evaluate. Prior to surgery, 1 applicator dose each day for 2 weeks before operation. Discontinue for at least 2 weeks after surgery.

*Special care*: hypertension, severe kidney disease receiving dialysis, Raynaud's disease, diabetes, multiple sclerosis, asthma, varicose veins, elevated levels of prolactin (a hormone) in the blood (hyperprolactinemia). Risk of thrombosis increases with smoking, age and obesity. Blood pressure, breasts and pelvic organs should be checked during period of treatment.

*Avoid use*: pregnancy, heart and circulatory diseases, angina, sickle cell anaemia, pulmonary hypertension. Also hormone-dependent cancers, undiagnosed vaginal bleeding, chorea, liver disease, history of cholestatic jaundice of pregnancy, infectious hepatitis, Dublin–Johnson syndrome, Rotor syndrome, recent trophoblastic disease.

*Possible interaction*: phenytoin, carbamazepine, tetracyclines, primidone, chloral hydrate, glutethimide, phenylbutazone, rifampicin, griseofulvin, ampicillin, dichloralphenazone, ethosuximide, barbiturates, St John's Wort.

*Side effects*: feeling of bloatedness due to fluid retention, leg pains, breast enlargement, erosion of cervix, muscular cramps, weight gain, breakthrough bleeding, depression, headaches, vaginal discharge, loss of libido, nausea, brown patches on skin (chloasma). Stop drug immediately in event of pregnancy.

*Manufacturer*: Organon.

## OVRANETTE

*Description*: a hormonal combined oestrogen/progestogen preparation, available as sugar-coated, beige tablets containing 30μg of ethinylestradiol and 150μg levonorgestrel.

*Used for*: oral contraception.

*Dosage*: 1 tablet each day for 21 days starting on first day of period followed by 7 tablet-free days.

*Special care*: hypertension, severe kidney disease receiving dialysis, Raynaud's disease, diabetes, multiple sclerosis, asthma, varicose veins, elevated levels of prolactin (a hormone) in the blood (hyperprolactinemia). Risk of thrombosis increases with smoking, age and obesity. Blood pressure, breasts and pelvic organs should be checked during period of treatment.

*Avoid use*: pregnancy, heart and circulatory diseases, angina, sickle cell anaemia, pulmonary hypertension. Also hormone-dependent cancers, undiagnosed vaginal bleeding, chorea, liver disease, history of cholestatic jaundice of pregnancy, infectious hepatitis, Dublin–Johnson syndrome, Rotor syndrome, recent trophoblastic disease.

*Possible interaction*: phenytoin, carbamazepine, tetracyclines, primidone, chloral hydrate, glutethimide, phenylbutazone, rifampicin, griseofulvin, ampicillin, dichloralphenazone, ethosuximide, barbiturates, St John's Wort.

*Side effects*: feeling of bloatedness due to fluid retention, leg pains, breast enlargement, erosion of cervix, muscular cramps, weight gain, breakthrough bleeding, depression, headaches, vaginal discharge, loss of libido, nausea, brown patches on skin (chloasma). Stop drug immediately in event of pregnancy, if frequent, severe headaches occur or signs of thromboses, severe pain in upper abdominal region, enlarged liver, jaundice, rise in blood pressure, severe depression, increased number of fits. Drug should be discontinued 6 weeks before major planned surgery and re-started 2 weeks afterwards, as

long as woman is fully mobile. Should be discontinued during long periods of immobility.
*Manufacturer*: Wyeth.

## OVYSMEN

*Description*: a hormonal combined oestrogen/progestogen preparation available as white tablets containing 35µg of ethinylestradiol and 500µg of norethisterone marked C over 535.
*Used for*: oral contraception.
*Dosage*: 1 tablet each day for 21 days starting on 1st or 5th day of period followed by 7 tablet-free days.
*Special care*: hypertension, severe kidney disease receiving dialysis, Raynaud's disease, diabetes, multiple sclerosis, asthma, varicose veins, elevated levels of prolactin (a hormone) in the blood (hyperprolactinemia). Risk of thrombosis increases with smoking, age and obesity. Blood pressure, breasts and pelvic organs should be checked during period of treatment.
*Avoid use*: pregnancy, heart and circulatory diseases, angina, sickle cell anaemia, pulmonary hypertension. Also hormone-dependent cancers, undiagnosed vaginal bleeding, chorea, liver disease, history of cholestatic jaundice of pregnancy, infectious hepatitis, Dublin–Johnson syndrome, Rotor syndrome, recent trophoblastic disease.
*Possible interaction*: phenytoin, carbamazepine, tetracyclines, primidone, chloral hydrate, glutethimide, phenylbutazone, rifampicin, griseofulvin, ampicillin, dichloralphenazone, ethosuximide, barbiturates, St John's Wort.

*Side effects*: feeling of bloatedness due to fluid retention, leg pains, breast enlargement, erosion of cervix, muscular cramps, weight gain, breakthrough bleeding, depression, headaches, vaginal discharge, loss of libido, nausea, brown patches on skin (chloasma). Stop drug immediately in event of pregnancy, if frequent, severe headaches occur or signs of thromboses, severe pain in upper abdominal region, enlarged liver, jaundice, rise in blood pressure, severe depression, increased number of fits. Drug should be discontinued 6 weeks before major planned surgery and re-started 2 weeks afterwards, as long as woman is fully mobile. Should be discontinued during long periods of immobility

*Manufacturer*: Janssen-Cilag.

## OXIS TURBOHALER

*Description*: a selective ß2-agonist available as a powder for use with a breath-activated inhaler device, in 2 strengths, containing 6µg and 12µg of formoterol fumarate.

*Used for*: asthma, to relieve bronchospasm when corticosteroids are not sufficiently effective. Exercise-induced asthma.

*Dosage*: adults, bronchospasm, 6 to 12µg once or twice each day, inhaled in morning and/or at night. The maximum maintenance dose is 48mg in divided doses each day. Exercise-induced asthma, 12µg prior to starting activity. Additional doses up to 72µg each day in divided doses can be occasionally given, but consult manufacturer's literature and according to medical advice. Children, aged over 6 years, bronchospasm, 12μg once or twice each day inhaled in morning and/or at night. Maximum daily dose is 24μg, divided. Exercise-induced asthma, 12μg inhaled before starting activity.

*Special care*: pregnancy, severe and acute asthma, severe heart failure, subvalvular aortic stenosis (narrowed aorta), toxicosis of thyroid gland, aneurysm, diabetes, hypertrophic, obstructive, cardiomyopathy (enlarged, damaged heart muscle), severe high blood pressure, phaeochromocytoma (adrenal gland tumour), arrhythmias of tachycardic origin, ischaemic heart disease, prolongation of QT interval (part of ECG).

*Avoid use*: children aged under 6 years, breastfeeding. Not for acute asthma attacks. Do not reduce or stop prescribed steroids.

*Possible interaction*: drugs that prolong QT interval, antiarrhythmics, ß-blockers, anaesthetics, MAOIs, sympathomimetics.

*Side effects*: headache, tremor, palpitations. In rare cases, disturbed sleep, low blood potassium levels, agitation, rash, muscular cramps.

*Manufacturer*: AstraZeneca.

## OXPRENOLOL *SEE*: TRASICOR, TRASIDREX.

## OXYBUTYNIN *SEE*: CYSTRIN.

## OXYTETRACYCLINE *SEE*: TERAMYCIN, TRIMOVATE.

# P

**PACLITAXEL *SEE*: TAXOL.**

**PAMIDRONATE *SEE*: AREDIA.**

**PANTOPRAZOLE *SEE*: PROTIUM.**

**PARACETAMOL *SEE*: CALPOL, PARAMAX, SOLPADOL.**

**PARADICHLOROBENZENE *SEE*: CERUMOL.**

**PARAMAX**

*Description*: an NSAID combining an analgesic and anti-emetic preparation available as scored, white tablets containing 500mg of paracetamol and 5mg of metoclopramide hydrochloride, marked PARAMAX. Also **PARAMAX SACHETS**, effervescent powder with same quantities of drugs.

*Used for*: migraine.

*Dosage*: adults over 20 years, 2 tablets when attack starts followed by 2 every 4 hours up to maximum dose of 6 in 24 hours. Children aged 12 to 19 years, 1 tablet at start of attack to maximum dose of 3 in 24 hours.

*Special care*: pregnancy, breast-feeding, liver or kidney disorder, recent surgery to gastrointestinal tract, phaeochromocytoma (adrenal gland tumour).

*Avoid use*: children aged under 12 years, breast cancer which is prolactin-dependent.

*Possible interaction*: phenothiazines, anticholinergics, butyrophenones.

*Side effects*: drowsiness, raised blood levels of prolactin, diarrhoea, extrapyramidal reactions (characterized by reflex-type muscle movements and spasms).

*Manufacturer*: Sanofi-Synthelabo.

## PARIET

*Description*: a proton pump inhibitor which inhibits secretion of gastric acid, available as enteric-coated tablets in 2 strengths containing 10mg and 20mg of rabeprazole sodium, marked E241 and E243, respectively.

*Used for*: ulcers, gastro-oesophageal reflux disease (GORD), long-term treatment of GORD, in conjunction with antibiotics for elimination of *H. pylori* in stomach ulcer disease.

*Dosage*: adults, for duodenal ulcer, 20mg once per day in the morning for 4 to 8 weeks; for gastric ulcer, 20mg once per day in the morning for 6 to 12 weeks; for GORD, 20mg once each day in the morning for 4 to 8 weeks. Long-term maintenance treatment of GORD, 10 or 20mg once each day. Symptoms of GORD, 10mg once each day for 1 month. Triple therapy with antibiotics to eliminate *H. pylori,* 20mg of Pariet, 500mg of clarithromycin, 1g of amoxicillin, all twice each day for 1 week. Take Pariet tablet whole before eating food.

*Special care*: ensure there is no malignancy prior to treatment,

severe liver disorder. Patients receiving long-term treatment must be monitored.
*Avoid use*: pregnancy, breastfeeding, children.
*Possible interaction*: digoxin, ketoconazole.
*Side effects*: gastrointestinal upset, rash, headache, weakness.
*Manufacturer*: Eisai/Janssen.

## PAROXETINE *SEE*: SEROXAT.

## PARVOLEX

*Description*: an amino acid preparation used to treat drug overdose and available as a solution in ampoules for injection containing 200mg of acetylcysteine per ml. Acetylcysteine acts to protect the liver from damage.
*Used for*: paracetamol overdose.
*Dosage*: consult manufacturer's instructions.
*Special care*: history of bronchospasm or asthma. Vomiting should be induced if patient is treated within 4 hours of overdose. Plasma concentrations of potassium require monitoring. Patients who have chronic alcohol problem, malnourishment or who are on drugs that induce liver enzymes may be more at risk if overdose of paracetamol is taken.
*Possible interaction*: metals and rubber.
*Side effects*: rash, slow heartbeat, liver impairment, fainting, allergic reactions, anaphylaxis, cardiac or respiratory arrest.
*Manufacturer*: Celltech.

## PENBRITIN

*Description*: an antibiotic, broad-spectrum penicillin preparation available as black/red capsules containing 250mg of ampicillin, marked with strength and name. *Also*, **PENBRITIN INJECTION** available as powder in vials containing 500mg of ampicillin sodium.

*Used for*: ear, nose, throat and respiratory infections, soft tissue infections. Infections of urinary tract and gonorrhoea.

*Dosage*: adults, capsules, 250mg to 1g every 6 hours; injection, 500mg by intravenous or intramuscular injection, 4, 5 or 6 times each day; for meningitis, 2g every 6 hours by intravenous route. Children, aged under 10 years, capsules, half adult dose. Injection, half adult dose; for meningitis, 150mg per kg of body weight by intravenous route in divided doses.

*Special care*: patients with glandular fever.

*Side effects*: gastro-intestinal upset, hypersensitivity reactions. In rare cases, pseudomembranous colitis.

*Manufacturer*: GlaxoSmithKline.

## PEPCID

*Description*: an H2 blocker available as square, beige tablets and square, brown tablets containing 20mg and 40mg of famotidine respectively, both marked with strength and name.

*Used for*: treatment of stomach and duodenal ulcers, prevention of relapse of duodenal ulcers. Prevention and treatment of reflux disease of stomach and oesophagus (GORD), treatment of Zollinger-Ellison syndrome.

*Dosage*: treatment of ulcers, 40mg taken at night for 4 to 8 weeks; prevention of relapse of duodenal ulcer, 20mg taken at night. Gastro-oesophageal reflux disease, 20mg twice each day for 6 weeks to 3 months (or 40mg, if damage or ulceration is present). Prevention, 20mg twice each day. Zollinger-Ellison syndrome, 20mg every 6 hours at first adjusted according to response to a maximum dose of 800mg each day.
*Special care*: pregnancy, stomach cancer or kidney disease.
*Avoid use*: children, breastfeeding.
*Side effects*: nausea, diarrhoea, constipation, rash, joint pains, cholestatic jaundice, abdominal pains, angioedema (widespread swelling due to fluid retention), gastrointestinal upset, dry mouth, disturbances in central nervous system, abnormal liver enzymes, headache, anorexia, anaphylaxis, dizziness, weariness. In rare cases, enlargement of breasts in males (reversible), heart block, death of epidermal skin cells.
*Manufacturer*: M.S.D.

## PERDIX

*Description*: an ACE inhibitor, moexipril hydrochloride, which blocks the enzyme, ACE, stopping the formation of angiotensin II which constricts blood vessels. This produces dilatation, decreasing blood pressure. It is available as scored, pink, film-coated tablets in 2, respectively.
*Used for*: high blood pressure, either as sole therapy or with calcium antagonists or diuretics.
*Dosage*: adults, 7.5 kg once each day to start, increased to

15 to 30mg (maximum 30mg). If diuretic is being used, cease use 2 to 3 days before therapy, then begin with 3.75mg once daily, afterwards adjusting according to response. Resume diuretic once established, if required. If nifedipine is used, start with 3.75mg also. For the elderly, start with 3.75mg once each day.

*Special care*: liver or kidney disorder, narrowing of renal artery or aorta, undergoing anaesthesia or surgery, collagen-vascular disease.

*Avoid use*: children, pregnancy, breastfeeding, past angioedema (widespread swelling due to fluid retention) – cease use if symptoms develop.

*Possible interaction*: NSAIDs, lithium, drugs altering potassium levels, neuroleptics, tricyclic antidepressants (TCADs), antihypertensives, antidiabetics.

Side effects: rash, headache, cough, tiredness, flushing, dizziness.

*Manufacturer*: Schwarz.

## PERGOLIDE *SEE*: CELANCE.

## PERIACTIN

*Description*: an antihistamine and serotonin antagonist available as scored, white tablets containing 4mg of cyproheptadine hydrochloride, marked MSD 62.

*Used for*: migraine, allergies and itchy skin conditions.

*Dosage*: adults, migraine, 1 tablet with a further one taken after 30 minutes, if necessary to a maximum dose of 2 in 4 to 6 hours. Maintenance dose is 1 tablet every 4 to 6 hours. Allergies/skin disorders, 1 tablet 3 to 4 times daily. Children, for skin conditions and allergies only, aged 2 to 6 years, 1/2 tablet; aged 7 to 14 years, 1 tablet; all doses 3 times each day.

*Special care*: pregnancy, asthma, overactive thyroid gland, epilepsy, high blood pressure, raised pressure within the eye, heart and circulatory disease.

*Avoid use*: newborn babies, elderly or debilitated patients, breastfeeding, enlarged prostate gland, stomach ulcer causing narrowing, obstruction of stomach/duodenal outlet, acute asthma attack, retention of urine.

*Possible interaction*: depressants of central nervous system, MAOIs, alcohol.

*Side effects*: anticholinergic effects, drowsiness, excitation in children, impaired reactions.

*Manufacturer*: M.S.D.

## PERINDOPRIL *SEE*: COVERSYL.

## PERIOSTAT

*Description*: a tetracycline available as film-coated, white tablets containing 20mg of doxycycline hyclate marked PS20.

*Used for*: additional therapy in the treatment of periodontitis (inflammation of the tissues around the teeth).

*Dosage*: adults, 1 tablet twice each day taken at least 1 hour before eating a meal.

*Special care*: oral thrush, liver disorder, phototoxicity, pseudomembranous colitis.

*Avoid use*: children, pregnancy, breastfeeding, achlorhydria (abnormal absence of hydrochloric acid in gastric juice).

*Possible interaction*: phenytoin, penicillin, anticoagulants, oral contraceptives, antacids, carbamazepine, primidone, mineral supplements, methoxyflurane, barbiturates.

*Side effects*: hypersensitivity, oesophageal ulceration and oesophagitis, rash, photosensitivity, gastrointestinal upset, superinfections, blood disorders, increase in urea. Drug should be withdrawn in event of raised pressure within skull.

*Manufacturer*: CollaGenex.

## PERU BALSAM *SEE*: ANUSOL HC.

## PHENERGAN

*Description*: an antihistamine preparation of phenothiazine type available as film-coated, blue tablets in 2 strengths containing 10mg and 25mg of promethazine hydrochloride, marked PN10 and PN25, respectively. *Also,* **PHENERGAN ELIXIR,** containing 5mg of promethazine hydrochloride per 5ml. *Also,* **PHENERGAN INJECTION,** available in ampoules for injection containing 25mg of promethazine hydrochloride per ml.

*Used for*: allergies, nausea, vomiting, sedation.

*Dosage*: adults, tablets and elixir, 10 to 25mg 2 to 3 times each day. Injection, 25 to 50mg given by deep intramuscular injection. In emergency can be given diluted by slow intravenous injection. Children, tablets and elixir, allergies, aged 2 to 5 years, 5 to 15mg; aged 5 to 10 years, 10 to

25mg. If being given as 2 divided doses every 24 hours, the lowest dose should be used. Children, for travel sickness, aged 2 to 5 years, 5mg; aged 5 to 10 years, 10mg; aged over 10 years, 25mg. Dose to be taken the night before travelling and then repeated after 6 to 8 hours, if necessary. Children sedation, aged 2 to 5 years, 15 to 20mg; aged 5 to 10 years, 20 to 50mg. All to be given as single bedtime dose. Injection, aged over 5 years, 6.25 to 12.5mg by deep intramuscular injection.

*Avoid use*: children under 2 years (oral preparations), children aged under 5 years (injection), pregnancy, breastfeeding.

*Possible interaction*: MAOIs, depressants of central nervous system.

*Side effects*: extrapyramidal effects (affecting extrapyramidal structures associated with central nervous system, involving movements), disorientation, drowsiness, impairment of reactions, anticholinergic effects, sensitivity to light.

*Manufacturer*: R.P.R.

## PHENYLEPHRINE *SEE*: ISOPTO FRIN.

## PILOCARPINE *SEE*: MINIMS PILOCARPINE.

## PINDOLOL *SEE*: VISKALDIX, VISKEN.

## PIRITON

*Description*: an antihistamine preparation of the arylalkylamine type available as scored, yellow tablets containing 4mg of chlorphenamine maleate, all marked P. *Also,* **PIRITON SYRUP,** containing 2mg of chlorphenamine maleate per 5ml.

*Used for*: allergies

*Dosage*: adults and children over 12 years, 1 tablet every 4 to 6 hours to a maximum of 6 each day or 10ml, 4 to 6 hourly to a maximum of 60ml each day. Children, aged 6 to 12 years, ° tablet every 4 to 6 hours to a maximum of 3 each day. Syrup, aged 1 to 2 years, 2.5ml twice each day; aged 2 to 5 years, 2.5ml every 4 to 6 hours to a maximum daily dose of 15ml; aged 6 to 12 years, 5ml every 4 to 6 hours to a daily maximum of 30ml.

*Special care*: pregnancy, breastfeeding, high blood pressure, raised intraocular pressure or BPH, asthma, liver disorder, thyrotoxicosis (toxicity of thyroid gland), epilepsy.

*Possible interaction*: MAOIs, phenytoin, alcohol, depressants of central nervous system.

*Side effects*: impaired reactions, blurring of vision, sleepiness, dizziness, stimulation of central nervous system.

*Manufacturer*: GlaxoSmithKline.

## PIROXICAM *SEE*: FELDENE, FELDENE GEL.

## PLANTAGO OVATA *SEE*: MANEVAC.

## PLENDIL

*Description*: an antihypertensive class II calcium antagonist available as film-coated sustained-release tablets in

3 strengths, all containing felodipine. Yellow tablets contain 2.5mg, pink tablets contain 5mg, red tablets contain 10mg, all marked with strength and A/FL, A/FM and A/FE, respectively.

*Used for*: prevention of stable, chronic angina, high blood pressure.

*Dosage*: adults, 5mg once each day increasing if necessary to a usual maintenance dose of 5 to 10mg. The maximum daily dose is 20mg. Elderly patients should be started on 2.5mg.

*Special care*: breastfeeding, severe disorder of left ventricle of heart.

*Avoid use*: children, pregnancy, uncompensated heart failure, aortic stenosis (narrowing of aorta), within 1 month of heart attack, heart shock.

*Possible interaction*: phenytoin, itraconazole, phenobarbital, cimetidine, erythromycin, ketoconazole, other inhibitors or inducers of CYP3A4, carbamazepine, grapefruit juice.

*Side effects*: flushing, swelling of ankles, worsening of angina, weariness, giddiness, headache, slight swelling of gums, vomiting, palpitations.

*Manufacturer*: AstraZeneca.

## POLOXAMER '188' *SEE*: CODALAX.

## POLYETHYLENE GLYCOL *SEE*: MOVICOL.

## POLYFAX

*Description*: a preparation of peptide antibiotics available as an ointment containing 10,000 units polymyxin B sulphate and 500 units bacitracin zinc per gram.

*Used for*: eye infections including conjunctivitis, keratitis, styes, blepharitis. Prevention of infection after removal of foreign objects from the eye or surgery. Also, impetigo, infected burns and skin infections.

*Dosage*: apply thinly at least twice each day.

*Special care*: patients with extensive, open wounds.

*Side effects*: skin sensitization, toxic effects on kidneys.

*Manufacturer*: PLIVA.

## POLYMYXIN B *SEE*: NEOSPORIN, OTOSPORIN, POLYFAX.

## POLYTRIM

*Description*: A combined antibacterial preparation available in the form of eyedrops containing 1mg trimethoprim and 10,000 units polymyxin B sulphate per ml. Also, **POLYTRIM OINTMENT** containing 5mg trimethoprim and 10,000 units polymyxin B sulphate/gram.

*Used for*: bacterial eye infections.

*Dosage*: apply 3 or 4 times each day, continuing for 2 days after symptoms have cleared.

*Manufacturer*: PLIVA.

## POLYVINYL ALCOHOL *SEE*: HYPOTEARS, LIQUIFILM TEARS.

## POTASSIUM CHLORIDE *SEE*: BURINEX K, MOVICOL.

## POWERGEL

*Description*: an NSAID available as a gel containing 2.5% ketoprofen.

*Used for*: soft tissue injuries, strains and sprains – to relieve pain and inflammation.

*Dosage*: adults, 5 to 10cm of gel applied over affected area and rubbed in, 2 to 3 times each day for up to 10 days. Area should then be massaged for a short time.

*Special care*: pregnancy, breastfeeding, kidney disorders.

*Avoid use*: children, allergy to NSAID or aspirin, asthma.

*Side effects*: mild irritation where gel is applied.

*Manufacturer*: Menarini

## PRAVASTATIN *SEE*: LIPOSTAT.

## PRAZOSIN *SEE*: HYPOVASE.

## PREDNISOLONE *SEE*: PREDSOL.

## PREDSOL

*Description*: a steroid colorectal agent available as an enema containing 20mg of prednisolone as disodium phosphate. *Also*, **PREDSOL SUPPOSITORIES** containing 5mg prednisolone (as disodium phosphate).

*Used for*: enema, rectosigmoidal disease in Crohn's

disease and ulcerative colitis; suppositories, proctitis (inflammation of rectum) and anal disorders resulting from Crohn's disease (a disorder of the intestine or part of digestive tract in which there is inflammation and ulceration).

*Dosage*: adults, enema, 1 at night for 2, 3 or 4 weeks; suppositories, 1 every night and morning after passing stool.

*Special care*: pregnancy, breastfeeding; short-term use only.

*Avoid use*: children, bacterial, fungal, tuberculous or viral infections.

*Side effects*: systemic glucocorticoid effects, e.g. mood swings, euphoria and depression, changes as in Cushing's syndrome, peptic ulcer, hyperglycaemia, osteoporosis.

*Manufacturer*: Celltech.

## PREDSOL EAR DROPS

*Description*: a corticosteroid preparation available as ear drops containing 0.5% prednisolone sodium phosphate. *Also,* **PREDSOL-N,** combined corticosteroid and antibiotic ear drops containing 0.5% prednisolone sodium phosphate and 0.5% neomycin sulphate.

*Used for*: Predsol, non-infected, inflamed ear conditions. Predsol-N, short-term treatment of ear inflammation where prevention of infection is also considered to be necessary.

*Dosage*: Predsol, 2 to 3 drops into ear every 2 to 3 hours until condition improves, then reduce frequency of use. Withdraw after 1 week if no improvement has occurred. Predsol-N, 2 to 3 drops 3 to 4 times each day.

*Special care*: pregnancy, long-term use in babies. Do not use unless necessary.
*Avoid use*: perforated ear drum, conditions in which tuberculous, fungal or viral infection is present or if there is discharge of pus.
*Side effects*: cross-resistance to neomycin, sensitisation. Increased risk of deafness.
*Manufacturer*: Celltech.

## PREDSOL EYE DROPS

*Description*: a corticosteroid preparation available as eye drops containing 0.5% prednisolone sodium phosphate. *Also,* **PREDSOL-N,** eye drops containing 0.5% prednisolone sodium phosphate and 0.55 neomycin sulphate.
*Used for*: Predsol, inflammatory conditions of the eye in which no infection is present. Predsol-N, similar conditions where prevention of infection is also necessary.
*Dosage*: Predsol, 1 to 2 drops every 1 to 2 hours until condition improves, then reduce frequency of use. Withdraw if condition has not responded after 1 week. Predsol-N, 1 to 2 drops up to 6 times each day.
*Special care*: pregnancy, long-term use in babies.
*Avoid use*: glaucoma, eye infections of tubercular, fungal or viral origin or those producing pus, dendritic ulcer, patients wearing soft contact lenses.
*Side effects*: sensitisation, corneal thinning, cataracts, raised pressure within eye.
*Manufacturer*: Celltech.

## PREMARIN

*Description*: an oestrogen preparation available as sugar-coated, oval, maroon tablets and sugar-coated, oval, yellow tablets containing 0.625mg and 1.25mg of conjugated oestrogens, respectively. Also, **PREMARIN VAGINAL CREAM** containing 0.625mg per g of conjugated oestrogens.

*Used for*: tablets, hormone replacement therapy for menopausal women who have had a hysterectomy. Prevention of osteoporosis following menopause. Cream, atrophic vaginitis and urethritis, Kraurosis vulvae (a disease of the external genital area, characterized by degeneration of tissues and itching, affecting elderly women).

*Dosage*: tablets, 0.625mg to 1.25mg each day at first, then using lowest dose that is effective, for maintenance. Cream, 1 to 2g applied daily to affected area or intra-vaginally for 3 weeks, using applicator, followed by 1 week without treatment.

*Special care*: high blood pressure, severe kidney disease receiving dialysis, Raynaud's disease, diabetes, multiple sclerosis, asthma, varicose veins, elevated levels of prolactin (a hormone) in the blood (hyperprolactinemia). Risk of thrombosis increases with smoking, age and obesity. Blood pressure, breasts and pelvic organs should be checked during period of treatment.

*Avoid use*: pregnancy, heart and circulatory diseases, angina, sickle cell anaemia, pulmonary hypertension. Also hormone-dependent cancers, undiagnosed vaginal bleeding, chorea, liver disease, history of cholestatic jaundice of pregnancy, infectious hepatitis, Dublin–Johnson syndrome, Rotor syndrome, recent trophoblastic disease.

*Possible interaction*: phenytoin, carbamazepine, tetracyclines, primidone, chloral hydrate, glutethimide, phenylbutazone, rifampicin, griseofulvin, ampicillin, dichloralphenazone, ethosuximide, barbiturates, St John's Wort.

*Side effects*: feeling of bloatedness due to fluid retention, leg pains, breast enlargement, erosion of cervix, muscular cramps, weight gain, breakthrough bleeding, depression, headaches, vaginal discharge, loss of libido, nausea, brown patches on skin (chloasma). Stop drug immediately in event of pregnancy.

*Manufacturer*: Wyeth.

## PREMIQUE

*Description*: an oestrogen/progestogen compound available as sugar-coated, blue, oval tablets containing 0.625mg of conjugated oestrogens and 5mg medroxyprogesterone acetate.

*Used for*: hormone replacement therapy for menopausal symptoms, prevention of postmenopausal osteoporosis for women with an intact uterus.

*Dosage*: 1 tablet every day starting on the first day of cycle or at any time if menstruation is not regular.

*Special care*: high blood pressure, severe kidney disease receiving dialysis, Raynaud's disease, diabetes, multiple sclerosis, asthma, varicose veins, elevated levels of prolactin (a hormone) in the blood (hyperprolactinemia).

Risk of thrombosis increases with smoking, age and obesity. Blood pressure, breasts and pelvic organs should be checked during period of treatment.

*Avoid use*: pregnancy, heart and circulatory diseases, angina, sickle cell anaemia, pulmonary hypertension. Also hormone-dependent cancers, undiagnosed vaginal bleeding, chorea, liver disease, history of cholestatic jaundice of pregnancy, infectious hepatitis, Dublin–Johnson syndrome, Rotor syndrome, recent trophoblastic disease.

*Possible interaction*: phenytoin, carbamazepine, tetracyclines, primidone, chloral hydrate, glutethimide, phenylbutazone, rifampicin, griseofulvin, ampicillin, dichloralphenazone, ethosuximide, barbiturates, St John's Wort.

*Side effects*: feeling of bloatedness due to fluid retention, leg pains, breast enlargement, erosion of cervix, muscular cramps, weight gain, breakthrough bleeding, depression, headaches, vaginal discharge, loss of libido, nausea, brown patches on skin (chloasma). Stop drug immediately in event of pregnancy.

*Manufacturer*: Wyeth.

## PREMPAK-C

*Description*: an oestrogen and progestogen preparation available in the form of sugar-coated oval tablets in 2 strengths, 28 maroon or 28 yellow containing 0.625mg or 1.25mg conjugated oestrogens respectively. Also, 12 sugar-coated brown tablets containing 0.15mg norgestrel in same pack.

*Used for*: hormone replacement therapy in women who have

not had a hysterectomy, for menopausal symptoms, prevention of osteoporosis following menopause.

*Dosage*: 1 maroon or yellow tablet for 16 days then 1 maroon or 1 yellow tablet and 1 brown tablet for 12 days, starting on first day of period if present.

*Special care*: high blood pressure, severe kidney disease receiving dialysis, Raynaud's disease, diabetes, multiple sclerosis, asthma, varicose veins, elevated levels of prolactin (a hormone) in the blood (hyperprolactinemia). Risk of thrombosis increases with smoking, age and obesity. Blood pressure, breasts and pelvic organs should be checked during period of treatment.

*Avoid use*: pregnancy, heart and circulatory diseases, angina, sickle cell anaemia, pulmonary hypertension. Also hormone-dependent cancers, undiagnosed vaginal bleeding, chorea, liver disease, history of cholestatic jaundice of pregnancy, infectious hepatitis, Dublin–Johnson syndrome, Rotor syndrome, recent trophoblastic disease.

*Possible interaction*: phenytoin, carbamazepine, tetracyclines, primidone, chloral hydrate, glutethimide, phenylbutazone, rifampicin, griseofulvin, ampicillin, dichloralphenazone, ethosuximide, barbiturates, St John's Wort.

*Side effects*: feeling of bloatedness due to fluid retention, leg pains, breast enlargement, erosion of cervix, muscular cramps, weight gain, breakthrough bleeding, depression, headaches, vaginal discharge, loss of libido, nausea, brown patches on skin (chloasma). Stop drug immediately in event of pregnancy.

*Manufacturer*: Wyeth.

## PRESCAL

*Description*: an antihypertensive preparation which is a class II calcium antagonist, available as scored yellow tablets containing 2.5mg of isradipine marked NM and CIBA.

*Used for*: high blood pressure.

*Dosage*: 1 tablet in the morning and at night, increasing after 3 or 4 weeks to 2 twice each day if needed. Maximum dose is 4 tablets twice each day. Elderly, half a tablet twice each day at first.

*Special care*: pregnancy, breastfeeding, sick sinus syndrome, diabetes, low blood pressure, weak heart.

*Avoid use*: children, narrowed aorta (aortic stenosis), within 1 month of heart attack, heart shock, patients who have had more than 1 heart attack.

*Possible interaction*: drugs affecting P450, cimetidine, anticonvulsants, rifampicin, grapefruit juice.

*Side effects*: rapid heartbeat, palpitations, headache, giddiness, worsening of angina, flushing, fluid retention in hands and feet, pain in abdomen, raised levels of transaminase enzymes in blood, gain in weight, tiredness, skin rashes.

*Manufacturer*: Novartis.

## PRESERVEX

*Description*: an NSAID and phenyloxyacetic acid available as film-coated, white tablets containing 100mg of aceclofenac.

*Used for*: rheumatoid arthritis, ankylosing spondylitis, osteoarthritis.

*Dosage*: adults, 1 tablet in the morning and at night.
*Special care*: liver, kidney or heart disease, gastrointestinal disorders.
*Avoid use*: children, pregnancy, breastfeeding, stomach ulcer, moderate to serious kidney disease, bleeding in gastrointestinal tract, allergy to aspirin or NSAID.
*Possible interaction*: corticosteroids, methotrexate, lithium, ciclosporin, diuretics, quinolone antibiotics, digoxin, antidiabetics, other NSAIDs.
*Side effects*: itching, rise in liver enzymes, dizziness, gastrointestinal disturbance.
*Manufacturer*: UCB.

## PROCHLORPERAZINE MALEATE *SEE*: BUCCASTEM.

## PROFLEX

*Description*: an NSAID available as a cream containing 5% ibuprofen.
*Used for*: strains, sprains, rheumatic and muscular aches and pains.
*Dosage*: adults, apply 4 to 10cm of cream to skin over affected area every 4 hours, 3 to 4 times each day.
*Avoid use*: pregnancy, known allergy to anti-inflammatory drugs or aspirin.
*Side effects*: skin reddening.
*Manufacturer*: Novartis Consumer.

## PROGYNOVA

*Description*: an hormonal oestrogen preparation available in the form of beige, sugar-coated tablets, containing 1mg and blue, containing 2mg of oestradiol valerate, respectively.

*Used for*: menopausal symptoms, prevention of post-menopausal osteoporosis.

*Dosage*: women, menopausal symptoms, 1mg or 2mg each day, using lowest dose that is effective. Prevention of osteoporosis, 2mg each day. Women who have not had a hysterectomy require a progestogen for 12 days out of every month.

*Special care*: high blood pressure, severe kidney disease receiving dialysis, Raynaud's disease, diabetes, multiple sclerosis, asthma, varicose veins, elevated levels of prolactin (a hormone) in the blood (hyperprolactinemia). Risk of thrombosis increases with smoking, age and obesity. Blood pressure, breasts and pelvic organs should be checked during period of treatment.

*Avoid use*: pregnancy, heart and circulatory diseases, angina, sickle cell anaemia, pulmonary hypertension. Also hormone-dependent cancers, undiagnosed vaginal bleeding, chorea, liver disease, history of cholestatic jaundice of pregnancy, infectious hepatitis, Dublin–Johnson syndrome, Rotor syndrome, recent trophoblastic disease.

*Possible interaction*: phenytoin, carbamazepine, tetracyclines, primidone, chloral hydrate, glutethimide, phenylbutazone, rifampicin, griseofulvin, ampicillin, dichloralphenazone, ethosuximide, barbiturates, St John's Wort.

*Side effects*: feeling of bloatedness due to fluid retention, leg pains, breast enlargement, erosion of cervix, muscular cramps, weight gain, breakthrough bleeding, depression, headaches, vaginal discharge, loss of libido, nausea, brown patches on skin (chloasma). Stop drug immediately in event of pregnancy.
*Manufacturer*: Schering H.C.

## PROPAFENONE *SEE*: ARYTHMOL.

## PROPECIA

*Description*: a selective 5-alpha reductase inhibitor available as film-coated, octagonal-shaped, brown tablets, marked P and PROPECIA, containing 1mg of finasteride.
*Used for*: alopecia androgenetica (abnormal loss of hair connected with male hormones, androgens).
*Dosage*: males only, 1 tablet each day for 3 to 6 months or continuously.
*Special care*: females should not handle tablets, especially if broken, as drug may be absorbed through skin – poses risk in pregnancy.
*Side effects*: reduced libido, impotence, low volume of ejaculate, allergic reactions and nettle rash, enlargement of breasts and tenderness, pain in testicles. Any adverse side effects should be reported to the Committee on the Safety of Medicines (CSM).
*Manufacturer*: M.S.D.

## PROPINE

*Description*: a sympathomimetic preparation available as eyedrops containing 0.1% dipivefrin hydrochloride.

*Used for*: high pressure within eye, open angle glaucoma.

*Dosage*: adults, 1 drop into eye every 12 hours.

*Special care*: patients without whole or part of lens (aphakia) e.g. as in surgical removal of cataracts, narrow angle between iris and cornea of eye.

*Avoid use*: children, closed angle glaucoma, wearing soft contact lenses.

*Side effects*: short-lived stinging, allergic responses, increased blood flow. In rare cases, raised blood pressure.

*Manufacturer*: Allergan.

## PROPANOLOL *SEE*: BETA-PROGRANE, INDERAL.

## PROSCAR

*Description*: a preparation which is a selective 5-alpha reductase inhibitor available as film-coated, apple-shaped blue tablets containing 5mg of finasteride marked with name and MSD 72.

*Used for*: benign enlargement of the prostate gland, to lessen retention of urine and need for corrective operation.

*Dosage*: 1 tablet each day for at least 6 months, then continuing long-term if condition is responding.

*Special care*: obstruction or disease of genital/urinary tract. Presence of cancer should be eliminated before treatment begins and during therapy. Women may absorb drug via semen through sexual intercourse or by handling tablets—risk in pregnancy.

*Avoid use*: patients with prostate cancer.

*Side effects*: decreased libido, impotence, reduced volume of ejaculate possibly affecting fertility, allergic reactions and nettle rash, enlarged, tender breasts, pain in testicles.

*Manufacturer*: M.S.D.

## PROSTIN E2

*Description*: a prostaglandin preparation available as white, vaginal tablets containing 3mg of dinoprostone marked 715 and UPJOHN. **PROSTIN E2 1MG SOLUTION**, alcoholic solution in ampoules containing 1mg of dinoprostone per ml. *Also,* **PROSTIN E2 VAGINAL GEL**, in 2 strengths containing 1mg and 2mg of dinoprostone per 3g of gel. *Also,* **PROSTIN E2 10MG SOLUTION,** alcoholic solution available in ampoules for injection containing 10mg of dinoprostone per ml.

*Used for*: all preparations except Prostin E2 10mg Solution, induction of labour. Prostin E2 10mg Solution, to terminate pregnancy.

For *Dosages etc.* consult manufacturer's literature.

*Manufacturer*: Pharmacia.

## PROTHIADEN

*Description*: a TCAD preparation available as brown/red capsules containing 25mg of dosulepin hydrochloride marked P25. *Also,* **PROTHIADEN TABLETS,** sugar-coated red tablets containing 75mg of dosulepin hydrochloride, marked P75.

*Used for*: depression and anxiety.

*Dosage*: adults, 75 to 150mg each day either as divided doses or taken as single dose at night. Elderly patients, 50 to 75mg each day increasing slowly, if required, but only under strict medical advice.

*Special care*: patients with psychoses or suicidal tendencies, elderly persons, pregnant and nursing mothers, people with cardiac disorders, epilepsy, hyperthyroidism, urine retention, closed angle glaucoma, liver disease, tumours of adrenal gland, diabetes

*Avoid use*: children, patients with recent heart attack, heart arrhythmias, heart block, porphyria (rare blood disorder).

*Possible interaction*: alcohol, barbiturate drugs, local anaesthetics (containing adrenaline or noradrenaline), antihypertensive and sympathomimetic drugs, anticholinergic drugs, cimetidine, oestrogens.

*Side effects*: anticholinergic effects including urine retention, dry mouth, constipation, blurred vision, rapid heartbeat, palpitations, nervousness, insomnia, sweating, dizziness, fatigue, weight changes, jaundice, blood changes, allergic skin rashes, changes in libido, breast enlargement and impotence.

*Manufacturer*: Abbott.

## PROTIUM

*Description*: a proton pump inhibitor available as enteric-coated, yellow tablets in 2 strengths containing 20 and

40mg of pantoprazole, as sodium sesquihydrate, marked P20 and P40, respectively. *Also,* **PROTIUM IV,** available as a powder in vials for reconstitution and injection containing 40mg of pantoprazole as sodium.

*Used for*: ulcers in the stomach or duodenum, prevention of ulceration caused by NSAID treatment, reflux oesophagitis (GORD) and its prevention, with antibiotics, to eliminate *H. pylori* bacteria in patients with gastritis or duodenal ulcer.

*Dosage*: adults, tablets, ulcer treatment, 40mg each day taken in the morning – for 2 weeks in case of duodenal ulcer (continued for another 2 weeks if not healed) and for 4 weeks in case of stomach ulcer (continued for another 4 weeks if not healed). Ulceration caused by NSAID, 20mg each day. GORD, 20 to 40mg taken in the morning for 2 weeks to 1 month, continuing for a further 4 weeks, if needed. Maintenance dose is 20mg each day and patient should be re-assessed after 1 year and risk/benefit analysis performed. Triple therapy to eliminate *H. pylori,* 40mg 2 times each day with 250mg of clarithromycin and 400mg of metronidazole twice each day for 1 week. Or, with 500mg of clarithromycin and 1g of amoxicillin 2 times each day for 1 week. Injection, 40mg by intravenous infusion or slow intravenous injection over 2 to 15 minutes once each day for up to 1 week. Patients should be transferred to tablets as soon as possible.

*Special care*: pregnancy, breastfeeding, severe liver disorders-liver enzymes should be monitored and treatment withdrawn if these are raised.

*Avoid use*: children.
*Side effects*: diarrhoea, dizziness, rash, headache.
*Manufacturer*: Abbott.

## PROZAC

*Description*: an antidepressant preparation which is a 5HT reuptake inhibitor, promoting the availability of this neurotransmitter. It is available as capsules in 2 strengths: yellow/green capsules containing 20mg fluoxetine hydrochloride marked with name and strength; yellow capsules containing 60mg of fluoxetine hydrochloride. *Also*, **PROZAC LIQUID**, a syrup containing 20mg of fluoxetine hydrochloride per 5ml.
*Used for*: depression which may be accompanied by anxiety, especially when sedation is not needed. Obsessive-compulsive disorders, bulimia nervosa (eating disorder), pre-menstrual dysphoric disorder (PMDD).
*Dosage*: adults, depression and PMDD, 20mg each day; obsessive compulsive disorder, 20 to 60mg each day; bulimia nervosa, 60mg each day. Maximum in all cases is 80mg daily and doses may be adjusted up or down to achieve best result.
*Special care*: pregnancy, breastfeeding, heart disease, history of fits, previous mania or hypomania diabetes, liver disease, history of bleeding disorders. Evaluate carefully before treating for PMDD and discuss risks and benefits.
*Avoid use*: children, unstable epilepsy.
*Possible interaction*: vinblastine, MAOIs, clozapine, lithium, tramadol, vinblastine, carbamazepine, TCADs, flecainide,

carbamazepine, encainide, phenytoin, tryptophan, haloperidol, drugs affecting platelets or ECT, diazepam, warfarin, St John's Wort.

*Side effects*: sleep abnormalities, sweating, anorexia, euphoria, baldness, anxiety, abnormal milk production, disturbance of vision, headache, sexual dysfunction, priapism (abnormal, persistent and painful erection of penis), dizziness, gastrointestinal upset, frequent urination and urine retention, drowsiness, anxiety, weakness, fever, convulsions. sensitivity to light, muscle and joint pains, chills, short-lived disorders of movement, liver function abnormalities. In rare cases, bleeding, serotonin syndrome. Withdraw drug if allergic reactions or rash occur.

*Manufacturer*: Dista.

## PSEUDOEPHEDRINE *SEE*: DIMOTANE PLUS, SUDAFED, SUDAFED PLUS.

## PULMICORT

*Description*: a bronchodilator corticosteroid preparation in 3 strengths delivering 100µg, 200µg, and 400µg of budesonide per metered dose aerosol, suitable for use with a Turbohaler. *Also*, **PULMICORT LS** delivering 50µg of budesonide per metered dose, for use with Nebuhaler. *Also,* **PULMICORT INHALER** for use with a NebuChamber or Nebuhaler delivering 200µg budesonide per metered dose. *Also,* **PULMICORT RESPULES** available at strength of 0.5mg and 1mg of budesonide per 2ml available in ampoules for nebulization. *Also,* **PULMICORT L.S,** delivering 50μg of budesonide per metered dose as an aerosol for use with Nebuhaler.

*Used for*: all except Pulmicort Respules, bronchial asthma. Pulmicort Respules, asthma in which some other breath-actuated inhalers have failed to control; croup.

*Dosage*: adults, Pulmicort, severe attack, 200 to 1600μg in 2 divided doses each day; less severe attack, 200 to 800μg. Both when starting therapy or when reducing steroids taken orally. For mild to moderate asthma in patients not on steroids, 200 to 400μg as on evening dose. Patients taking inhaled steroids twice each day, up to 800μg as single evening dose; if changing to once a day, start with same total daily dose and then reduce until maintenance is achieved. Pulmicort Inhaler, 1 puff 2 times each day for mild to moderate asthma; up to 8 puffs each day for severe asthma. Pulmicort Respules, in order of 1 to 2mg 2 times each day but more if very severe; usual maintenance is in order of 0.5 to 1mg twice each day. Children, Pulmicort, severe asthma at start of treatment and during reduction of steroids taken by mouth, 200 to 800μg each day in 2 divided doses. Mild to moderate asthma in patients not on steroids or on steroids inhaled 2 times each day, 200 to 400μg taken as single evening dose. If changing to once a day regimen, start with same total daily dose and then reduce until maintenance is achieved. Pulmicort Inhaler, 1 to 2 puffs 2 times each day, or up to 4, in severe cases. Pulmicort L.S. 1 to 8 puffs each day. Pulmicort Respules, asthma, aged 3 months to 12 years,

0.5 to 1mg twice each day with maintenance dose of 0.25 to 0.5mg twice each day. Croup, 2mg nebulised and administered as single dose; or 1mg nebulised followed by a second 1mg dose, 30 minutes later.

*Special care*: pregnancy, breastfeeding, quiescent pulmonary tuberculosi, those transferring from other (systemic) steroids, viral or fungal respiratory injections. Risk of suppression of adrenal glands with long-term treatment, also, systemic steroid effects. Height of children should be monitored and systemic steroid may be needed in event of surgery or stress.

*Avoid use*: active pulmonary tuberculosis.

*Side effects*: candidiasis of throat and mouth, dryness and hoarseness. In rare cases, allergic reactions, skin effects, paradoxical bronchospasm, angioedema (widespread swelling due to fluid retention).

*Manufacturer*: AstraZeneca.

## PYLORID

*Description*: an H2 blocker and cytoprotectant available as octagonal, film-coated, pale blue tablets containing 400mg of ranitidine bismuth citrate, marked with logo.

*Used for*: duodenal and stomach ulcer, prevention of relapse of stomach ulcer, with antibiotic treatment to eradicate *H. pylori*.

*Dosage*: adults, duodenal and stomach ulcer, 1 tablet 2 times each day taken with food for 1 to 2 months (duodenal ulcer) and for 2 months (stomach ulcer). With antibiotics to eliminate *H. pylori,* triple therapy, 400mg with 500mg of clarithromycin and 1g of amoxicillin, all 2 times each day for 1 week. Or, same dose of Pylorid and clarithromycin but with 400 or 500mg of metronidazole 2 times each day for 1 week. Or same dose of Pylorid and metronidazole but with 250mg of clarithromycin, all 2 times each day for 1 week. Dual therapy, 400mg of Pylorid 2 times each day with 500mg of amoxicillin 4 times each day for 2 weeks. To heal ulcer completely, continue with 400mg of Pylorid twice daily for 1month. Treatment should be for a maximum period of 16 weeks in any 1 year.

*Special care*: pregnancy, breastfeeding, elderly patients, kidney disease, porphyria (inherited, metabolic disorder involving porphyrins). Possibility of malignancy should be excluded before starting treatment.

*Avoid use*: children, moderate to severe kidney disorders.

*Side effects*: headache, slow heartbeat, gastrointestinal upset, slight anaemia, alteration in liver enzymes, blackening of stools and tongue. In rare cases, blood changes, allergic reactions, effects on breasts in males, muscle and bone disorders, confusion, pancreatitis, hepatitis.

*Manufacturer*: GlaxoSmithKline.

**PYRAZINAMIDE *SEE*: RIFATER.**

**QUINAPRIL *SEE*: ACCUPRO, ACCURETIC.**

# R

**RABEPRAZOLE *SEE*: PARIET.**

**RAMIPRIL *SEE*: TRIAPIN, TRITACE.**

**RANITIDINE *SEE*: ZANTAC.**

**RANITIDINE BISMUTH CITRATE *SEE*: PYLORID.**

**RAPITIL**

*Description*: an NSAID available as eye drops containing 2% nedocromil sodium.

*Used for*: allergic and other forms of conjunctivitis.

*Dosage*: adults, allergic conjunctivitis, 1 drop twice each day into both eyes increasing to 1 drop 4 times each day, if needed. If treating seasonal conjunctivitis, do not use for more than 12 weeks. Vernal keratoconjunctivitis, 1 drop in both eyes 4 times each day. Children aged over 6 years, use as for adults to treat seasonal allergic conjunctivitis only.

*Special care*: pregnancy.

*Avoid use*: children aged under 6 years, wearers of soft contact lenses.

*Side effects*: short-lived irritation, taste changes.

*Manufacturer*: R.P.R.

## RELAXIT

*Description*: a faecal softener and osmotic preparation available as a micro-enema containing 450mg of sodium citrate, 75mg of sodium lauryl sulphate, 5mg of sorbic acid in a glycerol and sorbitol solution.

*Used for*: constipation.

*Dosage*: adults and children over 3 years, 1 enema inserted to complete extent of applicator nozzle. Children aged under 3 years, 1 enema with applicator nozzle inserted to half its length.

*Manufacturer*: Crawford.

## RELIFEX

*Description*: an NSAID and naphthylalkanone available as film-coated, red tablets containing 500mg of nabumetone, coded RELIFEX 500. *Also*, **RELIFEX SUSPENSION** containing 500mg of nabumetone per 5ml.

*Used for*: rheumatoid arthritis and osteoarthritis.

*Dosage*: adults, 2 tablets or 10ml as 1 dose at bedtime. An extra 1 to 2 tablets or 5–10ml may be taken in the morning, if symptoms are severe. Elderly, 1 to 2 tablets or 5–10ml each day.

*Special care*: elderly, liver or kidney disease, history of stomach ulcer.

*Avoid use*: children, pregnancy, breastfeeding, active stomach ulcer, severe liver disease, allergy to aspirin or NSAIDs.

*Possible interaction*: sulphonylurea hypoglycaemics, hydantoin, anticoagulants taken by mouth, anticonvulsants.

*Side effects*: headache, dizziness, gastrointestinal upset, skin rash, sedation.
*Manufacturer*: Meda.

## RETROVIR

*Description*: a nucleoside reverse transcriptase inhibitor available as capsules in 2 strengths, both containing zidovudine. White capsules, marked 100 and Y9C contain 100mg; blue/white capsules, marked 250 and H2F contain 250mg. All capsules also marked Wellcome and with blue band. *Also,* **RETROVIR SYRUP,** a light yellow, sugar-free liquid containing 50mg of zidovudine per 5ml supplied with oral syringe. *Also,* **RETROVIR INFUSION,** a solution in vials containing 10mg of zidovudine per ml.
*Used for*: combined with other retroviral drugs to treat HIV infections; as sole therapy in HIV-positive, pregnant women more than 14 weeks into pregnancy and their newborn babies, to prevent mother-child transmission.
*Dosage*: adults, capsules and syrup, 500 to 600mg each day in 2 to 3 divided doses. Infusion, 1 to 2mg per kg of body weight every 4 hours by slow intravenous infusion over 1 hour; patients should be given oral preparations as soon as possible. Children, capsules and syrup, aged 3 months to 12 years, 360 to 480mg per $m^2$ of body surface area in 3 to 4 divided doses each day with a maximum dose of 200mg every 6 hours. Infusion, 80 to 160mg per $m^2$ of body surface area every 6 hours. In adults and children combined with other retrovirals. Prevention of mother-child

transmission, capsules, syrup, infusion: mother, 100mg 5 times each day taken by mouth until labour starts then 2mg per kg of body weight by intravenous infusion over 1 hour during labour and delivery, continuing with 1mg per kg of body weight until baby is delivered and cord is clamped. Baby, 2mg per kg of body weight by mouth or 1.5mg per kg of body weight by intravenous infusion over half an hour, both every 6 hours and starting within 12 hours of birth, continuing for 6 weeks. If caesarian birth or false labour, consult manufacturer's literature.

*Special care*: elderly, pregnant women during first 14 weeks of pregnancy (treatment not usually given unless benefit to mother greatly outweighs risk to foetus), liver or kidney disorders. Dosages may require adjusting if bone marrow suppression or anaemia occurs. Blood tests must be carried out every week in those receiving infusion and every 2 weeks in those taking oral preparations during initial 3 months of treatment. These should continue to be carried out every month in patients with advanced HIV.

*Avoid use*: breastfeeding, low white blood cell counts or haemoglobin levels, newborn babies with high levels of bilirubin in blood or raised transaminase levels.

*Possible interaction*: ribavirin, probenecid, some drugs affecting liver function, phenytoin, stavudine, chronic use of analgesics, especially paracetamol, other drugs suppressing bone marrow or nephrotoxic preparations. Patients should be carefully warned about taking other drugs.

*Side effects*: gastrointestinal upset, insomnia, blood changes (leucopenia, thrombocytopenia, anaemia, pancytopenia), muscle pains and muscle disease, rash, heart muscle disease, raised liver enzymes, enlargement of liver with steatosis, lactic acid acidosis, headache, pancreatitis, cough, shortness of breath, anxiety, depression, sensation of numbness/tingling/pins-and-needles, pigmentation affecting skin and nails, fits.

*Manufacturer*: GlaxoSmithKline.

## RHEUMOX

*Description*: a benzotriazine available as dark/light orange capsules marked WYETH and RHEUMOX containing 300mg of azapropazone dihydrate. *Also,* **RHEUMOX TABLETS,** film-coated, scored, oblong tablets containing 600mg of azapropazone dihydrate.

*Used for*: ankylosing spondylitis, rheumatoid arthritis, acute gout which has not responded to other treatments.

*Dosage*: adults, ankylosing spondylitis and rheumatoid arthritis, 1.2g each day in 2 or 4 divided doses; elderly, 300mg every morning and night to a maximum daily dose of 600mg. Acute gout, adults, 1.8g each day in divided doses for up to 4 days, then 1.2g each day until symptoms improve. Elderly, 1.8g in divided doses for 24 hours, then 1.2g each day for up to 4 days, then gradually reducing to 600mg daily as symptoms improve.

*Special care*: elderly or patients who are debilitated, asthma, high blood pressure, kidney disorders, allergy to aspirin or anti-inflammatories. Patients taking drug long-term should be regularly assessed and should be advised to avoid exposure to direct sunlight as far as possible.

*Avoid use*: children, pregnancy, breastfeeding, severe liver or kidney disease, blood changes, ulcerative colitis, previous stomach ulcer, porphyria (an inherited, metabolic disorder involving porphyrins).

*Possible interaction*: hypoglycaemics, phenytoin, methotrexate, cimetidine, lithium, anticoagulants, digoxin.

*Side effects*: fluid retention, sensitivity to light. Withdraw drug in the event of bleeding in gastrointestinal tract, positive Coombs test or alveolitis (inflammation of alveoli of lungs).

*Manufacturer*: Goldshield.

## RHINOLAST

*Description*: an antihistamine preparation available as a metered dose nasal spray delivering 0.1% azelastine hydrochloride.

*Used for*: rhinitis (running, irritated nose and sneezing) caused by allergy.

*Dosage*: adults, 1 application per nostril twice each day.

*Special care*: pregnancy, breastfeeding.

*Avoid use*: children.

*Side effects*: nasal irritation, effect on taste.

*Manufacturer*: Viatris.

## RIFADIN

*Description*: an antibiotic and antimalarial preparation available as capsules in 2 strengths, blue/red, containing

150mg and red, containing 300mg of rifampicin. *Also*, **RIFADIN SYRUP** containing 100mg of rifampicin per 5ml. *Also*, **RIFADIN INFUSION,** available as a powder in a vial containing 600mg of rifampicin, with 10ml solvent in an ampoule.

*Used for*: prevention of meningococcal meningitis in people not showing symptoms who are carriers of *N. meningitidis*, treatment of carriers of *Haemophilus influenzae*, additional therapy for brucellosis, Legionnaire's disease and serious staphylococcal infections, tuberculosis and mycobacterial infections, leprosy.

*Dosage*: adults, meningitis, 600mg twice each day for 2 days; influenza, 20mg per kg of body weight each day for 4 days; brucellosis, 600 to 1200mg each day as 2 to 4 doses; tuberculosis, 8 to 12mg per kg of body weight each day as single dose taken thirty minutes before or 2 hours after a meal; leprosy, 600mg once each month or 10mg per kg of body weight each day as one dose. Children: meningitis, aged 3 months to 1 year, 5mg per kg of body weight twice each day for 2 days; aged 1 to 12 years, 10mg per kg of body weight twice each day for 2 days; influenza, 20mg per kg of body weight each day for 4 days to a daily maximum of 600mg, newborn infants, 10mg per kg of body weight each day for 4 days; tuberculosis, 10 to 30mg per kg of body weight each day to a daily maximum of 600mg; leprosy, as adult dose.

*Special care*: pregnancy, breastfeeding, elderly, poorly nourished or the very young, liver disorders – function should be monitored.

*Avoid use*: jaundice.

*Possible interaction*: digitalis, hypoglycaemics, ciclosporin, analgesics, corticosteroids, anticoagulants, oral contraceptives, dapsone, quinidine, phenytoin, narcotics.

*Side effects*: rashes, gastrointestinal upset, flu-like symptoms, upset liver function, orange discolouration of urine, secretions and soft contact lenses.

*Manufacturer*: Aventis.

## RIFAMPICIN *SEE*: RIFADIN, RIFATUR, RIFINAH, RIMACTAZID.

## RIFATER

*Description*: a compound drug the components of which are derived from isonicotinic acid and nicotinic acid, available as sugar-coated, pink tablets containing 50mg of isoniazid, 300mg of pyrazinamide and 120mg of rifampicin.

*Used for*: pulmonary tuberculosis in the initial intensive phase.

*Dosage*: adults, a single dose should be taken either thirty minutes before or 2 hours after a meal; patients weighing over 65kg, 6 tablets per day; weighing 50 to 64kg, 5 tablets; weighing 40 to 49kg, 4 tablets; weighing under 40 kg, 3 tablets each day, to continue for 2 months followed by rifampicin/isoniazid compound. For the initial period, the additional use of ethambutol or streptomycin given intramuscularly, is advised.

*Special care*: elderly, pregnancy, breastfeeding, people who are malnourished, history of epilepsy, gout, liver disease (function should be monitored), haemoptysis (coughing up blood).

*Avoid use*: children, jaundice.

*Possible interaction*: digitalis, hypoglycaemics, ciclosporin, corticosteroids, analgesics, anticoagulants, oral contraceptives, dapsone, quinidine, phenytoin, narcotics.

*Side effects*: rashes, gastro-intestinal upset, flu-like symptoms, upset liver function, orange discolouration of urine, secretions and soft contact lenses.

*Manufacturer*: Aventis.

## RIFINAH

*Description*: a combined rifamycin and isonicotinic acid available as tablets in 2 strengths. Pink '150' tablets contain 150mg of rifampicin and 100mg of isoniazid. Oblong, orange '300' tablets contain 300mg of rifampicin and 150mg of isoniazid.

*Used for*: tuberculosis.

*Dosage*: adults, weighing under 50kg, 3x Rifinah '150' tablets each day; weighing over 50kg, 2x Rifinah '300' tablets each day. All to be taken as single dose either 30 minutes before or 2 hours after a meal.

*Special care*: pregnancy, breastfeeding, elderly, malnourished patients, porphyria (inherited metabolic disorder involving porphyrins), liver disorder (function should be monitored).

*Avoid use*: children, jaundice.

*Possible interaction*: digitalis, hypoglycaemics, ciclosporin, corticosteroids, analgesics, anticoagulants, oral contraceptives, dapsone, quinidine, phenytoin, narcotics.

*Side effects*: rashes, gastro-intestinal upset, flu-like symptoms, upset liver function, orange discolouration of urine, secretions and soft contact lenses.

*Manufacturer*: Aventis.

## RIMACTAZID

*Description*: a combined rifampicin/isonicotinic acid preparation available as sugar-coated tablets in 2 different strengths. Red tablets, marked CG and EL contain 150mg of rifampicin and 100mg of isoniazid; orange tablets, marked CG and DH, contain 300mg of rifampicin and 150mg of isoniazid.

*Used for*: tuberculosis, some infections caused by mycobacteria.

*Dosage*: adults, continuous treatment, 2x Rimactazid 300 once each day if weighing over 50kg; 3x Rimactazid 150 each day if weighing under 50kg. Intermittent treatment, weighing over 50kg, 2x Rimactazid 300 two to three times each week; weighing under 50kg, 3x Rimactazid 150 two or three times each week. All to be taken as a single dose thirty minutes before breakfast.

*Special care*: pregnancy, breastfeeding, undernourished patients, elderly, liver disease (monitor function), porphyria (an inherited metabolic disorder), epilepsy. Blood counts should be monitored

*Avoid use*: children, acute liver disorders, previous hepatitis caused by drugs, inflammation of peripheral nerves.

*Possible interaction*: digitalis, hypoglycaemics, ciclosporin, corticosteroids, anticoagulants, oral contraceptives, dapsone, quinidine, phenytoin, narcotics, analgesics. Other drugs being taken may require to be adjusted

*Side effects*: rashes, gastro-intestinal upset, flu-like symptoms, upset liver function, orange discolouration of urine and secretions.

*Manufacturer*: Swedish Orphan.

## RITALIN CD

*Description*: a central nervous system stimulant and controlled drug available as scored, white tablets containing 10mg of methylphenidate hydrochloride, marked AB and CG.

*Used for*: Attention-deficit hyperactivity disorder in children.

*Dosage*: children aged over 6 years, 5mg once or twice each day increasing, if required at weekly intervals, by increments of 5 to 10mg each day, to a daily maximum of 60mg in divided doses. If no improvement has been noticed within 4 weeks then the drug should be withdrawn.

*Special care*: must be prescribed only under specialist supervision by expert in behavioural disorders in children, pregnancy, breastfeeding, patients who are emotionally unstable, high blood pressure, epilepsy, psychosis. Weight, height and blood pressure should be monitored and blood counts performed if treatment is long-term. Drug should be stopped carefully.

*Avoid use*: heart arrhythmias, toxicity of thyroid gland, family history of Tourette's syndrome or tics, severe agitation, anxiety or tension, glaucoma, serious angina.

*Possible interaction*: guanethidine, anticonvulsants, phenylbutazone, anticoagulants, TCAD1 pressor agents, alcohol, MAOIs.

*Side effects*: insomnia, gastrointestinal upset, appetite loss, nervousness, headache.

*Manufacturer*: Cephalon.

## ROFECOXIB *SEE*: VIOXX.

## CD ROHYPNOL

*Description*: a hypnotic, controlled drug and intermediate-acting benzodiazepine, available as scored, oval, grey-green coloured tablets containing 1mg of flunitrazepam, marked 542.

*Used for*: short-term treatment of severe or disabling insomnia, to induce sleep at unusual times.

*Dosage*: adults, 1/2 to 1 tablet at bedtime (elderly, 1/2 tablet).

*Special care*: chronic liver, kidney or lung disease, acute, narrow-angle glaucoma, elderly persons, bereavement. May impair dexterity and judgement. Should not be used as sole therapy for depression or anxiety. To be withdrawn gradually.

*Avoid use*: children, pregnancy, breastfeeding, labour, acute lung disease, depression of the respiration, obsessional and phobic states, chronic psychosis. Also, myasthenia gravis, severe liver disorders, sleep apnoea syndrome

*Possible interaction*: anticonvulsants, CNS depressants, alcohol.

*Side effects*: confusion, vertigo, drowsiness, ataxia, light-headedness, gastro-intestinal upsets, skin rashes, weakness in muscles, hypotension, disturbance in vision. Urine retention, changes in libido, impaired ability to perform tasks and in exercise of judgement; rarely, jaundice and effects on blood. Dependence is possible especially at higher doses and with longer treatment periods.

*Manufacturer*: Roche.

# S

## SALAMOL INHALER

*Description*: a preparation which is a bronchodilator and selective ß2-agonist available as a metered dose aerosol for delivering 100µg of salbutamol per dose. *Also,* **SALAMOL EASI-BREATHE,** for use with a breath-activated inhaler delivering 100µg of salbutamol per dose. *Also,* **SALAMOL STERI-NEB** available as a preservative-free solution for nebulization containing 2.5mg and 5mg salbutamol as sulphate per 2.5ml, as single dose units.

*Used for*: Salamol Inhaler and Easi-Breathe, prevention of asthma caused by exercise, treatment of asthma and chronic bronchitis. Salamol Steri-Neb, severe bronchospasm and acute severe asthma which has failed to respond to other drugs.

*Dosage*: Salamol inhaler and Easi-Breathe, adults, for attack, 1 or 2 puffs; prevention, 2 puffs before exercise. Maximum dose is 8 puffs every 24 hours. Children, acute attack, 1 or 2 puffs; prevention, 2 puffs before exercise. Maximum dose, 8 puffs in 24 hours. Salamol Steri-Neb, adults and children, 2.5mg nebulized 3 or 4 times each day increasing to 5mg, 3 to 4 times daily, if needed.

*Special care*: pregnancy, weak heart, heart arrhythmias, angina, high blood pressure, over-active thyroid gland.

*Possible interaction*: ß-blockers, sympathomimetics.

*Side effects*: headache, dilation of peripheral blood vessels, tremor, low blood potassium levels. Any adverse side effects using inhaler should be reported to the Committee on the Safety of Medicines (CSM).

*Manufacturer*: Ivax.

## SALBUTAMOL *SEE*: AIROMIR, SALAMOL, VENTOLIN, VOLMAX.

## SALCATONIN *SEE*: CALSYNAR.

## SALMETEROL *SEE*: SERETIDE, SEREVENT.

## SANDRENA

*Description*: an oestrogen preparation available as a gel in 2 strengths containing 0.5 and 1mg of oestradiol as hemihydrate.

*Used for*: HRT to treat symptoms of the menopause.

*Dosage*: women, 1mg applied once each day either to the left or right thigh on alternate days at first. Then adjust after 2 to 3 months to maintenance in order of 0.5 to 1.5mg each day. In women retaining womb, a progestogen should be added for 10 to 12 days of each cycle.

*Special care*: high blood pressure, severe kidney disease receiving dialysis, Raynaud's disease, diabetes, multiple sclerosis, asthma, varicose veins, elevated levels of prolactin (a hormone) in the blood (hyperprolactinemia). Risk of thrombosis increases with smoking, age and obesity. Blood pressure, breasts and pelvic organs should be checked during period of treatment.

*Avoid use*: pregnancy, heart and circulatory diseases, angina, sickle cell anaemia, pulmonary hypertension. Also hormone-dependent cancers, undiagnosed vaginal bleeding, chorea, liver disease, history of cholestatic jaundice of pregnancy, infectious hepatitis, Dublin–Johnson syndrome, Rotor syndrome, recent trophoblastic disease.

*Possible interaction*: phenytoin, carbamazepine, tetracyclines, primidone, chloral hydrate, glutethimide, phenylbutazone, rifampicin, griseofulvin, ampicillin, dichloralphenazone, ethosuximide, barbiturates, St John's Wort.

*Side effects*: feeling of bloatedness due to fluid retention, leg pains, breast enlargement, erosion of cervix, muscular cramps, weight gain, breakthrough bleeding, depression, headaches, vaginal discharge, loss of libido, nausea, brown patches on skin (chloasma). Stop drug immediately in event of pregnancy.

*Manufacturer*: Organon.

## SECTRAL

*Description*: an antiarrhythmic, antianginal preparation which is a cardioselective ß-blocker available as capsules in 2 strengths, both containing acebutolol (as hydrochloride). White/buff contain 100mg and pink/buff contain 200mg both marked with strength and SECTRAL. *Also*, **SECTRAL TABLETS**, white, film-coated, containing 400mg of acebutolol as hydrochloride, marked SECTRAL 400.

*Used for*: heart arrhythmias, angina, high blood pressure.

*Dosage*: adults, arrhythmias, maintenance dose of 400 to 1200mg in 2 or 3 divided doses each day. Angina, 400mg once each day taken with breakfast or 200mg twice each day with a maximum of 1.2g daily. High blood pressure, same starting dose as for angina, increasing if necessary after 2 weeks to 400mg twice each day.

*Special care*: pregnancy, breast-feeding, liver or kidney disease, diabetes, metabolic acidosis, poor cerebral blood supply, history of bronchospasm, those undergoing anaesthesia; patients with weak hearts should be treated with digitalis and diuretics. Drug should be stopped gradually.

*Avoid use*: children, patients with asthma, heart diseases including heart block, heart shock, slow heartbeat rate, heart failure.

*Possible interaction*: cardiac depressants, anaesthetics, reserpine, sedatives, class II calcium antagonists, antihypertensives, sympathomimetics, cimetidine, indometacin, ergotamine, class I antiarrhythmic drugs, verapamil, clonidine withdrawal, hypoglycaemics, rifampicin, warfarin, ibuprofen.

*Side effects*: sleep disturbance, cold feet and hands, slow heartbeat, fatigue on exercise, wheeziness, heart failure, gastro-intestinal disorders; dry eyes or skin rash (stop use gradually), hair loss, low blood pressure, thrombocytopenia (abnormal decline in blood platelets causing increased likelihood of bleeding).

*Manufacturer*: Akita.

## SECURON

*Description*: a class I calcium antagonist available as film-coated, scored, white tablets containing 120mg of verapamil hydrochloride and marked with KNOLL, strength and tablet name. *Also,* **SECURON SR,** available as green, sustained-release, film-coated, oblong tablets containing 240mg of verapamil hydrochloride, marked with logo. *Also,* **HALF SECURON SR**, white, film-coated, sustained-release tablets containing 120mg of verapamil hydrochloride marked 120 SR and company name. *Also*, **SECURON IV** available as a solution in ampoules containing 2.5mg of verapamil hydrochloride per ml.

*Used for*: Securon tablets, supraventricular tachycardia (rapid heart beat), angina, high blood pressure. Other preparations, angina, high blood pressure, prevention of second heart attack in patients who do not have heart failure and who are not on diuretics and in whom **ß**-blockers cannot be used.

*Dosage*: adults, tachycardias, Securon Tablets, 40 to 120mg 3 times each day. Angina, Securon SR, Half Securon SR or Securon Tablets, 80 to 120mg 3 times each day. Hypertension, Securon SR or Half Securon SR, start with 120mg once each day then 240mg once each day with a maximum of 480mg in divided doses daily. Securon Tablets, 120mg twice each day at first increasing to 160mg twice daily if needed. Maximum dose is 480mg in divided doses daily. Secondary prevention of heart attack, Securon SR and Half Securon SR, start at least 1 week after first heart attack, 360mg each day in divided doses. Securon IV, consult manufacturer's literature.

*Special care*: pregnancy, breastfeeding, liver or kidney disorders, heart conduction disturbances, bradycardia (slow heartbeat), 1st degree heart block. Patients with weak hearts require digitalis and/or diuretics.

*Avoid use*: children, some kinds of heart block, heart shock, sick sinus syndrome, serious bradycardia, heart attack with bradycardia, severe low blood pressure or failure of left ventricle, uncompensated heart failure, low blood pressure below certain level, some types of heart flutter or fibrillation (Securon IV must not be used and oral preparations should be used very cautiously).

*Possible interaction*: digoxin, ß-blockers (Securon IV must not be used), cimetidine, muscle relaxant drugs, inhaled anaesthetics, ciclosporin, rifampicin, antihypertensives, lithium, antiarrhythmics, carbamazepine, theophylline, phenobarbital, phenytoin, alcohol, grapefruit juice.

*Side effects*: constipation. In rare cases, vomiting, reversible liver dysfunction, swelling of ankles due to fluid retention, nausea, headaches, fatigue, dizziness, allergic reactions, hypotension, abnormal enlargement of breasts, increased growth of gum tissues, flushes, decrease in heart rate and motility of heart muscle, 2nd or 3rd degree heart block, low blood pressure.

*Manufacturer*: Abbott.

**SENNA *SEE*: MANEVAC, SENOKOT.**

## SENOKOT

*Description*: a bowel stimulant available as brown tablets containing standardised senna equivalent to 7.5mg total sennosides, marked with sword and tablet name. *Also,* **SENOKOT GRANULES,** comprising standardised senna equivalent to 15mg total sennosides per 5ml spoonful; **SENOKOT SYRUP,** containing standardised senna equivalent to 7.5mg total sennosides per 5ml.

*Used for*: constipation.

*Dosage*: adults, 2 to 4 tablets or 5 to 10ml spoonfuls of granules or 10 to 20ml of syrup; all doses taken at bedtime. Children, aged 2 to 6 years, 2.5 to 5ml of syrup; aged over 6 years, half adult dose. All doses to be taken in the morning.

*Manufacturer*: R&C.

## SEPTRIN

*Description*: an antibiotic preparation combining a folic acid inhibitor and sulfonamide available as white tablets containing 80mg trimethoprim and 400mg sulfamethoxazole, marked with maker's name, tablet name and Y2B. *Also,* **SEPTRIN ADULT SUSPENSION** containing quantities as tablets per 5ml. *Also,* **SEPTRIN FORTE TABLETS,** scored, white tablets containing 160mg of trimethoprim and 800mg of sulfamethoxazole. *Also,* **SEPTRIN PAEDIATRIC SUSPENSION**, sugar-free, containing 40mg of trimethoprim and 200mg of sulfamethoxazole per 5ml. Also, **SEPTRIN FOR INFUSION** available in ampoules containing 80mg of trimethoprim and 400mg of sulfamethoxazole per 5ml.

*Used for*: infections of skin, gastro-intestinal, respiratory (acute flare-ups of chronic bronchitis) and urinary tracts, acute inflammation and infections of middle ear, all where this combination is deemed to be preferable. Also, prevention of pneumonitis caused by *P. carinii*, treatment of nocardiosis, prevention and treatment of toxoplasmosis.

*Dosage*: adults, tablets and adult suspension, 2 tablets or 10ml every 12 hours; for pneumonitis, nocardiosis and toxoplasmosis, manufacturer's literature should be consulted. Septrin Forte, 1 tablet every 12 hours. Children, Paediatric Suspension, 6 weeks to 5 months, 2.5ml; 6 months to 5 years, 5ml; over 6 years, 10ml, all twice each day. Infusion, adults and children, manufacturer's literature should be consulted.

*Special care*: pregnancy, breastfeeding, elderly, kidney disorders (lower doses or greater intervals), deficiency in G-6-PD or folate, asthma or severe allergies. Regular blood tests should be carried out in patients taking the drug long-term.

*Avoid use*: newborn babies, severe liver or kidney disorders, porphyria (inherited metabolic disorder involving porphyrins), blood changes.

*Possible interaction*: procainamide, digoxin, pyrimethamine, phenytoin, thiazides, anticonvulsants, amantadine, ciclosporin, folate inhibitors, hypoglycaemics, anticoagulants, lamivudine.

*Side effects*: vomiting, nausea, inflammation of tongue, liver and blood changes, skin rashes, folate deficiency. In rare cases, erythema multiformae (allergic disorder affecting

skin and mucous membranes), Stevens–Johnson syndrome, exfoliative dermatitis, Lyell syndrome, lack of coordination, vertigo, muscle and joint disorders, fits, inflammation of peripheral nerves.
*Manufacturer*: GlaxoSmithKline.

## SERETIDE ACCUHALER

*Description*: a combined selective ß2-agonist and corticosteroid preparation for use with breath-activated inhaler, available in 3 strengths, each delivering 50μg of salmeterol and 100, 250 or 500μg of fluticasone proprionate. *Also,* **SERETIDE EVOHALER,** for use with metered dose inhaler in 3 strengths delivering 25μg of salmeterol and 50, 125 or 250μg of fluticasone proprionate.
*Used for*: regular asthma treatment where long-acting **ß**2-agonist and inhaled corticosteroid is considered to be the best option for the patient.
*Dosage*: adults, Accuhaler, 1 puff 2 times each day using lowest effective (corticosteroid) dose; Evohaler, 2 puffs twice each day. Children, Accuhaler only, aged over 4 years, 1 puff of lowest dose corticosteroid (Seretide 100) each day.
*Special care*: pregnancy, breastfeeding, serious heart and circulatory diseases, pulmonary tuberculosis, toxicity of thyroid gland, low blood potassium levels, diabetes. Children being treated long-term should have weight and height monitored; systemic effects and suppression of adrenal glands possible with long-term treatment – function must be checked. Treatment should be stopped

in the event of paradoxical bronchospasm. In event of stress or surgery, additional steroid treatment may be needed.

*Avoid use*: children aged under 4 years.

*Possible interaction*: ß-blockers.

*Side effects*: hoarseness, thrush affecting mouth and throat, tremor, muscle cramps/ pains, joint pains, palpitations, heart arrhythmias, allergic reactions, headaches. Any adverse side effects should be reported to the Committee on the Safety of Medicines (CSM).

*Manufacturer*: A & H.

## SEREVENT

*Description*: a bronchodilator and selective ß2-agonist available as a metered dose aerosol delivering 25µg of salmeterol (as xinafoate) per dose. *Also*, **SEREVENT DISKHALER**, using disks containing 4 x 50µg blisters salmeterol (as xinafoate) with breath-activated delivery system. *Also*, **SEREVENT ACCUHALER**, breath-activated inhaler delivering 50µg of salmeterol as xinafoate per dose.

*Used for*: asthma (including that induced by exercise or occurring at night), chronic obstructive pulmonary disease (COPD) for those requiring long-term treatment. Generally combined with anti-inflammatory therapy.

*Dosage*: adults, Serevent, asthma, 2 puffs twice each day, 4 puffs if exceptionally severe; COPD, 2 puffs twice each day. Serevent Diskhaler, 1 blister twice each day or 2 if very severe; COPD, 1 blister twice each day. Children, Serevent, age over 4 years, 2 puffs twice each day. Serevent Diskhaler, 1 blister twice each day.

*Special care*: pregnancy, breastfeeding, thyrotoxicosis, severe asthma or worsening condition – oral steroids or high doses of inhaled steroids may be required. Steroid therapy should be continued.

*Avoid use*: children under 4 years, acute asthma attack. Do not start treatment if patient is getting significantly worse.

*Possible interaction*: steroids, ß-blockers, diuretics, xanthines.

*Side effects*: paradoxical bronchospasm, low blood potassium levels. In rare cases, skin effects, pain in chest, joints and muscles, headache, palpitations, tremor, irritation of throat.

*Manufacturer*: A & H.

## SEROXAT

*Description*: an antidepressant available as film-coated, oval, scored tablets in 2 strengths; white, containing 20mg and blue, containing 30mg of paroxetine (as hydrochloride). Marked with strength and tablet name.

*Used for*: depression and depressive illness with anxiety, obsessive compulsive disorder, panic disorder, social phobia, generalised anxiety, post-traumatic stress disorder.

*Dosage*: adults, depression, social phobia, 20mg once each day at first, taken with breakfast. Then increasing gradually, if necessary, every 2 or 3 weeks by 10mg to a maximum daily dose of 50mg. Obsessive compulsive disorder, post-traumatic stress disorder, same starting dose then increase by 10mg once each week to 40mg each day. Maximum is 50mg each day. Generalised anxiety, 20mg each day. Elderly persons start with dose of 20mg once each day increasing gradually by weekly increments of 10mg to maximum of 40mg daily, if needed.

*Special care*: pregnancy, breastfeeding, glaucoma, serious liver or kidney disorders, diabetes, bleeding disorders, electroconvulsive treatment, heart disease or disease of arteries of heart, epilepsy (if symptoms worsen, stop treatment), history of mania/hypomania. Drug should be gradually stopped.

*Avoid use*: children.

*Possible interaction*: sumatriptan, enzyme inhibitors and inducers, anticonvulsants, warfarin, tramadol, procyclidine, tryptophan, other neuroleptics, drugs that increase bleeding, drugs affecting liver enzymes, phenytoin, MAOIs, lithium, St John's Wort.

*Side effects*: dry mouth, sweating, sleepiness, insomnia, tremor, nausea, weakness, effects on sexual habits, impairment of muscle tone, effects/symptoms arising after drug is withdrawn.

*Manufacturer*: GlaxoSmithKline.

## SERTRALINE *SEE*: LUSTRAL

## SLIDENAFIL *SEE*: VIAGRA.

## SIMVASTATIN *SEE*: ZOCOR.

## SINEQUAN

*Description*: a TCAD preparation available as tablets in

different strengths, all containing doxepin (as hydrochloride). Red capsules contain 10mg, coded SQN; red/blue contain 25mg, coded SQN 25; blue contain 50mg, coded SQN 50; blue/yellow contain 75mg, coded SQN 75. All are marked PFIZER.

*Used for*: depression.

*Dosage*: adults, 10 to 100mg 3 times each day or a maximum of 100mg as a single bedtime dose.

*Special care*: patients with psychoses or suicidal tendencies, elderly persons, pregnant and nursing mothers, people with cardiac disorders, epilepsy, hyperthyroidism, urine retention, closed angle glaucoma, liver disease, tumours of adrenal gland, diabetes

*Avoid use*: children, patients with recent heart attack, heart arrhythmias, heart block, porphyria (rare blood disorder).

*Possible interaction*: alcohol, barbiturate drugs, local anaesthetics (containing adrenaline or noradrenaline), antihypertensive and sympathomimetic drugs, anticholinergic drugs, cimetidine, oestrogens.

*Side effects*: anticholinergic effects including urine retention, dry mouth, constipation, blurred vision, rapid heartbeat, palpitations, nervousness, insomnia, sweating, dizziness, fatigue, weight changes, jaundice, blood changes, allergic skin rashes, changes in libido, breast enlargement and impotence

*Manufacturer*: Pfizer.

**SODIUM ACID PHOSPHATE *SEE*: CARBALAX.**

**SODIUM ALGINATE *SEE*: GASTROCOTE, GAVISCON LIQUID.**

**SODIUM ALKYLSULPHOACETATE *SEE*: MICRALAX.**

**SODIUM BICARBONATE *SEE*: CARBALAX, GASTROCOTE, GAVISCON, MOVICOL.**

**SODIUM CHLORIDE *SEE*: MINIMS ARTIFICIAL TEARS, MOVICOL.**

**SODIUM CITRATE *SEE*: MICRALAX, RELAXIT.**

**SODIUM CLODRONATE *SEE*: BONEFOS.**

**SODIUM FUSIDATE *SEE*: FUCITHALMIC.**

**SOFRADEX**

*Description*: a compound preparation combining a corticosteroid, aminoglycoside and antibiotic available in the form of drops containing 0.05% dexamethasone, 0.5% framycetin sulphate and 0.005% gramicidin. Also, **SOFRADEX OINTMENT** containing 0.05% dexamethasone, 0.5% framycetin sulphate and 0.005% gramicidin.

*Used for*: inflammation and infection of outer ear. Inflammation of eye and prevention of infection – short term only, blepharitis (inflammation of hair follicles of eye lashes which may be caused by infection).

*Dosage*: drops, ear, apply 2 to 3 drops 3 or 4 times each day;

ointment, ear, apply once or twice daily. Drops, eye, 1 or 2 drops up to 6 times each day or more frequently if necessary. Ointment, eye, apply 2 or 3 times each day or at night if drops are being used as well.

*Special care*: long-term use in pregnancy or infants.

*Avoid use*: perforated eardrum (if for ear infections), eye infections producing pus or those with tuberculous, fungal or viral origin, glaucoma.

*Side effects*: superinfection, use in eyes may lead to thinning of cornea, fungal infection, cataract, rise in pressure within eye.

*Manufacturer*: Florizel.

## SOFRAMYCIN

*Description*: an antibiotic aminoglycoside preparation available in the form of drops containing 0.5% framycetin sulphate. Also, **SOFRAMYCIN OINTMENT** containing 0.5% framycetin sulphate.

*Used for*: drops, eye infections, styes, blepharitis (inflammation and infection of hair follicles of eye lashes), conjunctivitis. Ointment, bacterial infections of skin.

*Dosage*: eyes, apply 1 or 2 drops at 1 or 2 hourly intervals, as needed; apply ointment 2 or 3 times each day or at night if drops are being used. Skin, apply ointment to affected area up to 3 times each day.

*Special care*: use on more extensive, damaged areas of skin.

*Side effects*: sensitisation, ototoxicity (damage to organs of balance and hearing).

*Manufacturer*: Florizel.

## SONATA

*Description*: a hypnotic preparation available as capsules in 2 strengths, both containing zaleplon. Light brown/white capsules with gold banding contain 5mg and white with pink banding contain 10mg. All are marked with strength and W.

*Used for*: severe and disabling insomnia which is causing distress.

*Dosage*: adults, 10mg at bedtime, or during night if at least 4 hours is available for sleeping. Treatment period must not exceed 2 weeks. Elderly patients, 5mg.

*Special care*: elderly, previous drug or alcohol abuse, impaired respiration, mild to moderate liver disorders, depression.

*Avoid use*: children, pregnancy, breastfeeding, severely insufficient respiration, serious liver disorders, myasthenia gravis, sleep apnoea, suicide risk, psychoses.

*Possible interaction*: narcotic analgesics, ketoconazole, other inducers of CYP3A4, alcohol, anxiolytics, sedatives, anticonvulsants, erythromycin, phenobarbital, cimetidine, antipsychotics, anaesthetics, rifampicin, antidepressants, antihistamines, carbamazepine, hypnotics.

*Side effects*: disturbance to CNS, dizziness, headache, amnesia, weakness, sleepiness, rebound insomnia, impaired reactions, anxiety, tolerance and dependence. withdraw if paradoxical psychiatric disturbance occurs. Any adverse side effects should be reported to the Committee on the Safety of Medicines (CSM).

*Manufacturer*: Wyeth.

## SORBIC ACID *SEE*: MICRALAX, RELAXIT.

## SORBITOL *SEE*: RELAXIT.

## SOLATOL HYDROCHLORIDE *SEE*: BETA-CARDONE.

## SPIRONOLACTONE *SEE*: ALDACTIDE, ALDACTONE.

## STARIL

*Description*: an antihypertensive and ACE inhibitor available as diamond-shaped, white tablets in 2 strengths containing 10mg and 20mg of fosinopril sodium marked with star, 158 and SQUIBB and with star, 609 and SQUIBB, respectively.

*Used for*: heart failure, in combination with diuretic treatment, high blood pressure.

*Dosage*: adults, 10mg once each day at first with this also being the usual maintenance dose. If necessary, increase dose carefully to maximum daily dose of 40mg, (after 4 weeks in cases of high blood pressure). If being used for high blood pressure, any diuretic should be stopped a few days before treatment starts but can be resumed after 4 weeks, if needed.

*Special care*: congestive heart failure, kidney or liver disorders, receiving dialysis, renovascular hypertension, depletion of fluid or salts.

*Avoid use*: children, pregnancy, breastfeeding.

*Possible interaction*: antacids, potassium-sparing diuretics, potassium supplements, lithium, NSAIDs, antihypertensives, desensitising therapy, high-flux dialysis membranes.

*Side effects*: chest, skeletal and muscle pains, rash, gastrointestinal upset, fatigue, dizziness, palpitations, cough, disturbance of sense of taste. If angioneurotic oedema occurs, withdraw drug.

*Manufacturer*: BMS.

## STERCULIA *SEE*: NORMACOL, NORMACOL PLUS.

## STIEMYCIN

*Description*: an antibiotic and alcohol-based solution containing 2% erythromycin.

*Used for*: acne.

*Dosage*: adults, apply twice each day in the morning and evening after washing.

*Side effects*: possible slight irritation and dryness of skin at site of application.

*Manufacturer*: Stiefel.

## STILNOCT

*Description*: a hypnotic preparation available as film-coated, white tablets in 2 strengths containing 5mg and 10mg (oblong, scored tablets, marked SN 10) of zolpidem hemitartrate.

*Used for*: insomnia – short-term treatment only.

*Dosage*: adults, 10mg, elderly persons, 5mg; both taken at bedtime.

*Special care*: pregnancy, breastfeeding, previous alcohol or drug abuse, liver disorders, depression. Rebound insomnia, symptoms of dependence and withdrawal may occur on stopping the drug – patient should be monitored for these.

*Avoid use*: children, psychoses, obstructive sleep apnoea, depressed respiration, severe liver disorders, acute lung insufficiency, myasthenia gravis.

*Possible interaction*: other depressants of the CNS, alcohol.

*Side effects*: dizziness, headache, gastrointestinal upset. In rare cases, confusion, loss of memory, depression, tremor, disturbed perception.

*Manufacturer*: Sanofi-Synthelabo.

## STUGERON

*Description*: an antihistamine preparation available as scored, white tablets marked JANSSEN S/15, containing 15mg of cinnarizine. *Also*, **STUGERON FORTE,** cream/orange capsules containing 75mg of cinnarizine.

*Used for*: Stugeron, vestibular disorders (affecting organs of balance in inner ear), motion sickness. Stugeron Forte, peripheral vascular disorders including Raynaud's disease (a disorder of the circulation in which there is periodic interruption in the blood supply to outlying parts of the body, due to spasm in the small arteries involved, affecting fingers, toes, ears, nose), intermittent claudication (poor circulation to legs causing cramping pains).

*Dosage*: Stugeron, adults, vestibular disorders, 2 tablets 3 times each day; motion sickness, 2 tablets 2 hours before travelling then 1 tablet every 8 hours during journey. Stugeron Forte, adults, 1 capsule 3 times each day at first, then 1 capsule 2 to 3 times daily as maintenance dose.

*Special care*: pregnancy, breastfeeding, elderly, liver or kidney disorders, enlarged prostate gland, epilepsy, glaucoma, low blood pressure, Parkinson's disease. Patients should be warned not to drive or operate machinery due to possible drowsiness.

*Avoid use*: children.

*Possible interaction*: alcohol, anticholinergics, depressants of CNS.

*Side effects*: rash, drowsiness, anticholinergic effects, allergic reactions, gastrointestinal upset, blood disorders, CNS effects.

*Manufacturer*: Janssen-Cilag.

## SUCRALFATE *SEE*: ANTEPSIN.

## SUDAFED

*Description*: a sympathomimetic available as film-coated, brown tablets, marked SUDAFED and containing 60mg of pseudoephedrine hydrochloride. *Also,* **SUDAFED ELIXIR,** a liquid containing 30mg of pseudoephedrine hydrochloride per 5ml. *Also,* **SUDAFED PLUS,** combining an antihistamine and sympathomimetic available as scored, white tablets marked M2A, containing 2.5mg of triprolidine hydrochloride and 60mg of pseudoephedrine hydrochloride. *Also,* **SUDAFED PLUS SYRUP,** a liquid containing 1.25mg of triprolidine hydrochloride and 30mg of pseudoephedrine hydrochloride per 5ml.

*Used for*: Sudafed, Sudafed Elixir, blocked, stuffy nose. Sudafed Plus, Sudafed Plus Syrup, hayfever (allergic rhinitis).

*Dosage*: adults, all preparations, 1 tablet or 10ml 4 times each day.Children, Sudafed Elixir, Sudafed Plus Syrup, aged 2 to 5 years, 2.5ml; aged 6 to 12 years, 5ml; all 4 times each day.

*Special care*: overactive thyroid gland, diabetes, enlarged prostate gland, raised pressure within eye.

*Avoid use*: children aged under 2 years, severe high blood pressure, diseased coronary arteries.

*Possible interaction*: depressants of CNS, MAOIs, furazolidone, sympathomimetics.

*Side effects*: rash, drowsiness. In rare cases, hallucinations, disturbed sleep.

*Manufacturer*: Warner Lambert.

## SULFAMETHOXAZOLE *SEE*: SEPTRIN.

## SULPHUR *SEE*: ACTINAC.

## SURGAM SA

*Description*: an NSAID which is a propionic acid, available as sustained-release maroon/pink capsules enclosing white pellets containing 300mg of tiaprofenic acid, marked with logo and SURGAM SA. *Also*, **SURGAM TABLETS**, white, containing 200mg and 300mg of tiaprofenic acid, marked with logo on one side and name and strength on the reverse.

*Used for*: acute disorders of joints, skeleton and muscles including osteoarthritis, rheumatoid arthritis, lumbago, ankylosing spondylitis, injuries to soft tissues.

*Dosage*: adults, capsules, 2 as a single daily dose; tablets, 600mg as divided doses each day.

*Special care*: pregnancy, breastfeeding, elderly, heart failure, liver or kidney disorders (monitor function), known allergy to aspirin or NSAID.

*Avoid use*: children, previous stomach ulcer, bladder disease or disorders of prostate gland, previous disorders of the urinary system.

*Possible interaction*: sulfonamides, hypoglycaemics, diuretics, anticoagulants, hydantoins.

*Side effects*: headache, gastrointestinal upset, sleepiness, rash. Withdraw if cystitis and haematuria (blood in urine) occur or frequent urination, urination at night.

*Manufacturer*: Aventis Pharma.

## SURMONTIL

*Description*: a TCAD preparation available as white tablets in strengths of 10mg and 25mg containing trimipramine (as maleate), both marked with strength and SURMONTIL. *Also*, **SURMONTIL CAPSULES**, white/green containing 50mg of trimipramine as maleate, marked SU50.

*Used for*: depression and/or anxiety, agitation, disturbance of sleep.

*Dosage*: adults, mild or moderate symptoms, 50 to 75mg as single dose, 2 hours before going to bed. Continue for a minimum of 3 weeks. Moderate to severe symptoms, 75mg each day at first under specialist supervision, gradually increasing according to need. Usual dose is in the order of 150 to 300mg each day for 1 month to 6 weeks, then reducing for maintenance once condition improves. Elderly, 10 to 25mg, 3 times each day.

*Special care*: patients with psychoses or suicidal tendencies, elderly persons, pregnant and nursing mothers, people with cardiac disorders, epilepsy, hyperthyroidism, urine retention, closed angle glaucoma, liver disease, tumours of adrenal gland, diabetes.

*Avoid use*: children, patients with recent heart attack, heart arrhythmias, heart block, porphyria (rare blood disorder).

*Possible interaction*: alcohol, barbiturate drugs, local anaesthetics (containing adrenaline or noradrenaline), antihypertensive and sympathomimetic drugs, anticholinergic drugs, cimetidine, oestrogens.

*Side effects*: anticholinergic effects including urine retention, dry mouth, constipation, blurred vision, rapid heartbeat, palpitations, nervousness, insomnia, sweating, dizziness, fatigue, weight changes, jaundice, blood changes, allergic skin rashes, changes in libido, breast enlargement and impotence.

*Manufacturer*: Aventis.

## SYNALAR

*Description*: a potent topical steroid preparation available as cream and ointment containing 0.025% fluocinolone acetonide. *Also,* **SYNALAR 1:4**, a moderately potent steroid cream and ointment containing 0.00625% of fluocinolone acetonide. *Also*, **SYNALAR CREAM 1:10**, a mildly potent steroid cream containing 0.0025% of fluocinolone acetonide. *Also,* **SYNALAR C** a combined potent steroid, antibacterial, antifungal cream and ointment containing 0.025% fluocinolone acetonide and 3% clioquinol. *Also,* **SYNALAR N**, a potent steroid and antibacterial cream and ointment containing 0.025% fluocinolone acetonide and 0.5% neomycin sulphate. Also, **SYNALAR GEL** containing 0.025% fluocinolone acetate.

*Used for*: Synalar steroid preparations, skin conditions responsive to steroid treatment; Synalar combined preparations, infected skin conditions responsive to steroid treatment. Synalar Gel, skin conditions of the scalp responsive to steroid treatment.

*Dosage*: apply thinly 2 or 3 times each day and rub in. Synalar Gel, rub into scalp in the morning and at night at first and then once or twice each week for maintenance.

*Special care*: should not be used on face or on children for more than 5 days. Should be stopped gradually.

*Avoid use*: children aged under 4 years, prolonged or extensive use especially pregnant women or continual use as a preventative. Should not be used to treat acne, leg ulcers, scabies, peri-oral dermatitis, tuberculous skin conditions, skin disorders caused by viruses, ringworm, any untreated bacterial or fungal skin infections.

*Side effects*: thinning of skin, adrenal gland suppression, hair growth, Cushingoid type symptoms (Cushing's syndrome).

*Manufacturer*: GP Pharma.

## SYNFLEX

*Description*: an NSAID and propionic acid, available as blue tablets containing 275mg of naproxen sodium marked SYNTEX.

*Used for*: period pain, pain following operations, migraine, acute gout, osteoarthritis, rheumatoid arthritis, ankylosing spondylitis, other disorders of the skeleton and muscles.

*Dosage*: adults and children aged over 16 years, usual dose, period pain and gout, usually 2 at start then 1 tablet every 6 to 8 hours, as needed but with a maximum of 4 each day on subsequent days. Musculoskeletal disorders, arthritis, ankylosing spondylitis and post-operative pain, 2 tablets twice each day. Migraine, 3 tablets as first dose then 1 or 2 tablets 6 to 8-hourly with a daily maximum of 5.

*Special care*: pregnancy, breastfeeding, elderly, liver or kidney disorders – monitoring required if drug taken long-term, history of lesions in gastro-intestinal tract, heart failure, asthma. Patients taking drug long-term require careful monitoring, as do patients with coagulation disorders.

*Avoid use*: children under 16 years, known allergy to NSAID or aspirin, previous or current stomach ulcer.

*Possible interaction*: sulphonylureas, corticosteroids, cardiac glycosides, anticoagulants, furosemide, ß-blockers, quinolones, mifepristone, ACE inhibitors, ciclosporin, hydantoins, lithium probenecid, methotrexate.

*Side effects*: blood changes, headache, gastrointestinal intolerance, vertigo, rash, tinnitus.

*Manufacturer*: Roche.

## SYNPHASE

*Description*: a combined oestrogen/progestogen oral contraceptive preparation available as: 7 blue tablets containing 35µg ethinylestradiol and 0.5mg of norethisterone; 9 white tablets containing 35µg of ethinylestradiol and 1mg of norethisterone; 5 blue tablets containing 35µg of ethinylestradiol and 0.5mg of norethisterone, respectively. All are marked Searle and BX.

*Used for*: oral contraception.

*Dosage*: 1 tablet each day starting on 1st day of period then 7 tablet-free days.

*Special care*: hypertension, severe kidney disease receiving dialysis, Raynaud's disease, diabetes, multiple sclerosis, asthma, varicose veins, elevated levels of prolactin (a hormone) in the blood (hyperprolactinemia). Risk of thrombosis increases with smoking, age and obesity. Blood pressure, breasts and pelvic organs should be checked during period of treatment.

*Avoid use*: pregnancy, heart and circulatory diseases,

angina, sickle cell anaemia, pulmonary hypertension. Also hormone-dependent cancers, undiagnosed vaginal bleeding, chorea, liver disease, history of cholestatic jaundice of pregnancy, infectious hepatitis, Dublin–Johnson syndrome, Rotor syndrome, recent trophoblastic disease.

*Possible interaction*: phenytoin, carbamazepine, tetracyclines, primidone, chloral hydrate, glutethimide, phenylbutazone, rifampicin, griseofulvin, ampicillin, dichloralphenazone, ethosuximide, barbiturates, St John's Wort.

*Side effects*: feeling of bloatedness due to fluid retention, leg pains, breast enlargement, erosion of cervix, muscular cramps, weight gain, breakthrough bleeding, depression, headaches, vaginal discharge, loss of libido, nausea, brown patches on skin (chloasma). Stop drug immediately in event of pregnancy, if frequent, severe headaches occur or signs of thromboses, severe pain in upper abdominal region, enlarged liver, jaundice, rise in blood pressure, severe depression, increased number of fits. Drug should be discontinued 6 weeks before major planned surgery and re-started 2 weeks afterwards, as long as woman is fully mobile. Should be discontinued during long periods of immobility.

*Manufacturer*: Pharmacia.

## SYSCOR MR

*Description*: a class II calcium antagonist available as film-coated, sustained-release tablets in 3 strengths containing 10mg, 20mg and 30mg of nisoldipine.

*Used for*: prevention of stable, chronic angina, mild to moderate high blood pressure.

*Dosage*: adults, 10mg once each day taken in the morning at first, to be swallowed without chewing before food. Then, increase to a maintenance dose in order of 20 to 40mg once each day. The maximum is 40mg once daily.

*Special care*: low blood pressure, heart failure producing symptoms.

*Avoid use*: children, pregnancy, breastfeeding, impaired liver function, aortic stenosis (narrowing of aorta), heart shock, within 1 week of heart attack, malignant high blood pressure.

*Possible interaction*: carbamazepine, ß-blockers, cimetidine, quinidine, azole antifungals, rifampicin, phenytoin, grapefruit juice.

*Side effects*: weakness, dizziness, fluid retention, pains in chest, tingling/numbness/'pins-and-needles' sensation, headache, tremor, muscle pains, shortness of breath, nervousness, rapid heartbeat, skin reactions, flushes, frequent urination, high levels of ALT, CPK, AST (drug should be stopped if these do not fall again).

*Manufacturer*: Forest.

# T

## TAGAMET

*Description*: an H2 blocker available as film-coated, green tablets in 3 strengths, all containing cimetidine. Green containing 200mg; green, oblong containing 400mg; green, oval containing 800mg. All are marked SK&F; 200 and 400mg ones are marked TAGAMET; 800mg ones are marked T800. *Also,* **TAGAMET EFFERVESCENT**, white effervescent tablets containing 400mg of cimetidine. *Also,* **TAGAMET SYRUP** containing 200mg of cimetidine per 5ml. *Also*, **TAGAMET INJECTION** containing 200mg of cimetidine per 2ml, in ampoules.

*Used for*: duodenal and benign stomach ulcers, recurrent ulcers, stomal ulcers, dyspepsia, oesophageal reflux and where gastric acid has to be reduced.

*Dosage*: adults, oral preparations, duodenal ulcer, 800mg at bedtime or 400mg twice each day for at least 4 weeks, then 400mg taken at bedtime (or twice each day) for maintenance. See manufacturer's literature for other conditions. Injection, according to manufacturer's literature, by intravenous injection or infusion, or intramuscularly. Children, oral preparations, aged over 1 year, 25 to 30mg per kg of body weight each day in divided doses. Injection, according to manufacturer's literature.

*Special care*: pregnancy, breastfeeding, impaired kidney function. Malignant disease should be excluded before starting treatment and patients receiving drug long-term require monitoring.

*Possible interaction*: theophylline, intravenous lidocaine, oral anticoagulants, phenytoin.

*Side effects*: rash, dizziness, tiredness, diarrhoea, confusion, depression, hallucinations, abnormal enlargement of breasts, liver damage which is reversible. In very rare cases, acute pancreatitis, leucopenia (decline in white blood cells), aplastic anaemia, pancytopenia (decline in all blood elements), thrombocytopenia (bleeding caused by decline in blood platelets), interstitial nephritis (kidney inflammation), fever, slowed heartbeat (bradycardia) and sinus bradycardia, muscle and joint pain, headache, heart block, rapid heartbeat, anaphylaxis.

*Manufacturer*: GlaxoSmithKline.

## TANATRIL

*Description*: an antihypertensive and ACE inhibitor, available as oblong, scored white tablets in 3 strengths containing 5mg, 10mg and 20mg of imidapril hydrochloride.

*Used for*: high blood pressure.

*Dosage*: adults, 5mg each day to begin with taken at same time daily, 15 minutes before eating meal. Then increase if needed after 3 weeks to 10mg once each day, taken in same way. The daily maximum is 20mg. Salt or volume depletion should be corrected before treatment starts and any diuretic being taken must be stopped 2 to 3 days beforehand. Elderly patients, 2.5mg once each day to begin with, then adjusted according to need to daily maximum of 10mg.

*Special care*: surgery, aortic stenosis (narrowing of aorta), impaired liver function, psoriasis, enlarged, damaged heart, haemodialysis or apheresis using high-flux membranes. In patients with heart failure, low blood sodium levels or volume depletion, there is risk of severe low blood pressure developing.

*Avoid use*: children, pregnancy, breastfeeding, angioedema (widespread swelling due to fluid retention), kidney failure, severely impaired kidney function, angioedema caused by previous ACE inhibitor treatment.

*Possible interaction*: immunosuppressants, sympathomimetics, corticosteroids, potassium supplements and potassium – sparing diuretics, antipsychotics, NSAIDs, oral hypoglycaemics, lithium, allopurinol, anaesthetics, cytostatics, rifampicin, narcotics, procainamide, desensitising treatment for insect stings and bites.

*Side effects*: gastrointestinal upset, severe low blood pressure, allergic reactions, dizziness, angioedema, cough, kidney failure, weariness.

*Manufacturer*: Trinity.

## TAVEGIL

*Description*: an antihistamine preparation of the arylalkylamine type, available as white, scored tablets containing 1mg of clemastine as hydrogen fumarate, marked TAVEGIL.

*Used for*: allergic rhinitis (runny, inflamed nose – hayfever), allergic skin reactions, nettle rash, angioneurotic oedema (widespread swelling due to fluid collection), allergic drug reactions.

*Dosage*: adults, 1 tablet, taken at night and in the morning. Children aged 3 to 6 years, 1/2 tablet; aged over 6 years, 1/2 to 1 tablet. All doses taken at night and in the morning.
*Special care*: pregnancy, breastfeeding, stomach ulcer causing narrowing, obstruction in pyloroduodenal region, glaucoma, obstructed neck of bladder, enlarged prostate gland, retention of urine.
*Possible interaction*: depressants of CNS, alcohol, MAOIs.
*Side effects*: sleepiness. In rare cases, stimulation of CNS, palpitations, dizziness, heartburn, gastrointestinal upset, weakness, rash, weariness, headache.
*Manufacturer*: Novartis Consumer.

## TAXOL

*Description*: a chemotherapeutic drug and taxane, available as a solution in vials containing 6mg of paclitaxel per ml.
*Used for*: with cisplatin, for treatment of advanced and residual cancer of the ovaries, secondary treatment of ovarian cancer with metastases (i.e. which has spread) resistant to treatment with platinum. Treatment of metastatic breast cancer where previous treatment with anthracycline has failed or cannot be used, with cisplatin in the treatment of non-small cell lung cancer when radiotherapy and surgery cannot be used.
*Dosage*: primary ovarian cancer, 135mg per square metre of body area by intravenous infusion lasting 24 hours, followed by 75mg of cisplatin per square metre of body area. Treatment to be repeated at 3 week intervals if well-tolerated by patient. Secondary ovarian cancer and breast

cancer, 175mg per $m^2$ by intravenous infusion over 3 hours, repeated at 3 week intervals if well-tolerated by patient. Non-small cell lung cancer, 175mg per $m^2$ by intravenous infusion over 3 hours, followed by 80mg of cisplatin per $m^2$. Then repeat at 3 week intervals if well-tolerated by patient.

*Special care*: abnormalities in heart conduction, disease of peripheral nerves, impaired liver function. Blood counts should be carried out pre-treatment with antihistamines, H2-antagonists and corticosteroids required but manufacturer's literature should be consulted. Taxol should always be given before cisplatin.

*Avoid use*: children, pregnancy, breastfeeding, if neutrophils are low, very poor liver function.

*Side effects*: peripheral nerve disease (reduce dose of taxol if severe), suppression of bone marrow, joint and muscle pain, high readings in liver function tests, hair loss, low blood pressure, gastrointestinal upset, slow heartbeat, retention of fluid, reactions at needle site. In rare cases, cardiovascular conduction disturbances, severe allergic reactions (resuscitation equipment should be available).

*Manufacturer*: BMS.

## TAXOTERE

*Description*: a chemotherapeutic and taxoid drug available as a solution in vials with diluent, in 2 strengths containing 20mg and 80mg of docetaxel.

*Used for*: locally advanced or metastatic breast cancer (i.e. cancer which has spread) which has not responded, or is resistant to other cytotoxic therapy which included an alkylating agent or anthracycline. Metastatic or locally advanced, non-small cell cancer of the lung which is resistant to other chemotherapy.

*Dosage*: breast cancer, 100mg per square metre of body area by intravenous infusion lasting 1 hour, repeated at 3 weekly intervals. If patient develops any of the following: serious peripheral nerve damage, severe neutropenia (marked decline in white blood cells called neutrophils), fever, severe skin reaction, then next dose should be reduced to 75mg per $m^2$ and then 55mg per $m^2$, if symptoms do not resolve. If they still persist, treatment should be stopped. Patient should also be given 8mg of dexamethasone twice each day for 3 days, beginning 1 day before treatment with Taxotere.

*Special care*: liver function tests must be carried out and blood counts monitored; if severe neutropenia (decrease in neutrophils – white blood cells) occurs, subsequent doses should be lessened. Patient requires monitoring during infusion for fluid retention and hypersensitive reactions.

*Possible interaction*: erythromycin, terfenadine, troleandomycin, ciclosporin, ketoconazole.

*Side effects*: anaemia, neutropenia, thrombocytopenia (decline in blood platelets causing bleeding), damage to peripheral nerves, joint and muscle pains, fluid retention, skin reactions, raised liver enzymes, inflammation of mucous membranes.

*Manufacturer*: Aventis.

## TEARS NATURALE

*Description*: a preparation of artificial tears available as a solution containing 0.1% dextran 70 and 0.3% hypromellose.

*Used for*: deficiency in tears/dry eyes.

*Dosage*: 1 to 2 drops into eyes, as needed.

*Manufacturer*: Alcon.

## TELFAST

*Description*: an antihistamine preparation available as film-coated, peach-coloured, capsule-shaped tablets containing 120mg of fexofenadine hydrochloride. *Also,* **TELFAST 180,** film-coated, peach-coloured, capsule-shaped tablets containing 180mg of fexofenadine hydrochloride.

*Used for*: Telfast, hayfever; Telfast 180, chronic nettle rash (urticaria).

*Dosage*: adults, 1 tablet each day.

*Special care*: pregnancy.

*Avoid use*: children, pregnancy.

*Side effects*: nausea, weariness, dizziness, headache.

*Manufacturer*: Aventis.

## TENORMIN

*Description*: a cardioselective ß-blocker, atenolol, available as film-coated tablets in 2 strengths, both containing atenolol. White, containing 25mg, marked with TENORMIN, 25 and S and orange, containing 100mg, marked with TENORMIN and S. *Also,* **TENORMIN LS,** available as scored, film-coated, orange tablets containing 50mg of atenolol. *Also,* **TENORMIN SYRUP**, a lemon-lime flavoured, sugar-free syrup containing 25mg of atenolol per 5ml. *Also*, **TENORMIN INJECTION,** a solution in ampoules containing 0.5mg of atenolol per ml in 10ml ampoules.

*Used for*: oral preparations, cardiac arrhythmias, early treatment of heart attack, angina, high blood pressure. Injection, heart attack only.

*Dosage*: adults, oral preparations, 50 to 100mg each day, reduced for the elderly or where there is reduced kidney function. Injection, according to manufacturer's literature by infusion or slow intravenous injection.

*Special care*: pregnancy, breastfeeding, liver or kidney disease, diabetes, metabolic acidosis, poor cerebral blood supply, history of bronchospasm, those undergoing anaesthesia; patients with weak hearts should be treated with digitalis and diuretics. Drug should be stopped gradually.

*Avoid use*: children, patients with asthma, heart diseases including heart block, heart shock, slow heartbeat rate, heart failure.

*Possible interaction*: cardiac depressants,anaesthetics, reserpine, sedatives, class II calcium antagonists, antihypertensives, sympathomimetics, cimetidine, indometacin, ergotamine, class I antiarrhythmic drugs, verapamil, clonidine withdrawal, hypoglycaemics, rifampicin, warfarin, ibuprofen.

*Side effects*: sleep disturbance, cold feet and hands, slow heartbeat, fatigue on exercise, wheeziness, heart failure, gastro-intestinal disorders; dry eyes or skin rash (stop use gradually), hair loss, low blood pressure, thrombocytopenia (abnormal decline in blood platelets causing increased likelihood of bleeding).

*Manufacturer*: AstraZeneca.

## TENOXICAM *SEE*: MOBIFLEX.

## TEOPTIC

*Description*: a ß-blocker available as eyedrops in 2 strengths containing 1% and 2% drops carteolol hydrochloride.

*Used for*: high pressure within the eye, open-angle glaucoma and some forms of secondary glaucoma.

*Dosage*: start with 1 drop of 1% solution in affected eye(s) twice each day. Use 2% solution if 1% is ineffective.

*Special care*: breastfeeding, 2nd or 3rd degree heart block, heart shock, diabetes, insufficiency of right ventricle due to congestive heart failure or pulmonary hypertension, sinus bradycardia (slow heartbeat).

*Avoid use*: children, pregnancy, insufficiency of heart function which is not controlled, asthma, COPD (chronic obstructive pulmonary disease), soft contact lenses.

*Possible interaction*: other ß-blockers.

*Side effects*: blurred vision, burning sensation, pain, irritation of the eye, vertigo, hyperaemia (greater than normal amount of blood in the vessels), discharge from eye, slow heartbeat, shortness of breath, effects on cornea and inflammation, headache, weariness, intolerance of light.

*Manufacturer*: Novartis.

## TERAZOSIN *SEE*: HYTRIN.

## TETRACYCLINE *SEE*: DETECLO.

## THREONINE *SEE*: CICATRIN.

## TILDIEM LA

*Description*: an antianginal and antihypertensive preparation and class III calcium antagonist, available as sustained-release capsules in 2 strengths containing diltiazem hydrochloride. Grey/pink contain 200mg and yellow/white contain 300mg.*Also,* **TILDIEM RETARD,** sustained-release, white tablets in 2 strengths containing 90mg and 120mg of diltiazem hydrochloride. *Also,* **TILDIEM TABLETS,** off-white tablets containing 60mg of diltiazem hydrochloride coded TIDIEM 60.

*Used for*: angina, mild to moderate high blood pressure. Tildiem tablets are for angina only.

*Dosage*: adults, Tildiem LA, 1 x 200mg to start taken before or with meal once each day. Then increase if required to 2 x 200mg taken in same way once each day or to 1 x 300mg. The maximum daily dose is 1 x 300mg plus 1 x 200mg once each day. Elderly patients, start with same dose taken in same way then increase if required to 1 x 300mg once each day. Tildiem Retard, angina, 1 x 90mg or 1 x 120mg twice each day to start, increasing if required to a maximum dose of 2 x 120mg twice each day. Elderly patients, 1 x 60mg tablet twice each day to start, then increasing to 1 x 90mg or 1 x 120mg twice each day.

For high blood pressure, 120mg twice each day to start then 2 x 90mg twice each day, if required. Elderly, 120mg each day to begin with then 120mg twice daily, if required. Tildiem tablets, 60mg 3 times each day to begin with, increasing if required to a maximum dose of 480mg each day as divided doses. Elderly, 60mg twice each day to begin with then increasing if required, as directed by physician.

*Special care*: check heart rate in elderly or cases of liver and kidney disorder. Monitor patients with mild bradycardia (slow heartbeat) or prolonged PR interval (part of ECG).

*Avoid use*: children, pregnancy, breastfeeding, serious bradycardia, heart block, sick sinus syndrome, failure of left ventricle.

*Possible interaction*: other antihypertensives, ß-blockers, heart depressants, digoxin, dantrolene infusion, ciclosporin, lithium cimetidine, theophylline, carbamazepine.

*Side effects*: swollen ankles due to fluid retention, 1st degree heart block, rashes, slow heartbeat, headache, nausea.

*Manufacturer*: Sanofi-Synthelabo.

## TILORYTH

*Description*: a macrolide antibiotic available as clear capsules enclosing enteric-coated granules containing 250mg of erythromycin, marked with strength and name.

*Used for*: infections responsive to erythromycin, including those of soft tissues and skin and acne.

*Dosage*: erythromycin-sensitive infections, adults, either

500mg every 12 hours taken before or with meals or 250mg every 6 hours. Skin and soft tissue infections and acne, usually 1 capsule twice each day for 4 weeks, then 1 capsule daily. Children, erythromycin-sensitive infections only, 30 to 50mg per kg of body weight each day in divided doses, either twice each day or every 6 hours.

*Special care*: myasthenia gravis, impaired liver function.

*Possible interaction*: ciclosporin, statins, astemizole, oral anticoagulants, valproate, bromocriptine, theophylline, disopyramide, ergot derivatives, hexobarbital, phenytoin, terfenadine, digoxin, midazolam, cisapride, carbamazepine, triazolam, alfentanil.

*Side effects*: cholestatic jaundice, allergic effects, gastrointestinal upset.

*Manufacturer*: Tilomed.

## TIMOLOL *SEE*: TIMOPTOL.

## TIMOPTOL

*Description*: a ß-blocker, available as eye drops in 2 strengths containing 0.25% and 0.5% timolol maleate, available in metered dose or unit dose format. *Also,* **TIMOPTOL-LA,** available as a gel-forming solution in 2 strengths containing 0.25% and 0.5% timolol as maleate.

*Used for*: ocular hypertension, certain glaucomas.

*Dosage*: adults, 1 drop of 0.25% solution twice each day into eye(s), increasing to 0.5% solution twice each day if required.

*Special care*: pregnancy, breastfeeding, withdraw gradually.

Patients should report any other eye symptoms. Heart function must be monitored after filtration procedures.

*Avoid use*: children, uncompensated heart failure, heart block, heart shock, asthma, sinus bradycardia, past obstructive lung disease, soft lenses.

*Possible interaction*: adrenaline, antihypertensives, verapamil, quinidine, diltiazem, clonidine, **ß**-blockers.

*Side effects*: eye irritation, allergic effects, systemic ß-blocker effects (e.g. cold hands and feet, tiredness, stomach upset, rash), bronchospasm, worsening of myasthenia gravis, gastrointestinal and CNS effects.

*Manufacturer*: M.S.D.

## TOFRANIL

*Description*: a TCAD antidepressant, available as sugar-coated, brown tablets containing 25mg of imipramine hydrochloride, all marked GEIGY. *Also*, **TOFRANIL SYRUP**, containing 25mg of imipramine hydrochloride per 5ml.

*Used for*: depression, night-time bedwetting in children.

*Dosage*: adults, 25mg up to 3 times each day at first, then increasing to 150 to 200mg each day by 7th day of treatment. The maintenance dose is in the order of 50 to 100mg each day. If patient is hospitalised, the dose may be 100mg 3 times each day with a maintenance of 100mg daily. Elderly patients should start with 10mg each day, then increasing to 30 to 50mg daily. Children, bedwetting only, using syrup, aged over 11 years, 10 to 15ml; aged 8 to 11 years, 5 to 10ml; aged 6 to 7 years, 5ml. All doses taken at bedtime for 3 months maximum period then drug is gradually stopped.

*Special care*: patients with psychoses or suicidal tendencies, elderly persons, pregnant and nursing mothers, people with cardiac disorders, epilepsy, hyperthyroidism, urine retention, closed angle glaucoma, liver disease, tumours of adrenal gland, diabetes

*Avoid use*: children, patients with recent heart attack, heart arrhythmias, heart block, porphyria (rare blood disorder).

*Possible interaction*: alcohol, barbiturate drugs, local anaesthetics (containing adrenaline or noradrenaline), antihypertensive and sympathomimetic drugs, anticholinergic drugs, cimetidine, oestrogens.

*Side effects*: anticholinergic effects including urine retention, dry mouth, constipation, blurred vision, rapid heartbeat, palpitations, nervousness, insomnia, sweating, dizziness, fatigue, weight changes, jaundice, blood changes, allergic skin rashes, changes in libido, breast enlargement and impotence.

*Manufacturer*: Novartis.

## TRANDATE

*Description*: an antianginal and antihypertensive preparation and α/ß-blocker, available as orange tablets in 4 strengths containing 50, 100, 200 and 400mg of labetalol hydrochloride marked with name and strength. *Also,* **TRANDATE INJECTION**, a solution in ampoules containing 5mg of labetalol hydrochloride per ml.

*Used for*: tablets, angina, high blood pressure. Injection, severe high blood pressure.

*Dosage*: adults, tablets, start with 100mg twice each day taken with food, increasing if required at intervals of 2 weeks to a maximum of 2.4g each day in 3 to 4 divided doses. Elderly start with 50mg twice each day. Injection, consult manufacturer's literature.

*Special care*: pregnancy, breast-feeding, liver or kidney disease, diabetes, metabolic acidosis, poor cerebral blood supply, history of bronchospasm, those undergoing anaesthesia; patients with weak hearts should be treated with digitalis and diuretics. Drug should be stopped gradually.

*Avoid use*: children, patients with asthma, heart diseases including heart block, heart shock, slow heartbeat rate, heart failure.

*Possible interaction*: cardiac depressants,anaesthetics, reserpine, sedatives, class 11 calcium antagonists, antihypertensives, sympathomimetics, cimetidine, indometacin, ergotamine, class I antiarrhythmic drugs, verapamil, clonidine withdrawal, hypoglycaemics, rifampicin, warfarin, ibuprofen.

*Side effects*: fluid retention, blocked, stuffy nose, dizziness, fatigue, failure to ejaculate, headaches. In rare cases, low blood pressure on rising up; drug should be withdrawn in event of liver reaction.

*Manufacturer*: Celltech.

**TRANDOLAPRIL *SEE*: GOPTEN, ODRIK.**

## TRANXENE

*Description*: a long-acting benzodiazepine, clorazepate potassium available as capsules in 2 strengths containing clorazepate potassium. Grey/pink, contain 15mg and grey/maroon, contain 7.5mg, all marked with TRANXENE, capsule strength and symbol.

*Used for*: anxiety whether or not depression is present.

*Dosage*: adults and children aged over 16 years, 7.5 to 22.5mg each day, elderly persons, 7.5mg each day. As single or divided doses.

*Special care*: chronic lung insufficiency, chronic liver or kidney disease, depression, glaucoma (acute, narrow angle), bereavement. Drug can affect dexterity and judgement. Long-term use is to be avoided and drug should be withdrawn gradually.

*Avoid use*: children, pregnancy, breastfeeding, labour, acute lung insufficiency, depression of respiration (except in cases of acute muscle spasms), sleep apnoea, severe liver insufficiency, myasthenia gravis (a severe autoimmune disorder). Also when treating anxiety, obsessional states or chronic psychosis.

*Possible interaction*: alcohol and other CNS depressants, anticonvulsants.

*Side effects*: vertigo, gastro-intestinal upsets, confusion, ataxia, drowsiness, light-headedness, hypotension, disturbance of vision, skin rashes. Also urine retention, changes in libido. Dependence a potential problem.

*Manufacturer*: Boehringer Ingelheim.

## TRASICOR

*Description*: a non-cardioselective ß-blocker available as film-coated tablets in 3 strengths containing oxprenolol hydrochloride. White, contain 20 and 40mg; yellow, contain 80mg; all marked with strength, CIBA and name.

*Used for*: heart arrhythmias, angina, high blood pressure, anxiety.

*Dosage*: adults, arrhythmias, 40 to 240mg 2 or 3 times each day; angina and high blood pressure, 80 to 160mg in 2 to 3 divided doses daily to a maximum of 320mg; anxiety, 40 to 80mg each day in 1 to 2 divided doses.

*Special care*: pregnancy, breastfeeding, liver or kidney disease, diabetes, metabolic acidosis, poor cerebral blood supply, history of bronchospasm, those undergoing anaesthesia; patients with weak hearts should be treated with digitalis and diuretics. Drug should be stopped gradually.

*Avoid use*: children, patients with asthma, heart diseases including heart block, heart shock, slow heartbeat rate, heart failure.

*Possible interaction*: cardiac depressants, anaesthetics, reserpine, sedatives, class II calcium antagonists, antihypertensives, sympathomimetics, cimetidine, indometacin, ergotamine, class I antiarrhythmic drugs, verapamil, clonidine withdrawal, hypoglycaemics, rifampicin, warfarin, ibuprofen.

*Side effects*: sleep disturbance, cold feet and hands, slow heartbeat, fatigue on exercise, wheeziness, heart failure, gastro-intestinal disorders; dry eyes or skin rash (stop use gradually), hair loss, low blood pressure, thrombocytopenia (abnormal decline in blood platelets causing increased likelihood of bleeding).

*Manufacturer*: Novartis.

## TRASIDREX

*Description*: a non-cardioselective ß-blocker and thiazide, available as sugar-coated, red tablets containing 160mg of oxprenolol hydrochloride in a sustained-release core and 0.25mg of cyclopenthiazide in a red outer coat. The tablet is marked NOVARTIS and TRASIDREX.

*Used for*: high blood pressure.

*Dosage*: adults, start with 1 tablet each morning increasing to 2 each day after 1 week, if necessary.

*Special care*: pregnancy, breastfeeding, patients with weak hearts should receive digitalis and diuretics, history of bronchospasm, liver or kidney disease, diabetes, metabolic acidosis, raised blood lipid levels, gout, weakness, insufficient cerebral blood supply, tendency to allergy. Persons undergoing general anaesthesia, may require drug to be withdrawn before planned surgery. Electrolyte levels should be monitored. Drug should be gradually withdrawn.

*Avoid use*: children, patients with obstructive airways disease or history of bronchospasm (asthma), various heart disorders including heart block, heart shock, heart failure, sick sinus syndrome, serious peripheral arterial disease, sinus bradycardia, Prinzmetal's angina, low blood pressure, severe heart muscle disease, uncompensated heart failure. Also, untreated tumour of adrenal gland (phaeochromocytoma), failure of right ventricle secondary to pulmonary hypertension, severe or progressive kidney failure, anuria.

*Possible interaction*: cardiac depressant anaesthetics, antihypertensives, ergot alkaloids, ibuprofen, sympathomimetics, verapamil, clonidine withdrawal, central nervous system depressants, class I antiarrhythmic drugs, diltiazem, cimetidine, reserpine. Also, indometacin, theophylline, class II calcium antagonists, hypoglycaemics, lithium, warfarin, digitalis, rifampicin. Also, amantadine, NSAIDs, potassium-sparing diuretics, potassium supplements, allopurinol.

*Side effects*: bradycardia, fatigue on exercise, cold hands and feet, disturbance of sleep, gastro-intestinal upset, low blood pressure, bronchospasm, heart failure, blood changes, baldness, thrombocytopenia (low levels of blood platelets), blood changes, sensitivity to light, gout. Withdraw drug gradually if skin rash or dry eyes occur.

*Manufacturer*: Novartis.

## TRAZODONE *SEE*: MOLIPAXIN.

## TRIAMCINOLONE *SEE*: AUREOCORT.

## TRIAPIN

*Description*: an antihypertensive preparation combining a class II calcium antagonist and ACE inhibitor, available as film-coated, bi-layered, brown tablets containing 5mg of felodipine in sustained-release form and 5mg of ramipril. All are marked HOE and 5. *Also,* **TRIAPIN MITE,** film-coated, bi-layered, orange tablets containing 2.5mg of felodipine in sustained-release form and 2.5mg of ramipril, all marked HOD and 2.5.

*Used for*: high blood pressure in patients whose condition is controlled by the same drugs in these proportions given separately.

*Dosage*: adults, 1 tablet once each day.

*Special care*: enlarged, obstructed heart, renovascular high blood pressure, narrowed aortic or mitral valve of heart, mild to moderate kidney or liver disorders with impaired function, narrowed renal arteries, collagen vascular disease. There is high risk of severe low blood pressure in patients with low blood sodium levels, volume depletion or heart failure treated with large doses of diuretics. Kidney function must be checked before treatment starts and then monitored as therapy proceeds.

*Avoid use*: children, pregnancy, breastfeeding, heart block (2nd or 3rd degree), heart shock, seriously impaired liver or kidney function, stroke, angina which is not stabilised, heart attack, heart failure which is untreated, previous angioneurotic oedema (widespread swelling due to fluid retention), haemodialysis or apheresis using high-flux membranes.

*Possible interaction*:potassium supplements and potassium-sparing diuretics, oral hypoglycaemics, insulin, corticosteroids, drugs affecting cytochrome P450, NSAIDs, procainamide, immunosuppressants, desensitisation treatment for insect stings and bites, heparin, grapefruit juice, theophylline, cytostatics, lithium, allopurinol.

Side *effects*: cough, overgrowth of gum tissue, liver or kidney failure, swelling of ankles, serious low blood pressure, dizziness, gastrointestinal upset, headache, rapid heartbeat, skin effects. Stop treatment immediately in event of angioedema. Effects on blood – agranulocytosis and neutropenia; patients should report signs of infection. Any adverse side effects should be reported to the Committee on the Safety of Medicines (CSM).

*Manufacturer*: Aventis.

## TRIDESTRA

*Description*: a combined oestrogen/progestogen preparation available as 70 white tablets containing 2mg of oestradiol valerate, 14 blue tablets containing 20mg of medroxyprogesterone acetate and 7 yellow tablets which are a placebo.

*Used for*: HRT to treat symptoms of menopause, prevention of osteoporosis after the menopause.

*Dosage*: women, 1 white tablet each day for 70 days then 1 blue tablet for 14 days followed by 1 yellow tablet for 7 days.

*Special care*: high blood pressure, severe kidney disease receiving dialysis, Raynaud's disease, diabetes, multiple sclerosis, asthma, varicose veins, elevated levels of prolactin (a hormone) in the blood (hyperprolactinemia). Risk of thrombosis increases with smoking, age and obesity. Blood pressure, breasts and pelvic organs should be checked during period of treatment.

*Avoid use*: pregnancy, heart and circulatory diseases, angina, sickle cell anaemia, pulmonary hypertension. Also hormone-dependent cancers, undiagnosed vaginal bleeding, chorea, liver disease, history of cholestatic jaundice of pregnancy, infectious hepatitis, Dublin–Johnson syndrome, Rotor syndrome, recent trophoblastic disease.

*Possible interaction*: phenytoin, carbamazepine, tetracyclines, primidone, chloral hydrate, glutethimide, phenylbutazone, rifampicin, griseofulvin, ampicillin, dichloralphenazone, ethosuximide, barbiturates, St John's Wort.

*Side effects*: feeling of bloatedness due to fluid retention, leg pains, breast enlargement, erosion of cervix, muscular cramps, weight gain, breakthrough bleeding, depression, headaches, vaginal discharge, loss of libido, nausea, brown patches on skin (chloasma). Stop drug immediately in event of pregnancy.

*Manufacturer*: Orion.

## TRIMETHOPRIM *SEE*: POLYTRIM, SEPTRIN.

## TRIMOVATE

*Description*: a combined preparation containing a moderately potent steroid with antibiotic and antifungal agents, available as a cream containing 0.05% clobetasone butyrate, 100,000 units of nystatin per gram and 3% oxytetracycline as calcium salt.

*Used for*: skin conditions in moist areas such as where 2 surfaces rub together, responsive to steroids and where infection is present or likely to develop.

*Dosage*: rub onto affected area up to 4 times each day for a maximum period of 1 week.

*Special care*: should not be used on face or on children for more than 5 days. Should be stopped gradually.

*Avoid use*: children, prolonged or extensive use especially pregnant women or continual use as a preventative. Should not be used to treat acne, leg ulcers, scabies, perioral dermatitis, tuberculous skin conditions, skin disorders caused by viruses, ringworm, any untreated bacterial or fungal skin infections.

*Side effects*: thinning of skin, adrenal gland suppression, hair growth, Cushingoid type symptoms (Cushing's syndrome).

*Manufacturer*: GlaxoSmithKline.

## TRINORDIOL

*Description*: a combined oestrogen/progestogen hormonal preparation available as sugar-coated tablets. 6 brown tablets contain 30μg of ethinylestradiol and 50μg of levonorgestrel, 5 white tablets contain 40μg of ethinylestradiol and 75μg of levonorgestrel, 10 sandy coloured tablets contain 30μg of ethinylestradiol and 125μg of levonorgestrel.

*Used for*: oral contraception.

*Dosage*: women, starting on 1st day of period, 1 tablet each day taken in order indicated on pack, then 7 days without tablets.

*Special care*: hypertension, severe kidney disease receiving dialysis, Raynaud's disease, diabetes, multiple sclerosis, asthma, varicose veins, elevated levels of prolactin (a hormone) in the blood (hyperprolactinemia). Risk of thrombosis increases with smoking, age and obesity. Blood pressure, breasts and pelvic organs should be checked during period of treatment.

*Avoid use*: pregnancy, heart and circulatory diseases, angina, sickle cell anaemia, pulmonary hypertension. Also hormone-dependent cancers, undiagnosed vaginal bleeding, chorea, liver disease, history of cholestatic jaundice of pregnancy, infectious hepatitis, Dublin–Johnson syndrome, Rotor syndrome, recent trophoblastic disease.

*Possible interaction*: phenytoin, carbamazepine, tetracyclines, primidone, chloral hydrate, glutethimide, phenylbutazone, rifampicin, griseofulvin, ampicillin, dichloralphenazone, ethosuximide, barbiturates, St John's Wort.

*Side effects*: feeling of bloatedness due to fluid retention, leg pains, breast enlargement, erosion of cervix, muscular cramps, weight gain, breakthrough bleeding, depression, headaches, vaginal discharge, loss of libido, nausea, brown patches on skin (chloasma). Stop drug immediately in event of pregnancy, if frequent, severe headaches occur or signs of thromboses, severe pain in upper abdominal region, enlarged liver, jaundice, rise in blood pressure, severe depression, increased number of fits. Drug should be discontinued 6 weeks before major planned surgery and re-started 2 weeks afterwards, as long as woman is fully mobile. Should be discontinued during long periods of immobility.

*Manufacturer*: Wyeth.

## TRINOVUM

*Description*: a combined oestrogen/progestogen hormonal preparation available as 7 white tablets, marked C535, containing 35µg of ethinylestradiol and 0.5mg of norethisterone; 7 light orange tablets, marked C735, containing 35µg of ethinylestradiol and 0.75mg of norethisterone; 7 peach-coloured tablets, marked C135, containing 35µg of ethinylestradiol and 1mg of norethisterone.

*Used for*: oral contraception.

*Dosage*: women, 1 tablet each day for 21 days, taken in order indicated on pack, then 7 days without tablets.

*Special care*: hypertension, severe kidney disease receiving dialysis, Raynaud's disease, diabetes, multiple sclerosis, asthma, varicose veins, elevated levels of prolactin (a hormone) in the blood (hyperprolactinemia). Risk of thrombosis increases with smoking, age and obesity. Blood pressure, breasts and pelvic organs should be checked during period of treatment.

*Avoid use*: pregnancy, heart and circulatory diseases, angina, sickle cell anaemia, pulmonary hypertension. Also hormone-dependent cancers, undiagnosed vaginal bleeding, chorea, liver disease, history of cholestatic jaundice of pregnancy, infectious hepatitis, Dublin–Johnson syndrome, Rotor syndrome, recent trophoblastic disease.

*Possible interaction*: phenytoin, carbamazepine, tetracyclines, primidone, chloral hydrate, glutethimide, phenylbutazone, rifampicin, griseofulvin, ampicillin, dichloralphenazone, ethosuximide, barbiturates, St John's Wort.

*Side effects*: feeling of bloatedness due to fluid retention, leg pains, breast enlargement, erosion of cervix, muscular cramps, weight gain, breakthrough bleeding, depression, headaches, vaginal discharge, loss of libido, nausea, brown patches on skin (chloasma). Stop drug immediately in event of pregnancy, if frequent, severe headaches occur or signs of thromboses, severe pain in upper abdominal region, enlarged liver, jaundice, rise in blood pressure, severe depression, increased number of fits. Drug should be discontinued 6 weeks before major planned surgery and re-started 2 weeks afterwards, as long as woman is fully mobile. Should be discontinued during long periods of immobility.

*Manufacturer*: Janssen-Cilag.

## TRIPROLIDINE *SEE*: SUDAFED PLUS.

## TRITACE

*Description*: an antihypertensive preparation and ACE inhibitor available as oblong tablets in 4 different strengths, all containing ramipril. White contain 1.25mg, marked with strength, HMN and logo; yellow, scored, contain 2.5mg marked with strength, HMR and logo; red, scored, contain 5mg marked with strength, HMP and logo; white, scored, contain 10mg, marked with HMO/HMO.

*Used for*: congestive heart failure (with diuretics and possibly digitalis); after heart attack in patients with heart failure, to prevent progression of disease. In patients with disease of the heart circulation, diabetes or at risk of heart and circulatory disease who are over 55 years old, to reduce risk of heart attack, stroke or revascularisation or other cardiovascular event. Mild to moderate high blood pressure.

*Dosage*: adults, heart failure, reduction of heart attack, stroke etc., start with 1.25mg each day, then gradually double dose every 1 to 2 weeks according to need, to a daily maximum of 10mg. Reduce dosage of any diuretic being taken 2 to 3 days before starting treatment which should begin under expert and close supervision. Following heart attack, start with 2.5mg twice each day during first 3 to 10 days after attack. Then, 5mg twice each day for 48 hours. If first dose is not tolerated well it should be reduced to 1.25mg twice each day for 2 days, then 2.5mg and 5mg, as before. Treatment should begin in hospital under close, expert supervision. High blood pressure, 1.25mg once each day to start, gradually increasing to maintenance dose of 2.5 to 5mg once each day. Any diuretic being taken should be stopped 2 to 3 days before beginning treatment with Tritace.

*Special care*: impaired liver function, blood changes, congestive heart failure, kidney dialysis – Tritace should not be given to those being dialysed with high-flux membranes, poor kidney function (reduce dose and monitor during treatment).

*Avoid use*: children, pregnancy, breastfeeding, narrowing of the aorta, past angioneurotic oedema (widespread swelling of soft tissues due to fluid collection), outflow obstruction.

*Possible interaction*: NSAIDs, lithium, antidiabetic agents, potassium supplements, potassium-sparing diuretics, antihypertensives.

*Side effects*: headache, fatigue, nausea, impaired kidney function, vomiting, dizziness, pains in abdomen, cough, diarrhoea, hypersensitivity reactions. In rare cases, fainting, angioneurotic oedema, low blood pressure causing symptoms.

*Manufacturer*: Aventis.

## TRUSOPT

*Description*: a carbonic anhydrase inhibitor available as eye drops containing 25 dorzolamide as hydrochloride.

*Used for*: either with or without ß-blockers in open-angle or pseudo-exfoliative glaucoma, high pressure within eye.

*Dosage*: adults, as sole therapy, 1 drop 3 times each day; in conjunction with ß-blockers, 1 drop twice each day.

*Special care*: history of kidney stones, closed angle glaucoma, previous eye surgery, chronic defects of cornea, impaired liver function, allergy to sulfonamides.

*Avoid use*: children, pregnancy, breastfeeding, hyperchloraemic acidosis, seriously impaired liver function, soft contact lenses (leave at least 15 minute interval before inserting).

*Possible interaction*: other eye drops – leave at least a 10-minute interval before inserting.

*Side effects*: blurred vision, nausea, bitter taste in mouth, weakness, stinging, dizziness, headache, numbness/tingling/'pins-and-needles' sensation, rash, nose bleeds, kidney stones, allergy, detached choroid, angioedema (widespread soft tissue swelling).

*Manufacturer*: M.S.D.

# U

## UCERAX TABLETS

*Description*: an antihistamine preparation, available as film-coated, scored, white, oblong tablets containing 25mg of hydroxyzine hydrochloride. *Also*, **UCERAX SYRUP** containing 10mg of hydroxyzine hydrochloride per 5ml.

*Used for*: anxiety, skin disorders, itching due to acute and chronic urticaria (nettle rash), skin disorders.

*Dosage*: adults, anxiety, 50 to 100mg 4 times each day; skin conditions, start with 25mg taken at night, then up to 25mg 3 or 4 times each day, if necessary. Children, for skin conditions only, aged 6 months to 6 years, start with 5 to 15mg taken at night, increasing to a maximum of 50mg each day in divided doses; aged over 6 years, 15 to 25mg at first taken at night, increasing to 50 to 100mg daily maximum dose, as divided doses.

*Special care*: impaired kidney function. Judgement and dexterity may be affected.

*Avoid use*: pregnancy, breastfeeding.

*Possible interaction*: depressants of the CNS, alcohol.

*Side effects*: anticholinergic effects, drowsiness. At high doses, involuntary muscle movements may occur.

*Manufacturer*: UCB.

# V

## VALLERGAN

*Description*: an anti-allergic preparation which is an antihistamine of the phenothiazine type, available as film-coated, blue tablets containing 10mg of alimemazine tartrate marked V10. *Also*, **VALLERGAN SYRUP** containing 7.5mg of alimemazine tartrate per 5ml. *Also*, **VALLERGAN FORTE SYRUP**, containing 30mg of alimemazine tartrate per 5ml.

*Used for*: itching, nettle rash, premedication before surgery.

*Dosage*: adults, itching and nettle rash, 10mg 2 or 3 times each day with a maximum of 100mg daily. Elderly persons, 10mg once or twice daily. Children, for itching and allergic conditions, aged over 2 years, 2.5 to 5mg 3 or 4 times each day. Premedication, consult manufacturer's literature.

*Avoid use*: pregnancy, breast-feeding, liver or kidney disorders, Parkinson's disease, epilepsy, phaeochromocytoma (adrenal gland tumour), underactive thyroid gland, myasthenia gravis, glaucoma, enlarged prostate gland.

*Possible interaction*: antihypertensives, hypoglycaemics, alcohol, sympathomimetics, anticholinergics, MAOIs, depressants of CNS.

*Side effects*: sleepiness, rash, drowsiness, impaired performance and reactions, heart disturbances, low blood pressure, depression of respiration. Anticholinergic and extrapyramidal effects, convulsions, raised levels of pro-

lactin in blood, jaundice, abnormally low level of white blood cells, jaundice, sensitivity to light (with high doses).
*Manufacturer*: Castlemead.

## VALOID

*Description*: an antihistamine preparation available as scored, white tablets containing 50mg of cyclizine hydrochloride, marked WELLCOME T4A. *Also,* **VALOID INJECTION,** a solution containing 50mg of cyclizine lactate per ml.

*Used for*: nausea and vomiting caused by narcotic pain relieving drugs, radiotherapy, anaesthetics; also due to vertigo and disorders of organs of balance, motion sickness. Also, to prevent vomiting during surgery.

*Dosage*: adults, 50mg 3 times each day either by mouth or by intravenous or intramuscular injection. Prevention of nausea following surgery, 50mg by slow intravenous infusion 20 minutes before operation finishes. Prevention of vomiting during surgery, 25mg intravenously before anaesthesia. Children, aged 6 to 12 years, 25mg by mouth up to 3 times each day.

*Special care*: breastfeeding, elderly, liver or kidney disorders, enlarged prostate gland, epilepsy, glaucoma, low blood pressure, Parkinson's disease. Patients should be warned not to drive or operate machinery due to possible drowsiness.

*Avoid use*: pregnancy, serious heart failure.

*Possible interaction*: alcohol, anticholinergics, depressants of CNS.

*Side effects*: rash, drowsiness, anticholinergic effects, allergic reactions, gastrointestinal upset, blood disorders, CNS effects.

*Manufacturer*: CeNeS.

## VANCOCIN

*Description*: an antibiotic glycopeptide preparation available as powder in vials for reconstitution and injection in 2 strengths, containing 500mg and 1g of vancomycin (as hydrochloride). *Also*, **VANCOCIN MATRIGEL** available as capsules in 2 strengths, both containing vancomycin as hydrochloride; peach/blue contain 125mg coded Lilly 3125; grey/blue containing 250mg coded Lilly 3126.

*Used for*: injection, potentially fatal infections caused by staphylococci which are resistant to other antibiotics. Vancocin Matrigel, staphylococcal enterocolitis and pseudomembranous colitis.

*Dosage*: adults, injection 500mg every 6 hours or 1g every 12 hours given by slow intravenous infusion over 1 hour. Children, 10mg per kg of body weight by slow intravenous infusion over 1 hour at 6 hourly intervals. Vancocin Matrigel, adults, 500mg each day for 7 to 10 days in divided doses with a daily maximum of 2g. Children, 40mg per kg of body weight for 7 to 10 days in 3 or 4 divided doses with a daily maximum of 2g.

*Special care*: elderly, pregnancy, patients with existing loss of hearing, impaired kidney function. Blood, kidney function and hearing should be carefully monitored during the course of treatment.

*Possible interaction*: drugs with toxic effects on central nervous system or kidneys, anaesthetics.

*Side effects*: chills, rashes, fever, nausea, allergic reactions, phlebitis, reduction in number of some white blood cells and rise in number of eosinophils, toxic effects on kidneys and organs of hearing and balance. Anaphylactoid allergic reactions, flushing, severe pain at injection site, with infusion. In the event of Stevens–Johnson syndrome, death of epidermal skin cells, bullous dermatosis (skin disorder), discontinue drug – specialist evaluation required before treatment can be resumed.

*Manufacturer*: Lilly.

## VANCOMYCIN *SEE*: VANCOCIN.

## VASCACE

*Description*: an antihypertensive which is an ACE inhibitor, available in the form of oval, film-coated, scored tablets in 4 strengths, all containing cilazapril and marked with strength and CIL. White, contain 0.5mg; yellow, contain 1mg; red, contain 2.5mg and brown, contain 5mg.

*Used for*: with digitalis and/or diuretics for treatment of chronic heart failure, high blood pressure.

*Dosage*: high blood pressure, 1mg once each day at first, adjusting according to need with a usual maintenance dose in the order of 2.5 to 5mg once daily. Any diuretic being taken should be withdrawn 2 or 3 days before treatment starts and initial dose should then be 0.5mg once each day. Elderly patients, 0.5mg to 1mg once each day to start, adjusting according to response and need. Heart failure, 0.5mg once each day, then adjusted according to response, with treatment closely supervised. The usual maintenance dose is in the order of 1 to 2.5mg each day with a daily maximum of 5mg.

*Special care*: impaired liver or kidney function, undergoing kidney dialysis, enlarged, damaged heart or obstruction of outflow, anaesthesia or surgery, suffering from lack of fluid or salt.

*Avoid use*: children, pregnancy, breastfeeding, ascites (abnormal collection of fluid in the peritoneal cavity – a complication of various diseases), angioedema (widespread soft tissue swelling due to fluid collection) after previous treatment with ACE inhibitors.

*Possible interaction*: NSAIDs, potassium-sparing diuretics, potassium supplements, tricyclics, cytostatics, lithium, immunosuppressants, procainamide, antihypertensives, allopurinol, neuroleptics, desensitising preparations, corticosteroids.

*Side effects*: nausea, headache, coughing, fatigue, rash, acid indigestion, giddiness. In rare cases, pancreatitis, changes in blood count, angioneurotic oedema – drug should be immediately stopped if this involves face or mouth.

*Manufacturer*: Roche.

## VENTOLIN

*Description*: a ß-agonist available in 5ml ampoules containing 1mg of salbutamol as sulphate per ml, for hospital use.

*Used for*: premature labour with no complicating features, to try to stop contractions.

*Dosage*: diluted solution given by intravenous infusion in first instance, as directed by obstetrician according to manufacturer's literature.

*Special care*: disease of heart circulation, diabetes, maternal thyrotoxicosis. Maternal and foetal heartbeat require careful monitoring.

*Avoid use*: Likelihood of miscarriage, placenta praevia, haemorrhage, toxaemia, umbilical cord compression, danger to mother or child if pregnancy continues.

*Possible interaction*: beta blockers.

*side effects*: rapid heart beat, anxiety, rise in blood sugar levels, headache, tremor, low blood potassium levels (hypokalaemia), pulmonary oedema (fluid on lungs).

*Manufacturer*: A & H.

## VERAPAMIL *SEE*: CORDILOX, SECURON

## VEXOL

*Description*: a corticosteroid preparation available as eye drops containing 1% rimexolone.

*Used for*: various inflammatory conditions of the eye that are responsive to steroids, inflammation arising after surgery.

*Dosage*: adults, post-operative treatment, 1 drop into conjunctival sac 4 times each day beginning 24 hours after operation on eye, continuing for 2 weeks. Conditions responsive to steroids, 1 drop into conjunctival sac at least

4 times each day, continuing for up to 4 weeks. Uveitis, 1 drop each hour during day for 1st week, then 2 hourly for 2nd week, then 4 times each day for 3rd week. In 4th week, 1 drop twice each day for 4 days and then 1 drop daily for final 3 days.

*Special care*: pregnancy, breastfeeding. Intraocular pressure must be carefully monitored and long-term use avoided.

*Avoid use*: bacterial, fungal or viral infections of the eye.

*Side effects*: raised intraocular pressure, pain, discomfort, short-lived blurring of vision, discharge, feeling of foreign object in eye. All adverse side effects should be reported to the Committee on the Safety of Medicines (CSM).

*Manufacturer*: Alcon.

## VIAGRA

*Description*: a phosphodiesterase type 5 inhibitor that increases blood flow into the penis available as blue, diamond-shaped, film-coated tablets in 3 strengths, all containing sildenafil as citrate. Available in 25mg, 50mg and 100mg strengths all marked VGR, PFIZER, and with strength.

*Used for*: male erectile dysfunction.

*Dosage*: men, 50mg by mouth about one hour before sexual activity. Alter subsequent dosage depending upon response (maximum dose 100mg). No more than one dose per day. For elderly 25mg to start; subsequent doses may go up to 100mg as daily maximum.

*Special care*: sickle cell anaemia, leukaemia, multiple myeloma (a form of cancer), severely impaired kidney function, impaired liver function, abnormal anatomy of the penis, bleeding disorders, stomach ulcer.

*Avoid use*: boys, existing heart conditions where sexual activity is not advised, severe liver disorders, recent stroke or heart attack, low blood pressure, hereditary degenerative disorders of the retina of the eye.

*Possible interactions*: amylnitrite, nitrates, ritonavir (do not use Viagra), other therapies for the same condition, cimetidine, α-blockers, protease inhibitors, erythromycin, inhibitors of CYP 3A4, ketoconazole, grapefruit juice.

*Side effects*: dizziness, gastrointestinal upset, headache, blocked nose, flushes, disturbance of vision, pain in eyes and blood shot eyes, allergic reactions. In rare cases, prolonged erection or priapism (painful, abnormal persistent erection requiring medical treatment), serious cardiovascular effects including heart attack, angina, rapid or slow heartbeat, low or high blood pressure, transient ischaemic attack, palpitations, arrhythmias, haemorrhage, fainting.

*Manufacturer*: Pfizer.

## VIBRAMYCIN

*Description*: a tetracycline antibiotic preparation available as green capsules containing 100mg of doxycycline (as hydrochloride), marked VBM 100 and Pfizer. *Also*, **VIBRAMYCIN-D**, off-white, dissolvable tablets containing 100mg of Vibramycin marked Pfizer and D-9.

*Used for*: lower respiratory tract infections, pneumonia, soft tissue, urinary tract infections, sexually transmitted diseases, eye infections, miscellaneous infections including amoebiasis. Also see manufacturer's literature. Prevention of malaria.

*Dosage*: adults, most infections, 200mg with food or drink on first day then 100 to 200mg daily. Sexually transmitted diseases and miscellaneous infections, as advised in manufacturer's literature. Prevention of malaria, 100mg each day starting 1 or 2 days before travelling and continue to take for 1 month after leaving malarial area. Capsules should be swallowed with plenty of water while standing or sitting up and not taken near to bedtime.

*Special care*: patients with impaired liver function.

*Avoid use*: children, pregnancy, breastfeeding.

*Possible interaction*: carbamazepine, oral contraceptives, antacids, phenytoin, mineral supplements, alcohol, barbiturates, methoxyflurane, anticoagulants, penicillin.

*Side effects*: superinfections, rash, inflammation of oesophagus and ulceration, liver disorders, gastrointestinal upset, sensitivity to light, allergic responses, blood disorders. Withdraw if intracranial hypertension occurs.

*Manufacturer*: Pfizer.

## VIOXX

*Description*: an NSAID and coxib available as tablets in 2 strengths containing rofecoxib; off-white, contain 12.5mg, marked MSD 74 and yellow, contain 25mg marked MSD 110. All are marked VIOXX. *Also,* **VIOXX SUSPENSION,** a liquid in 2 strengths containing 12.5mg and 25mg of rofecoxib per 5ml. *Also,* **VIOXX ACUTE,** available as tablets in 2 strengths containing rofecoxib. Yellow, contain 25mg, marked MSD 741 and orange, contain 50mg, marked MSD 744.

*Used for*: Vioxx and Vioxx suspension, relief of symptoms of osteo- and rheumatoid arthritis; Vioxx acute, acute pain, period pain.

*Dosage*: adults, Vioxx and Vioxx suspension, osteoarthritis, 12.5mg once each day to start, increasing to 25mg once daily, if needed. Rheumatoid arthritis, 25mg once each day. Vioxx acute, acute pain, only while symptoms occurring, 50mg once each day to start then reduce to 25mg once daily as soon as possible. Period pain, 25mg or 50mg once each day with 50mg maximum daily dose.

*Special care*: pregnancy, previous stomach ulcer or bleeding, impaired kidney or liver function, cirrhosis of liver, heart failure, fluid retention, high blood pressure, uncompensated heart failure, dehydration, malfunction of left ventricle, patients with previous ischaemic heart disease – stop Vioxx if condition worsens. Elderly patients and those with heart, kidney or liver disorders must be closely monitored. If symptoms of liver malfunction occur, tests must be performed.

*Avoid use*: children, breastfeeding, last 3 months of pregnancy, serious kidney or liver disorders, allergic reactions or asthma occurring with aspirin or anti-inflammatories, active stomach ulcer or bleeding in gastrointestinal tract, inflammation of bowel, serious congestive heart failure.

*Possible interaction*: ACE inhibitors, theophylline, ciclosporin, amitriptyline, methotrexate, tacrolimus, high dose NSAIDs and aspirin, warfarin, tacrine, midazolam, oral anticoagulants, zileuton, ß-blockers, rifampicin, lithium, diuretics.

*Side effects*: headache, gastrointestinal upset, stomach and abdominal pains, fluid retention, dizziness, high blood pressure, dizziness, itching, raised liver enzymes, decreased haemocrit. Any adverse side effects must be reported to the Committee on the Safety of Medicines (CSM).

*Manufacturer*: M.S.D.

## VIRGAN

*Description*: an antiviral preparation available as an eye gel containing 0.15% ganciclovir.

*Used for*: acute keratitis (inflammation of cornea) caused by herpes infection.

*Dosage*: adults, 1 drop 5 times each day until cornea is healed and then 1 drop 3 times each day for further 1 week after healing. Maximum period of use is 3 weeks.

*Avoid use*: children, pregnancy, breastfeeding.

*Side effects*: stinging in eye.

*Manufacturer*: Chauvin.

## VISCOTEARS

*Description*: an eye preparation available as a liquid gel containing 0.2% carbomer 980. *Also,* **VISCOTEARS SINGLE DOSE,** single dose eye drops as gel containing 0.2% carbomer 980.

*Used for*: deficiency in tears secretion.
*Dosage*: adults, 1 drop 3 to 4 times each day into eye.
*Special care*: pregnancy, breastfeeding, wearing soft contact lenses.
*Avoid use*: children.
*Side effects*: sticky eyelid, short-lived irritation and blurring of vision.
*Manufacturer*: Novartis.

## VISKALDIX

*Description*: a combined non-cardioselective ß-blocker and thiazide available as scored white tablets marked with name containing 10mg of pindolol and 5mg of clopamide.
*Used for*: high blood pressure.
*Dosage*: start with 1 tablet in the morning increasing if required, after 2 or 3 weeks, to 2 or a maximum of 3 each day.
*Special care*: pregnancy, breastfeeding, liver or kidney disease, diabetes, metabolic acidosis, poor cerebral blood supply, history of bronchospasm, those undergoing anaesthesia; patients with weak hearts should be treated with digitalis and diuretics. Drug should be stopped gradually.
*Avoid use*: children, patients with asthma, heart diseases including heart block, heart shock, slow heartbeat rate, heart failure.
*Possible interaction*: cardiac depressants,anaesthetics, reserpine, sedatives, class II calcium antagonists, antihypertensives, sympathomimetics, cimetidine, indometacin, ergotamine, class I antiarrhythmic drugs, verapamil,

clonidine withdrawal, hypoglycaemics, rifampicin, warfarin, ibuprofen.

*Side effects*: sleep disturbance, cold feet and hands, slow heartbeat, fatigue on exercise, wheeziness, heart failure, gastro-intestinal disorders; dry eyes or skin rash (stop use gradually), hair loss, low blood pressure, thrombocytopenia (abnormal decline in blood platelets causing increased likelihood of bleeding).

*Manufacturer*: Novartis.

## VISKEN

*Description*: an antianginal, antihypertensive preparation and non-cardioselective ß-blocker available as scored, white tablets in 2 strengths containing 5mg and 15mg of pindolol marked with name and strength.

*Used for*: angina, high blood pressure.

*Dosage*: adults, angina, ° to 1 tablet 3 times each day; high blood pressure, 10 to 15mg each day in divided doses at first, increasing weekly to a daily maximum of 45mg, if necessary.

*Special care*: pregnancy, breastfeeding, liver or kidney disease, diabetes, metabolic acidosis, poor cerebral blood supply, history of bronchospasm, those undergoing anaesthesia; patients with weak hearts should be treated with digitalis and diuretics. Drug should be stopped gradually.

*Avoid use*: children, patients with asthma, heart diseases including heart block, heart shock, slow heartbeat rate, heart failure.

*Possible interaction*: cardiac depressants,anaesthetics, reserpine, sedatives, class II calcium antagonists, antihypertensives, sympathomimetics, cimetidine, indometacin, ergotamine, class I antiarrhythmic drugs, verapamil, clonidine withdrawal, hypoglycaemics, rifampicin, warfarin, ibuprofen.

*Side effects*: sleep disturbance, cold feet and hands, slow heartbeat, fatigue on exercise, wheeziness, heart failure, gastro-intestinal disorders; dry eyes or skin rash (stop use gradually), hair loss, low blood pressure, thrombocytopenia (abnormal decline in blood platelets causing increased likelihood of bleeding).

*Manufacturer*: Novartis.

## VOLMAX

*Description*: a selective ß2-agonist available as white, hexagonal, continuous-release tablets in 2 strengths containing 4 and 8mg of salbutamol sulphate marked with strength.

*Used for*: bronchospasm occurring with reversible airways obstruction or asthma.

*Dosage*: adults, 8mg twice each day. Children, aged 3 to 12 years, 4mg twice each day.

*Special care*: pregnancy, diabetes, over-active thyroid gland.

*Avoid use*: children aged under 3 years.

*Possible interaction*: sympathomimetics, steroids, xanthines, **ß**-blockers, diuretics.

*Side effects*: headache, dilatation of peripheral blood vessels, nervousness, paradoxical bronchospasm, fine

tremor, low blood potassium levels, rapid heartbeat, hyperactive behaviour in children.
*Manufacturer*: A. & H.

## VOLTAROL

*Description*: an NSAID and phenylacetic acid diclofenac sodium, available as enteric-coated tablets in 2 strengths containing diclofenac sodium; yellow, contain 25mg and brown contain 50mg, both marked with name and strength on one side and GEIGY on the other. *Also*, **VOLTAROL DISPERSIBLE** available as pink, triangular tablets containing 50mg of diclofenac sodium marked V on one side and GEIGY on the other, for adding to water. *Also*, **VOLTAROL RETARD**, available as sustained-release red tablets containing 100mg of diclofenac sodium marked VOLTAROL R and GEIGY. *Also*, **VOLTAROL SUPPOSITORIES** available in 4 strengths containing 12.5mg, 25mg, 50mg and 100mg of diclofenac sodium. *Also*, **VOLTAROL RAPID**, sugar-coated tablets in 2 strengths containing diclofenac sodium; pale red, contain 25mg, marked DD CG; reddish-borown, contain 50mg, marked CG PP. *Also*, **VOLTAROL INJECTION** available as a solution in ampoules containing 25mg of diclofenac sodium per ml.
*Used for*: oral preparations and suppositories, rheumatoid arthritis, osteoarthritis, ankylosing spondylitis, chronic juvenile arthritis, acute gout, pain from minor surgery, dental and orthopaedic procedures or trauma. Voltarol Rapid also used for pyrophosphate arthropathy and

related disorders and migraine in adults. Injection, acute gout, osteo- and rheumatoid arthritis, acute pain after trauma, surgery, acute back pain, renal colic, fractures.

*Dosage*: adults, Voltarol tablets, 75 to 150mg in 2 or 3 divided doses each day; Voltarol dispersible, 100 to 150mg added to water in 2 or 3 divided doses each day. Maximum period of treatment is 3 months. Voltarol SR, 1 tablet once or twice each day taken with meals and swallowed whole. Voltarol Retard, 1 each day taken with meal and swallowed whole. Suppositories, 75 to 150mg in divided doses, inserted into rectum. Voltarol Rapid, 100 to 150mg each day in 2 or 3 divided doses; for migraine, 50mg at start of attack, repeated after 2 hours, if required, then 50mg every 4 to 6 hours, if needed to a daily maximum of 200mg. Voltarol injection, 75mg once or twice each day by deep intramuscular injection into gluteal muscle (buttock) to a daily maximum of 150mg. For pain after operation, 75mg by intravenous infusion given over 30 minutes to 2hours. If necessary, can be repeated after 4 to 6 hours to a maximum daily dose of 150mg. To prevent post-operative pain, 25 to 50mg by intravenous infusion over 15minutes to 1 hour then continuous infusion at rate of 5mg per hour to a daily maximum of 150mg. In all cases, treatment duration should be no more than 2 days and then patient should be transferred to tablets or suppositories. Children, Voltarol tablets for juvenile rheumatoid arthritis, aged over 12 months, 1 to 3mg per kg of body weight each day in divided doses. Suppositories, using 12.5mg or 25mg strength only, 1 to 3mg per kg of body weight each day in divided doses. Voltarol rapid, aged over 14 years only, 75 to 100mg each day in 2 to 3 divided doses.

*Special care*: elderly, pregnancy, breastfeeding, impaired liver, kidney or heart function, porphyria (inherited, metabolic disorder involving porphyrins), previous gastrointestinal lesions, blood abnormalities, asthma, high blood pressure, heart failure. Patients receiving long-term treatment should be monitored.

*Avoid use*: children (most preparations except where indicated above), allergy to aspirin or anti-inflammatory drugs, stomach ulcer. With suppositories or Rapid, proctitis (inflammation of anus and rectum). With intravenous route, risk of haemorrhage with surgery, low blood volume, bleeding tendency, asthma, cerebrovascular haemorrhage, dehydrated patients, moderate to severely impaired kidney function.

*Possible interaction*: lithium, anticoagulants, cardiac glycosides, diuretics, digoxin, methotrexate, salicylates, ciclosporin, oral hypoglycaemics, NSAIDs, steroids, mifepristone, quinolones, methotrexate, antihypertensives.

*Side effects*: headache, dizziness, stomach pain, rash, bleeding, gastrointestinal upset. In rare cases, abnormal kidney and liver function, pain and tissue death at injection site, blood changes, stomach ulcer, high blood pressure, hypersensitivity reactions, fits, nephrotic syndrome (a kidney disorder), aseptic meningitis, vasculitis (inflammation of blood vessels), papillary necrosis, congestive heart failure, pneumonitis.

*Manufacturer*: Novartis.

## VOLTAROL EMULGEL

*Description*: an NSAID available as an aqueous gel containing 1.16g of diclofenac diethyl-ammonium salt (equivalent to 1g of diclofenac sodium).

*Used for*: soft tissue rheumatism, osteoarthritis of superficial joints, strains, sprains, bruises.

*Dosage*: adults, 2 to 4g rubbed into area 3 to 4 times each day. Review use after 2 weeks, (4 weeks in case of osteoarthritis.

*Special care*: pregnancy, breastfeeding.

*Avoid use*: children, allergy to aspirin or anti-inflammatory drugs.

*Possible interaction*: other NSAIDs.

*Side effects*: itching, dermatitis, reddening of skin, hypersensitivity, sensitivity to light.

*Manufacturer*: Novartis.

## VOLTAROL OPHTHA

*Description*: an NSAID available as single dose eyedrops containing 0.1% diclofenac sodium.

*Used for*: reduction of miosis (excessive constriction of the sphincter muscle of the iris) in cataract surgery, post-operative inflammation, pain and discomfort, streaming, irritated eyes due to hayfever.

For *Dosages etc.* consult manufacturer's literature.

*Manufacturer*: Novartis.

# W

## WELLDORM

*Description*: a sedative and hypnotic available as film-coated, purple oval tablets containing 707mg of cloral betaine (equivalent to 414mg of chloral hydrate). *Also*, **WELLDORM ELIXIR**, a liquid containing 143.3mg of chloral hydrate per 5ml.

*Used for*: insomnia – short-term treatment only.

*Dosage*: adults, tablets, 1 or 2 tablets at bedtime to a maximum of 2g chloral hydrate equivalent per day. Elixir, 15 to 45ml at bedtime to a daily maximum of 2g. Children, 30 to 50mg per kg of body weight to a daily maximum of 1g.

*Avoid use*: pregnancy, breastfeeding, severe heart, kidney or liver disease, acute, intermittent porphyria, gastritis (stomach inflammation/irritation).

*Possible interaction*: anticoagulants, anticholinergics, CNS depressants, alcohol.

*Side effects*: headache, nausea, vomiting, flatulence, bloating, rashes, excitability. In rare cases, blood disorders, ketonuria (ketones in urine).

*Manufacturer*: S & N.

# X

## XALACOM

*Description*: a combined prostaglandin and ß-blocker available as eye drops containing 0.005% latanoprost and 0.5% timolol maleate.

*Used for*: open angle glaucoma, high pressure within eye that do not adequately respond to topical ß-blockers alone.

*Dosage*: adults, 1 drop into affected eye(s) once each day in morning.

*Special care*: certain other forms of glaucoma and eye disorders, toxicity of thyroid gland, diabetes. Allow at least 5 minutes before using other eye preparations.

*Avoid use*: children, pregnancy, breastfeeding, asthma, 2nd or 3rd degree heart block, uncompensated heart failure, heart shock, severe obstructive airways disease, slow heartbeat.

*Possible interaction*: parasympathomimetics, anti-arrhythmics, cardiac glycosides, calcium antagonists, antihypertensives, other topical eye preparations and glaucoma treatments.

*Side effects*: feeling of foreign particle in eye, blurring of vision, darkening of eye, short-lived epithelial erosion, other eye effects, curling and darkening of lashes and skin, worsening of asthma, breathlessness. Any adverse side effects should be reported to the Committee on the Safety of Medicines (CSM).

*Manufacturer*: Pharmacia.

## XALATAN

*Description*: a prostaglandin analogue available as eye drops containing 50μg of latanoprost per ml.

*Used for*: open angle glaucoma, high pressure within eye.

*Dosage*: adults, 1 drop into affected eye(s) each day in evening.

*Special care*: other forms of glaucoma and eye diseases and disorders, severe asthma.

*Avoid use*: pregnancy, breastfeeding.

*Possible interaction*: other glaucoma treatments and eye drops. Leave at least 5 minutes before using other eye drops.

*Side effects*: feeling of foreign object in eye, darkening of eye colour, blurring of vision, thickening and darkening of eyelashes, other eye effects. In rare cases, worsening of asthma and breathlessness, inflammation of iris, uveitis, macular oedema (fluid retention), darkening of skin around eye.

*Manufacturer*: Pharmacia.

## XATRAL XL.

*Description*: a selective α1-blocker available as sustained-release, layered, yellow/white tablets containing 10mg of alfuzosin hydrochloride. *Also*, **XATRAL**, available as film-coated, white tablets containing 2.5mg of alfuzosin hydrochloride.

*Used for*: benign prostatic hypertrophy (enlargement of prostate gland).

*Dosage*: men, Xatral XL, 1 tablet each day taken after a meal. Xatral, 1 tablet 3 times each day to a maximum of 4.

*Special care*: weak heart, high blood pressure, impaired liver or kidney function. Monitor blood pressure especially when starting treatment. Stop 24 hours before anaesthesia, or if angina worsens.

*Avoid use*: severely impaired liver function, (or any impairment of liver with Xatral XL), past orthostatic hypotension (low blood pressure on standing).

*Possible interaction*: antihypertensives, other α-blockers.

*Side effects*: gastrointestinal upset, headache, sleepiness, malaise, dizziness, vertigo, rapid heartbeat, orthostatic hypotension, chest pain, fatigue, rash, flushing, fluid retention, palpitations, fainting.

*Manufacturer*: Sanofi-Synthelabo.

## XEPIN

*Description*: an antipruritic and antihistamine preparation available as a cream containing 5% doxepin hydrochloride.

*Used for*: itching and eczema.

*Dosage*: adults, apply a thin layer to affected skin 3 to 4 times each day to a maximum of 3g per dose.

*Special care*: pregnancy, breastfeeding, serious liver disease, glaucoma, retention of urine, mania.

*Avoid use*: children.

*Possible interaction*: drugs metabolised by liver microsomal enzymes, cimetidine, MAOIs, depressants of CNS.

*Side effects*: dry mouth, local irritation of skin, drowsiness – patient should be warned that this may occur.
*Manufacturer*: CHS.

**XYLOMETAZOLINE *SEE*: OTRIVINE, OTRIVINE-ANTISTIN.**

# Z

## ZAPELON *SEE*: SONATA.

## ZANIDIP

*Description*: an antihypertensive and Class II calcium antagonist available as film-coated, yellow tablets containing 10mg of lercanidipine hydrochloride.

*Used for*: mild to moderate high blood pressure.

*Dosage*: adults, 1 each day taken at least a quarter of an hour before a meal. If necessary, increase to 2 tablets each day.

*Special care*: dysfunction of left ventricle of heart, sick sinus syndrome, ischaemic heart disease.

*Avoid use*: children, pregnancy, breastfeeding, recent heart attack, congestive heart failure that is not being treated, obstruction of left ventricle outflow, angina that is not stabilised, severely impaired kidney or liver function.

*Possible interaction*: erythromycin, digoxin, terfenadine, rifampicin, ß-blockers, cimetidine, carbamazepine, cimetidine, azole antifungals, fluoxetine, phenytoin, astemizole, grapefruit juice.

*Side effects*: headache, rapid heartbeat, weakness, dizziness, flushes, fluid retention in hands and feet.

*Manufacturer*: Napp.

## ZANTAC

*Description*: an H2 blocker available as film-coated, white tablets in 2 strengths containing 150mg and 300mg of ranitidine hydrochloride marked with GXEC2 or GXEC3, respectively. Also, **ZANTAC EFFERVESCENT**, white effervescent tablets containing 150mg and 300mg of ranitidine as hydrochloride. *Also*, **ZANTAC SYRUP**, containing 150mg of ranitidine as hydrochloride per 10ml with 7.5% ethanol, in a sugar-free syrup. *Also*, **ZANTAC INJECTION**, containing 50mg of ranitidine as hydrochloride per 2ml as a solution in ampoules.

*Used for*: duodenal, benign stomach and post-operative ulcers; ulcers due to NSAIDs, prevention of ulcers induced by NSAIDs, duodenal ulcers linked with *H. pylori*, dyspepsia, oesophageal reflux, management of healed oesophagitis, Z-E syndrome, reduction of stomach acid, prevention of haemorrhage in bleeding ulcers, to prevent aspiration of stomach acid during anaesthesia.

*Dosage*: adults, oral preparations, ulcers, 150mg 2 times each day or 300mg at bedtime. Take for 4 weeks then reduce to maintenance dose of 150mg at bedtime. Duodenal ulcer linked with *H. pylori*, 300mg at bedtime or 150mg twice each day for 4 weeks, combined with 750mg of amoxicillin 3 times each day and 500mg of metronidazole 3 times each day – both for first 2 weeks. Prevention of duodenal ulcers caused by NSAIDs, 150mg twice each day. Reflux oesophagitis, 150mg twice each day or 300mg at bedtime for up to 3 months. In severe cases, 150mg 4 times each day for 3 months. Healed oesophagitis, 150mg twice each day. Z-E syndrome, 150mg 3 times each day, increasing to 6g daily, if needed. Chronic episodes of acid indigestion, 150mg twice each day for 6 weeks. Prevention of haemorrhage, 150mg twice each day to replace injection once food is being taken by mouth. Children for stomach ulcers only, 2 to 4mg per kg of body weight twice each day to a daily maximum of 300mg. Injection, adults, 50mg by intramuscular or slow intravenous injection over 2 minutes or by intermittent intravenous infusion at rate of 25mg per hour for 2 hours. Dose may be repeated every 6 to 8 hours, as needed.

*Special care*: pregnancy, breastfeeding, acute porphyria (inherited metabolic disorder involving porphyrins), impaired kidney function. Malignancy must be excluded before treatment begins.

*Avoid use*: injection in children.

*Side effects*: dizziness, altered liver function, headache. In rare cases, hepatitis, changes in blood counts – leucopenia, thrombocytopenia, pancytopenia, agranulocytosis, hypersensitivity, confusion, rash, slow heartbeat, pancreatitis, breast symptoms.

*Manufacturer*: GlaxoSmithKline.

## ZESTRIL

*Description*: an antihypertensive preparation and ACE inhibitor available as tablets in 4 strengths, all containing lisinopril and marked with heart shape and strength. White, contain 2.5mg; scored, pink, contain 5mg; pink, contain 10mg; pink, contain 20mg. 10 and 20mg strengths are also marked with trade mark.

*Used for*: all grades of essential and renovascular high blood pressure, certain kidney complications of diabetes associated with high blood pressure.

*Dosage*: adults, high blood pressure, start with 2.5mg each day, increasing gradually to a maintenance dose of 10 to 20mg once each day, with a daily maximum of 40mg. Cease using diuretic, if possible, 2 to 3 days before treatment for hypertension and resume later, if needed. Kidney complications of diabetes, 2.5mg once each day to start then increase to 10mg or 20mg once each day to achieve desired blood pressure (value depending upon type of diabetes).

*Special care*: breastfeeding, renovascular hypertension, impaired kidney function (monitor before and during treatment), kidney dialysis, narrowed renal arteries causing lessened blood flow, serious congestive heart failure, anaesthesia.

*Avoid use*: children, pregnancy, angioneurotic oedema (widespread swelling due to fluid retention) from past treatment with ACE inhibitor, narrowing of aorta, enlargement of right ventricle.

*Possible interaction*: potassium supplements, potassium-sparing diuretics, lithium, antihypertensives, NSAIDs. antidiabetics.

*Side effects*: kidney failure, angioneurotic oedema, low blood pressure, gastrointestinal upset, dizziness, headache, fatigue, cough, nausea, palpitations, rash, weakness.

*Manufacturer*: AstraZeneca.

**ZIDOVINE *SEE*: RETROVIR.**

## ZIMOVANE

*Description*: an anxiolytic and cyclopyrrolone available as film-coated tablets in 2 strengths, both containing zopiclone. Blue, contain 3.75mg, marked Z and white, contain 7.5mg marked ZM.

*Used for*: insomnia, short-term treatment only especially when severe and debilitating.

*Dosage*: 1 x 7.5mg tablet at bedtime. Elderly, 1 x 3.75mg tablet at bedtime to start, increasing dose if necessary. Maximum period of treatment is 1 month.

*Special care*: insufficient liver or kidney function; patients should be checked for withdrawal symptoms on completing treatment.

*Avoid use*: children, pregnancy, breastfeeding, severely impaired liver function, respiratory failure, severe sleep apnoea (a condition in which person momentarily stops breathing during sleeping), myasthenia gravis.

*Possible interaction*: trimipramine, alcohol, other depressants of the CNS.

*Side effects*: gastrointestinal upset, metallic aftertaste, allergic reactions, psychological changes. In rare cases, lack of co-ordination, light headedness.

*Manufacturer*: R.P.R.

## ZINACEF

*Description*: an antibacterial and cephalosporin and antibacterial preparation available in vials in 3 strengths containing 250mg, 750mg and 1.5g of cefuroxime as sodium salt.

*Used for*: infections of soft tissue, the respiratory and urinary tracts, bones and joints, meningitis, gonorrhoea, other serious infections pending laboratory results, prevention of infection during surgery.
*Dosage*: see literature.
*Special care*: pregnancy, breastfeeding, allergy to beta-lactam antibiotics.
*Possible interaction*: aminoglycosides, loop diuretics.
*Side effects*: gastrointestinal upset,short-lived pain at injection site, hypersensitivity reactions, candidiasis when used long-term, blood cell changes (eosinophilia, leucopenia, neutropenia), fall in haemoglobin levels, positive Coombs test, short-lived rise in liver enzymes. In rare cases, thrombocytopenia (decline in blood platelets with increased likelihood of bleeding).
*Manufacturer*: GlaxoSmithKline.

## ZINC OXIDE *SEE*: ANUSOL-HC, ANUSOL.

## ZINERYT

*Description*: an antibiotic preparation available as an alcohol-based solution containing 4% erythromycin and zinc acetate 1.2% complex.
*Used for*: acne.
*Dosage*: apply twice each day to affected skin.
*Special care*: do not allow contact with mucous membranes or eyes.
*Side effects*: short-lived irritation.
*Manufacturer*: Yamanouchi.

## ZINNAT

*Description*: a cephalosporin and antibacterial available as film-coated white tables in 2 strengths containing 125mg and 250mg of cefuroxime as axetil, marked with strength and GLAXO. *Also*, **ZINNAT SUSPENSION**, available as a solution containing 125mg of cefuroxime as axetil per 5ml or as granules in sachets for reconstitution.

*Used for*: infections of the ear, nose and throat, respiratory or urinary tracts, skin and soft tissues, gonorrhoea.

*Dosage*: adults, bronchitis and most other conditions, usually 250mg twice each day after food, 500mg twice daily for severe infections and pneumonia and a 1g single dose each day for gonorrhoea. Urinary tract infections, 125mg twice each day but 250mg twice daily for pyelonephritis (a kidney infection). Children aged over 3 months, most infections, 125mg twice each day after food. Middle ear infections, aged 3 months to 2 years, 125mg; aged over 2 years, 250mg. Both twice each day.

*Special care*: pregnancy, breastfeeding, hypersensitivity to penicillin.

*Side effects*: pseudomembranous colitis, hypersensitivity reactions, headache, gastrointestinal upset, short-lived candidosis, eosinophilia (increase in number of eosinophils in blood – usually as inflammatory response), Positive Coombs test, increase in liver enzymes. In rare cases, Stevens–Johnson syndrome, erythema multiforme (skin disorder), toxic epidermal necrolysis (death of epidermal skin cells), interstitial nephritis (kidney disorder),

leucopenia (fall in number white blood cells), thrombocytopenia (decline in number of blood platelets).
*Manufacturer*: GlaxoSmithKline.

## ZIRTEK

*Description*: an antihistamine preparation available as film-coated, white oblong tablets containing 10mg of cetirizine hydrochloride marked Y/Y. *Also,* **ZIRTEK SOLUTION**, a banana-flavoured, sugar-free liquid containing 1mg of cetirizine dihydrochloride per ml.
*Used for*: allergic nettle rash, seasonal and perennial rhinitis (hayfever).
*Dosage*: adults, 1 tablet or 10ml each day. Children aged 2 to 6 years, for seasonal hayfever only, 5ml each day. Aged over 6 years, for seasonal hayfever only, as adult
*Special care*: pregnancy, insufficiency of kidneys.
*Avoid use*: breastfeeding.
*Side effects*: agitation, gastrointestinal upset, dizziness, headache, dry mouth, drowsiness.
*Manufacturer*: UCB.

## ZOCOR

*Description*: a lipid-lowering and statin available as film-coated tablets in 4 strengths, all containing simvastatin. Peach-coloured, oval. contain 10mg, marked ZOCOR 10; tan-coloured, oval, contain 20mg, marked ZOCOR 20; red, oval, contain 40mg, marked MSD 749; capsule-shaped, red, contain 80mg, marked 80 and 543.
*Used for*: primary high blood cholesterol levels, with di-

etary measures, lowering of blood lipid levels, to slow progression of coronary heart disease and atherosclerosis, to reduce risk of mortality, death from coronary disease, reduce risks for patients undergoing certain surgical heart procedures.

*Dosage*: adults, high blood lipid levels, start with 10mg taken at night, altered to match response at 4 week intervals, within the range 10 to 80mg. Coronary heart disease, start with 20mg as single nightly dose, then adjust every 4 weeks according to response to nightly maximum of 80mg. Certain high blood cholesterol conditions, 40mg as single nightly dose or 80mg each day in 3 divided doses.

*Special care*: past liver disease, check liver function.

*Avoid use*: children, pregnancy, breastfeeding; women should use non-hormonal contraception, liver disease.

*Possible interaction*: ciclosporin, macrolide antibiotics, erythromycin, digoxin, coumarin anticoagulants, clarithromycin, nefazodone, gemfibrozil, nicotinic acid, immunosuppressants, azole antifungals, protease inhibitors, other CYP3A4 inhibitors, grapefruit juice.

*Side effects*: headache, gastrointestinal upset, abdominal pain, weakness, muscle cramps and pains, anaemia, dizziness, baldness, weakness, numbness/tingling/'pins-and-needles sensation', peripheral nerve damage, pancreatitis. In rare cases, jaundice, hepatitis, muscle disease, disintegration of striated muscle fibres.

*Manufacturer*: M.S.D.

**ZOLPIDEM** ***SEE*****: STILNOCT.**

## ZOPICLONE *SEE*: ZIMOVANE.

## ZOVIRAX

*Description*: an antiviral DNA polymerase inhibitor available in shield-shaped, dispersible tablets in 2 strengths containing aciclovir. Blue, contain 200mg and pink, contain 400mg, both marked with triangle, strength and name. *Also*, scored, white, dispersible, elongated tablets containing 800mg of aciclovir, marked with strength and name. *Also* **ZOVIRAX SUSPENSION,** in 2 strengths containing 200mg and 400mg of aciclovir per 5ml. *Also,* **ZOVIRAX CREAM**, containing 5% aciclovir. *Also,* **ZOVIRAX OINTMENT,** containing 3% aciclovir. *Also*, **ZOVIRAX INFUSION**, available as a powder in vials in 2 strengths for reconstitution and injection containing 250 and 500mg of aciclovir.

*Used for*: tablets, suspension and cream, treatment and suppression of infections of skin and mucous membranes caused by herpes simplex; prevention of these infections in patients with low immunity. Treatment of infections caused by herpes zoster and varicella. Tablets, suspension and cream, treatment and suppression of genital herpes; prevention of genital herpes in patients with low immunity. Ointment, keratitis (eye inflammation) caused by herpes simplex. Infusion, consult manufacturer's literature.

*Dosage*: oral preparations, adults, treatment of herpes simplex, 200mg every 4 hours 5 times each day with break over night for 5 days. In severe cases, treatment period may need to be extended. Suppression of herpes simplex, 200mg 4 times each day every 6 hours or 400mg twice each day, for 6 months to 1 year, then evaluate. Patients with low immunity, treatment, 400mg every 4 hours, 5 times each day. Prevention, 200 to 400mg every 6 hours, 4 times each day. Herpes zoster or varicella, 800mg 5 times each day every 4 hours with break at night for 1 week. Genital herpes, 200mg every 4 hours, 5 times each day; patients with low immunity, 400mg every 4 hours, 5 times each day for at least 5 days. Suppression, 400mg twice each day or 200mg 4 times each day (possibly, 3 times or 2 times daily may be adequate, in some cases). Prevention in patients with low immunity, 200 to 400mg 4 times each day. Cream, apply 5 times each day every 4 hours for 5 days, possibly extending treatment period for further 5 days if healing is not complete. Ointment, insert 1 cm of ointment into lower conjunctival sac every 4 hours, 5 times each day with break at night and continue for 3 days beyond disappearance of symptoms. Infusion, consult manufacturer's literature. Children, oral preparations, herpes simplex, treatment and prevention, aged under 2 years, half adult dose; aged over 2 years, as for adults. Varicella, aged under 2 years, treatment, 200mg 4 times each day; aged 2 to 5 years, 400mg 4 times each day; aged over 6 years, 800mg 4 times each day. All treatments for 5 days. Genital herpes, treatment, aged under 2 years, 100mg every 4 hours 5 times each day; aged over 2 years, as for adults. All treatment for 5 days. Prevention, aged under 2 years, 100mg every 6 hours,

4 times each day; aged over 2 years, as for adults. Cream, as adult dose. Ointment and infusion, consult manufacturer's literature.

*Special care*: elderly, pregnancy, breastfeeding, severely impaired kidney function. Patients receiving infusion must be well hydrated.

*Possible interaction*: mycophenolate, probenecid, cimetidine.

*Side effects*: with oral preparations, sleepiness, dizziness, headaches, sensitivity to light, rash, fits, hallucinations, confusion. In rare cases, jaundice, hepatitis, haematological changes, short-lived rise in liver enzymes, creatinine and blood urea levels, acute kidney failure. With cream, slight flaking and skin dryness, short-lived irritation. Ointment, slight irritation and stinging, superficial punctate keratopathy (damage to cornea).

*Manufacturer*: GlaxoSmithKline.

## ZUCLOPENTHIXOL *SEE*: CLOPIXOL.

## ZUMENON

*Description*: a hormonal, oestrogen preparation available as film-coated tablets in 2 strengths, both containing oestradiol. White, contain 1mg and red, contain 2mg, both marked S and 379.

*Used for*: a hormonal replacement therapy for symptoms of the menopause, prevention of post-menopausal osteoporosis.

*Dosage*: women, symptoms, start with 1mg each day then

increase to 2mg strength, if necessary, but reducing again to 1mg strength as soon as possible. Commence on fifth day of menstruation (any time if absent). Prevention of osteoporosis, 2mg each day continuously. In women with intact womb, a progestogen should be taken for 10 to 14 days of each month.

*Special care*: high blood pressure, severe kidney disease receiving dialysis, Raynaud's disease, diabetes, multiple sclerosis, asthma, varicose veins, elevated levels of prolactin (a hormone) in the blood (hyperprolactinemia). Risk of thrombosis increases with smoking, age and obesity. Blood pressure, breasts and pelvic organs should be checked during period of treatment.

*Avoid use*: pregnancy, heart and circulatory diseases, angina, sickle cell anaemia, pulmonary hypertension. Also hormone-dependent cancers, undiagnosed vaginal bleeding, chorea, liver disease, history of cholestatic jaundice of pregnancy, infectious hepatitis, Dublin–Johnson syndrome, Rotor syndrome, recent trophoblastic disease.

*Possible interaction*: phenytoin, carbamazepine, tetracyclines, primidone, chloral hydrate, glutethimide, phenylbutazone, rifampicin, griseofulvin, ampicillin, dichloralphenazone, ethosuximide, barbiturates, St John's Wort.

*Side effects*: feeling of bloatedness due to fluid retention, leg pains, breast enlargement, erosion of cervix, muscular cramps, weight gain, breakthrough bleeding, depression, headaches, vaginal cervix, muscular cramps, weight gain, breakthrough bleeding, depression, headaches, vaginal discharge, loss of libido, nausea, brown patches on skin (chloasma). Stop drug immediately in event of pregnancy.

*Manufacturer*: Solvay.

# INDEX

## A

## B



## C

## D

## E



## F

## G



## H

## I

## J



## K



## L

## M



## N

## O



## P

## R

## S



## T

## U



## V

## W



## Z